Current Topics in Airway Management

Current Topics in Airway Management

Editor: Richard Wright

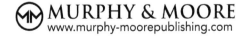

MURPHY & MOORE
www.murphy-moorepublishing.com

www.murphy-moorepublishing.com

MURPHY & MOORE

Cataloging-in-Publication Data

Current topics in airway management / edited by Richard Wright.
    p. cm.
Includes bibliographical references and index.
ISBN 978-1-63987-794-2
1. Airway (Medicine). 2. Trachea--Intubation. 3. Artificial respiration.
4. Anesthesiology. I. Wright, Richard.
RC732 .C87 2023
616.2--dc23

Murphy & Moore Publishing
1 Rockefeller Plaza,
New York City,
NY 10020, USA

ISBN 978-1-63987-794-2

Contents

Permissions

List of Contributors

Index

Preface

Airway management refers to the assessment, planning and series of medical procedures necessary to restore or preserve a person's breathing or ventilation. It could be necessary for people in a range of situations from simple choking to complex airway obstruction. Medical procedures involved in airway management include supplemental oxygen, positioning, and bag-mask ventilation with or without adjuncts. Mechanical ventilation and airway management of patients are essential techniques in emergency medicine, cardiopulmonary resuscitation, intensive therapy, and emergency medical services. Complicated cases wherein the patients' airways are severely compromised usually require advanced airway devices such as supraglottic devices, endotracheal tubes, or surgical airway devices. This book elucidates the concepts and innovative models around prospective developments with respect to airway management. It presents researches and studies performed by experts across the globe. The extensive content of this book provides the readers with a thorough understanding of the subject.

The researches compiled throughout the book are authentic and of high quality, combining several disciplines and from very diverse regions from around the world. Drawing on the contributions of many researchers from diverse countries, the book's objective is to provide the readers with the latest achievements in the area of research. This book will surely be a source of knowledge to all interested and researching the field.

In the end, I would like to express my deep sense of gratitude to all the authors for meeting the set deadlines in completing and submitting their research chapters. I would also like to thank the publisher for the support offered to us throughout the course of the book. Finally, I extend my sincere thanks to my family for being a constant source of inspiration and encouragement.

Editor

LMA Gastro™ airway is feasible during upper gastrointestinal interventional endoscopic procedures in high risk patients

Axel Schmutz[1]* ⓘ, Thomas Loeffler[1], Arthur Schmidt[2] and Ulrich Goebel[1]

Abstract

Background: Nonoperating room anesthesia during gastroenterological procedures is a growing field in anesthetic practice. While the numbers of patients with severe comorbidities are rising constantly, gastrointestinal endoscopic interventions are moving closer to minimally invasive endoscopic surgery. The LMA Gastro™ is a new supraglottic airway device, developed specifically for upper gastrointestinal endoscopy and interventions. The aim of this study was to evaluate the feasibility of LMA Gastro™ in patients with ASA physical status ≥3 undergoing advanced endoscopic procedures.

Methods: We analyzed data from 214 patients retrospectively who received anesthesia for gastroenterological interventions. Inclusion criteria were upper gastrointestinal endoscopic interventions, airway management with LMA Gastro™ and ASA status ≥3. The primary outcome measure was successful use of LMA Gastro™ for airway management and endoscopic intervention.

Results: Thirtyone patients with ASA physical status ≥3, undergoing complex and prolonged upper gastrointestinal endoscopic procedures were included. There were 7 endoscopic retrograde cholangiopancreatographies, 7 peroral endoscopic myotomies, 5 percutaneous endoscopic gastrostomies and 12 other complex procedures (e.g. endoscopic submucosal dissection, esophageal stent placement etc.). Of these, 27 patients were managed successfully using the LMA Gastro™. Placement of the LMA Gastro™ was reported as easy. Positive pressure ventilation was performed without difficulty. The feasibility of the LMA Gastro™ for endoscopic intervention was rated excellent by the endoscopists. In four patients, placement or ventilation with LMA Gastro™ was not possible.

Conclusions: We demonstrated the feasibility of the LMA Gastro™ during general anesthesia for advanced endoscopic procedures in high-risk patients.

Keywords: Achalasia, Endoscopic procedures, Endoscopic submucosal dissection, High-risk patients, Supraglottic airway device

* Correspondence: axel.schmutz@uniklinik-freiburg.de
[1]Department of Anesthesiology and Critical Care, Faculty of Medicine, Medical Center - University of Freiburg, University of Freiburg, Hugstetter Strasse 55, 79106 Freiburg im Breisgau, Germany

Background

Nonoperating room anesthesia in the gastroenterology suite is a growing field in anesthesiology practice [1, 2]. While the majority of gastrointestinal endoscopies are performed under conscious sedation by non-anesthesia personnel, there is a shift towards deep sedation or general anesthesia for advanced procedures and interventions [3]. Especially for patients with ASA physical status ≥3, high BMI, obstructive sleep apnea and severe comorbidities, the presence of an anesthesiologist is recommended [3–5]. General anesthesia is associated with shorter procedure times, higher complete resection rates, a decreased incidence of coughing and lower perforation rates [6–8]. From a practical point of view, securing an airway for complex procedures with a gastroscope in situ usually requires tracheal intubation. The numbers of patients with severe comorbidities presenting for upper gastrointestinal endoscopic interventions are rising, so the need for a fast and yet gentle and safe airway device is relevant.

Dual channel laryngeal masks, also referred to as "second-generation" supraglottic airway devices (2nd SAD), are defined by the presence of an accessory tube for gastric drainage. Shortly after the first commercially available 2nd SAD [9], there was a report of a modified, self-made laryngeal mask, which allowed passing instruments like a gastroscope through the accessory tube into the esophageus [10]. A modified laryngeal tube, the gastro-laryngeal tube (VBM Medizintechnik GmbH, Sulz am Neckar, Germany), has been described as an alternative airway device with a dedicated channel for an endoscope [11]. This approach was not developed further until 2017, when M. Skinner introduced a refined tool in advanced airway management for upper gastrointestinal endoscopy (i.e. the LMA® Gastro™ Airway[1]) [12, 13]. This silicone-based, cuffed LMA offers an additional and separate channel for the passage of instruments (such as an endoscope) of up to a width of 16 mm in diameter [14]. If the mask is placed correctly the endoscope is guided directly towards the upper oesophageal entrance and the airway is left unobstructed. Ventilatory parameters, especially peak airway pressure, are not altered due to insertion of the endoscope through the separate channel. The endoscope may glide easily through the channel, providing excellent conditions for the endoscopist in terms of endoscope movement, including rotation and interventions. To date, the new LMA Gastro™ Airway has only been evaluated in healthy patients for diagnostic upper gastrointestinal endoscopy, demonstrating good efficacy without any detrimental or harmful side effects [12].

It was the aim of this study to evaluate the feasibility of this tool not only in ASA I and II patients for diagnostic upper gastrointestinal endoscopy, who may not even require general anesthesia but in older and high risk patients, undergoing more complex and lengthy endoscopy and subsequently more challenging interventions under general anesthesia.

Methods

This retrospective cohort analysis was approved by the local Ethics Committee, University of Freiburg, Germany (approval number EK 37/19, date: March 19th 2019, PI: Axel Schmutz, MD). The study was conducted at the Department of Anesthesiology and Critical Care and the Department of Medicine II, Medical Centre – University of Freiburg, Faculty of Medicine, Freiburg, Germany. The study was registered in the German Clinical Trials Register (DRKS00017396), PI Axel Schmutz, MD, on May 23rd 2019. The study was planned and designed in accordance with the initiative for Strengthening the Reporting of Observational Studies in Epidemiology (STROBE), using the suggested checklist for epidemiological cohort studies [15]. The data of closed files between October 2018 and March 2019 was collected by chart review and entered into a database. 214 patients who underwent upper gastrointestinal endoscopic procedures and interventions were included; 31 patients were finally analyzed. Written informed consent was obtained from all subjects, a legal surrogate, or the parents or legal guardians. A priori sample size calculation was not applicable due to the retrospective study design.

High-risk patients undergoing elective upper gastrointestinal endoscopic procedures and interventions with the need for general anesthesia were analyzed. Inclusion criteria were airway management with LMA Gastro™, ASA status 3 or above, age 10 years and older, body weight above 30 kg. Patients fasted for at least 6 h for solids and at least two hours for clear fluids. It was our intention not to exclude any patients with esophageal reflux, esophageal strictures, cancer of the upper gastrointestinal tract or the stomach, achalasia, pancreatitis, upper GI bleeding, colitis, pyloric stenosis, morbid obesity etc.

Anesthetic management

After implementation of routine monitoring (ECG, non-invasive blood pressure, peripheral oxygen saturation) general anesthesia was induced using i.v. sufentanil (0.2–0.3 µg·kg^{-1} body weight (BW)) followed by remifentanil (0.1–0.5 µg·kg^{-1}·min^{-1}) and propofol 3.0–5.0 µg·ml^{-1} effect site concentration target-controlled infusion (Agilia™, Schnider model). Paralytic medication was not administered. Normocapnia and normoxia were achieved by positive pressure ventilation (pressure

---

[1]LMA is a registered trademark of The Laryngeal Mask Company Ltd., an affiliate of Teleflex Incorporated

controlled ventilation, positive endexspiratory pressure: of 3–5 mbar, respiratory rate: 10–18/min) with a F_IO_2 of 0.5 after insertion of the lubricated LMA Gastro™ Airway (Size 3, 4 or 5). The LMA cuff was filled with air until the indicator of the cuff pressure valve was in the "green zone" of the cuff pressure valve. This corresponds to a cuff pressure of 40 cm H_2O. (Cuff Pilot, embedded cuff monitoring system). According to our departmental standards a successful insertion was assumed by a square wave pattern capnography, symmetrical chest wall expansion and absence of an audible oral air leak with a cuff pressure between 20 and 40 cmH_2O. Haemodynamic shifts (mean arterial blood pressure ± 20% regarding baseline values) were treated with i.v. ephedrine/norepinephrine or urapidil respectively. After fixation of the LMA Gastro™ Airway, a well lubricated flexible endoscope was inserted into the gastric channel and advanced into the oesophagus. Anesthetic and endoscopic records and ward charts of patients were analyzed for periinterventional data regarding airway management, pharyngeal bleeding, sore throat, hoarseness and any other serious adverse events during or within 24 h after the endoscopic intervention.

If tracheal intubation was necessary, neuromuscular block was induced using an i.v. bolus of rocuronium bromide (0.6–1.0 mg·kg^{-1} body weight).

The combined outcome was defined as the feasibility to use the LMA Gastro™ successfully for both, the endoscopic intervention and a sufficient airway management in the defined high-risk patients. Secondary outcome parameters comprised (a) the ease of placement of the LMA Gastro™ or any additional attempts required to correctly place the device, (b) the need for any alternative airway devices (i.e. tracheal tube) in case of uncontrollable permanent airway leakage, (c) any form of dislocation associated with the endoscopic procedure, thus necessitating an alternative airway tool, other than the LMA Gastro™, (d) the incidence of pharyngeal bleeding during placement or after the removal of the LMA Gastro™, (e) any unwanted events during the endoscopic procedure with the main focus on regurgitation, aspiration or hypoxia, (f) duration of the endoscopic procedure, (g) sore throat and/or hoarseness and (h) the comfort of advancing and operating the endoscope through the gastric channel rated by the attending endoscopist after the procedure via a 5 point Likert-type scale (0 = not at all satisfied, 1 = slightly satisfied, 2 = moderately satisfied, 3 = very satisfied, 4 = completely satisfied).

The data was collected in a MS Excel™ (Microsoft, Redmond, USA) datasheet. Further statistical processing was performed using SPSS™ (IBM, Armonk, USA).

Results

Of 214 patients receiving anesthetic care in the gastroenterology suite, 75 patients were ventilated with the LMA Gastro™. Thirtyone cases were advanced procedures in high-risk patients lasting for a median of 60 min (Additional file 1: Figure S1). Patient characteristics, endoscopic interventions, duration of the procedures and the endoscopists' ratings are summarized in Table 1. These 31 endoscopic interventions were performed under general anesthesia, of which 27 finally were performed successfully with LMA Gastro™ (Fig. 1).

Procedures performed were endoscopic retrograde cholangiopancreatography (ERCP) (n = 7), peroral endoscopic myotomy (POEM) (n = 7) (Additional file 1: Figure S2), percutaneous endoscopic or fluoroscopic gastrostomy (PEG) (n = 5) (Fig. 2, Additional file 4), endoscopic submucosal dissection (ESD) and submucosal tunneling endoscopic resection (STER) (n = 6) or other advanced procedures (e.g. esophageal stent placement; Fig. 3; Additional file 2; endoscopic ultrasound probe, Fig. 4) in patients with considerable comorbidity (n = 6). The feasibility of the LMA Gastro™ for endoscopic intervention was rated as satisfactory by the four endoscopists (Table 1).

Table 1 Patient characteristics, endoscopic procedures (n = 31). Values are number (proportion) or median (IQR [range])

Age (yrs) median [IQR]	65 [31–72]
Sex	
male	23
female	8
ASA physical status[a]	
3	22 [71%]
4	9 [29%]
Body Mass Index median [IQR]	24 [20–25]
Reflux	9 [32%]
Results	
Endoscopic procedure	
PEG[b]	5 [16%]
ERCP[c]	7 [23%]
POEM[d]	7 [23%]
ESD[e], STER[f]	6 [19%]
other	6 [19%]
Ventilation and endoscopic procedure through LMA Gastro™ successful	27 [87%]
Duration of endoscopic procedure (min) median, [IQR]	60 [25–75]
Sore throat and/or hoarseness (in PACU)	4 [13%]
Rating of endoscopist[g], mean [range]	3.7 [3–4]

Abbreviations: [a]ASA physical status: ASA Physical Status Classification System [16]; [b]PEG, percutaneous endoscopic or fluoroscopic gastrostomy; [c]ERCP, endoscopic retrograde cholangiopancreatography; [d]POEM, peroral endoscopic myotomy; [e]ESD, Endoscopic submucosal dissection; [f]STER, submucosal tunneling endoscopic resection. [g]Rating of endoscopist Likert-type scale (0 = not at all satisfied, 1 = slightly satisfied, 2 = moderately satisfied, 3 = very satisfied, 4 = completely satisfied)

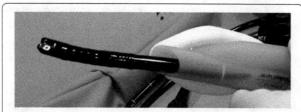

Fig. 1 Gastroduodenoscope passing through the gastric channel of a LMA Gastro™

Placement of the LMA Gastro™ was reported as easy. All LMA Gastro™ were positioned at the first insertion attempt. In four patients, ventilation with LMA Gastro™ was not possible and tracheal intubation was performed instead. In one of these patients tracheal intubation was performed through the LMA Gastro™ using a 5.0 mm I.D. (6.9 mm O.D) microlaryngoscopy tube (Fig. 5 a-c; Additional file 3). The tube was mounted on a fiberscope (Ambu® aScope™ 4 Broncho Slim 3.8). In two other patients, one additional attempt at LMA Gastro™ placement was necessary.

Positive pressure ventilation was performed without any difficulties. There were no detectable differences regarding peak airway pressures or tidal volumes after insertion of the flexible endoscope. No signs of hypoxia, regurgitation or aspiration were noted. Even complex interventions with considerable insufflation of CO_2 did not result in clinically significant hypercarbia.

One patient developed subcutaneous emphysema of the neck and left chestwall after endoscopic resection of an esophageal leiomyoma. This condition resolved spontaneously without any intervention.

There was not a single dislocation of the LMA Gastro™ due to endoscope movement through the designated channel.

Post interventional course
There were no clinically significant adverse events within the cohort. No patient had to be admitted to the intensive care unit unexpectedly. All but one patient were discharged from PACU to a regular ward. We did not observe any pharyngeal bleeding. One patient developed a minor uvular hematoma, possibly due to positioning, and had difficulties swallowing for two days following the intervention.

Discussion
In this retrospective analysis, we demonstrated the feasibility of the LMA Gastro™ airway as a valuable tool for advanced gastrointestinal endoscopic interventions under general anesthesia in high-risk patients.

The design of the LMA Gastro™ with its wide endoscope channel, an integrated bite block and an adjustable holder facilitates easy passage of a well lubricated endoscope (Fig. 2). The use of SAD usually reduces anesthetic dose requirements and decreases recovery time compared to tracheal intubation in nonendoscopic procedures. Furthermore, relaxation is not required. Compared to patients with orotracheal intubation, endoscopists estimated conditions with regard to access to the gastrointestinal tract as equal or better. The LMA Gastro™ aids the insertion of the gastroduodenoscope by guiding it into the upper esophagus. This may be the reason for the high degree of satisfaction we found in our setting.

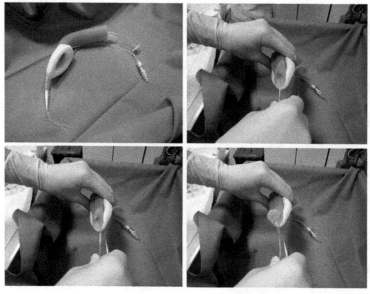

Fig. 2 Percutaneous endoscopic gastrostomy, "pull" technique

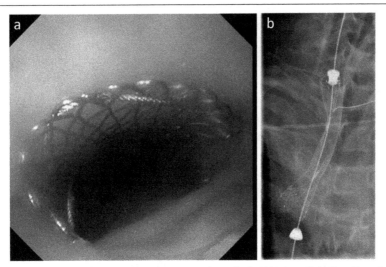

Fig. 3 Esophageal stent placement. **a** Endoscopic view through the gastric channel of a LMA Gastro™. **b** Chest X-ray: Esophageal stent placement, LMA Gastro™ in situ

We performed about 87% of all anesthetics for endoscopic intervention with the LMA Gastro™ successfully. Secondary conversion to an oral tracheal tube was required for four patients only, three of them with a history of major oral cancer and radiation therapy. Due to our experience, we would not recommend the use of LMA Gastro™ in this patient population because of the difficulties in positioning, risk of bleeding and an insufficient seal of the LMA with the periglottic structures.

The cuff of the LMA Gastro™ is more voluminous compared to first generation SAD [17]. Nevertheless, anesthesia providers reported insertion efforts similar to other second generation SADs. The pre-curved design and the bendability improved handling and enabled providers to insert the device in the supine and left lateral

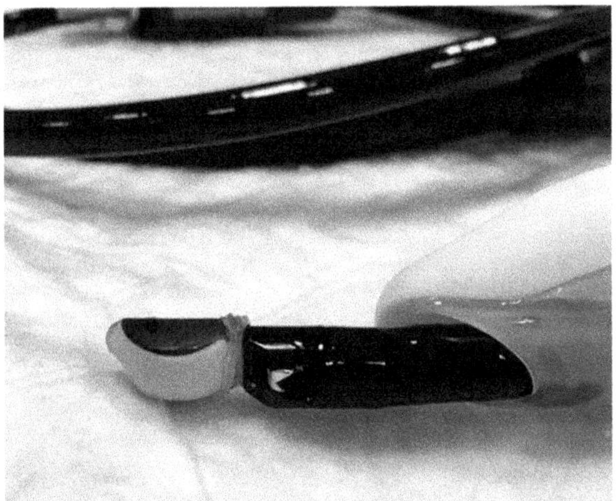

Fig. 4 Endoscopic ultrasound probe passing through the LMA Gastro™

position without any difficulties. Providers should be cautious during insertion, as the distal opening of the endoscope channel may entrap soft palate structures causing mucosal lacerations.

The increasing popularity of deep sedation in patients undergoing upper gastrointestinal procedures will account for a rising number of anesthesiologist guided deep sedation. Patients who have previously showed poor tolerance to endoscopy under conscious sedation and who subsequently need to undergo prolonged and repeated procedures may be of particular benefit from the use of the LMA Gastro™. Intolerance of conscious sedation is a significant factor in failure of endoscopic procedures [18].

In advanced procedures like peroral esophageal myotomy (POEM) or endoscopic submucosal dissection (ESD), minimal patient movement is preferred to limit adverse events like perforation or bleeding.

ERCP is most often performed in spontaneously breathing patients under deep sedation without airway protection in the prone position, thereby reducing the risk of aspiration. However, patients with ASA physical status III and above, patients with severe cardio-pulmonary comorbidity, morbid obesity, obstructive sleep apnoea or reflux represent a group with an increased risk of cardio-respiratory adverse events [19, 20] and therefore tracheal intubation during general anesthesia is a common technique for this population [21].

Although studies of airway management using first generation "classic" LMA during ERCP in adults [22] and during esophagogastroduodenoscopy in paediatric patients [23] have been performed, this technique is not commonly used. This accounts to an even lesser extent for long interventions in high-risk patients. The LMA

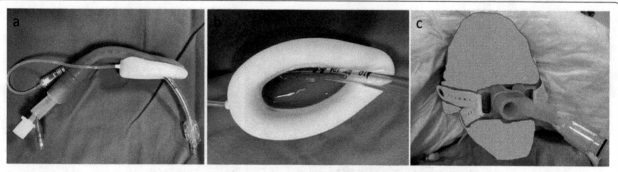

Fig. 5 a Microlaryngoscopy tube (5.0 mm I.D., 6.9 mm O.D) passing through the airway lumen of the LMA Gastro™. **b** proximal end of the LMA Gastro™ with ETT in place. Please notice the large gastric channel narrowing the airway lumen. **c** LMA Gastro™ with a microlaryngoscopy tube in tracheal position

Gastro™ may offer a suitable alternative for airway control during ERCP.

An additional indication to use the LMA Gastro™ may be transesophageal echocardiography (TEE) under deep sedation. We used TEE in a patient with a left ventricular assist device immediately before ERCP.

On principle, the LMA Gastro™ was not designed to facilitate tracheal intubation. The narrow internal diameter (ID) of the airway lumen prevents a tracheal tube from passing through. If tracheal intubation through a SAD is planned, we therefore recommend to either exchange the LMA Gastro™ for another SAD that will allow direct passage of an adult-sized ETT or using a microlaryngoscopy tube, a pediatric-sized standard ETT (5.0 mm ID) with an adult length, mounted over a bronchoscope and inserted through the LMA Gastro™ into the trachea.

We are fully aware, that some of our patients met the criteria for tracheal intubation. Recommendations for patients with achalasia undergoing POEM typically include rapid sequence induction followed by tracheal intubation [24–26]. In our approach, patients with no residual solid food during prior diagnostic esophagoscopy, after induction of anesthesia without face-mask ventilation and insertion of the LMA Gastro™, the endoscopist immediately advanced the gastroscope through the gastric channel into the esophagus and stomach and evacuated any residual esophageal content.

This study has several limitations. First, the retrospective design at a single university medical center limits our conclusions, so they may not be generalizable. Second, the data relied on provider documentation to identify the use and success of the airway device. Due to the retrospective nature of this study, the reasoning behind a provider's decision to perform tracheal intubation rather than use an SAD could not be assessed. Third, this is an observational study, not including a control group.

Our analysis should be considered as a pilot study for future randomized clinical trials with multicenter and

prospective design to clarify the role of SAD devices during general anesthesia for endoscopic procedures. Especially comparisons with alternative techniques using other airway devices and monitored anesthesia care without airway protection are needed to evaluate the risks and benefits of different techniques.

In conclusion, we demonstrated the feasibility of the LMA Gastro™ during general anesthesia for endoscopic procedures in high-risk patients.

Supplementary information

Additional file 1: Figure S1. CONSORT diagram of patient recruitment. **Figure S2**. Gastroduodenoscope with attachment cap for peroral endoscopic myotomy (POEM), passing through the gastric channel of a LMA Gastro™.

Additional file 2. Esophageal stent through LMA Gastro™. Access to the videos also via the following link: https://drive.google.com/drive/folders/1 mVOhwgJGT5y5I5WE-cTyQpitMEc7VS88?usp=sharing.

Additional file 3. Microlaryngoscopy tracheal tube through LMA Gastro™. Access to the videos also via the following link: https://drive.google.com/drive/folders/1mVOhwgJGT5y5I5WE-cTyQpitMEc7VS88?usp=sharing.

Additional file 4. Percutaneous endoscopic gastrostomy through LMA Gastro™. Access to the videos also via the following link: https://drive.google.com/drive/folders/1mVOhwgJGT5y5I5WE-cTyQpitMEc7VS88?usp=sharing.

Abbreviations

ASA: American society of anesthesiologists; BMI: Body mass index; CO_2: Carbon dioxide; ECG: Electrocardiogram; ERCP: Endoscopic retrograde cholangiopancreatography; ESD: Endoscopic submucosal dissection; ETT: Tracheal tube; F_iO_2: Fraction of inspired oxygen; ID: Internal diameter; LMA: Laryngeal mask airway; PEG: Percutaneous endoscopic or fluoroscopic gastrostomy; POEM: Peroral endoscopic myotomy; SAD: Supraglottic airway device; STER: Submucosal tunneling endoscopic resection; STROBE: Strengthening the Reporting of Observational Studies in Epidemiology; TEE: Transesophageal echocardiography

Acknowledgments

The authors would like to thank Dr. Helen Engelstaedter, Department of Anesthesia, Helios Rosmann Hospital, Breisach, GERMANY, for language editing and Susan Koehler, Department of Anesthesiology and Critical Care, Medical Center - University of Freiburg, GERMANY for administrative support.

LMA GastroTM airway is feasible during upper gastrointestinal interventional endoscopic procedures in high...

7

Authors' contributions

Study design: AxS, TL, protocol design: AxS, TL, advisor for study protocol and management of the study: AxS, TL, UG, data collection: AxS, TL, ArS, study conduct: AxS, TL, ArS, study monitoring: AxS, TL, ArS, data analysis: AxS, TL, ArS, UG, data evaluation: AxS, TL, ArS, UG, writing the manuscript: AxS, TL, ArS, UG, editing and approval of the manuscript: AxS, TL, ArS, UG. All authors read and approved the final manuscript.

Author details

[1]Department of Anesthesiology and Critical Care, Faculty of Medicine, Medical Center - University of Freiburg, University of Freiburg, Hugstetter Strasse 55, 79106 Freiburg im Breisgau, Germany. [2]Department of Medicine II, Faculty of Medicine, Medical Center - University of Freiburg University of Freiburg, Hugstetter Strasse 55, Freiburg im Breisgau 79106, Germany.

References

1. Gabriel RA, Burton BN, Tsai MH, Ehrenfeld JM, Dutton RP, Urman RD. After-hour versus daytime shifts in non-operating room anesthesia environments: National Distribution of case volume, patient characteristics, and procedures. J Med Syst. 2017;41:140.
2. Nagrebetsky A, Gabriel RA, Dutton RP, Urman RD. Growth of nonoperating room anesthesia Care in the United States: a contemporary trends analysis. Anesth Analg. 2017;124:1261–7.
3. Sidhu R, Turnbull D, Newton M, et al. Deep sedation and anaesthesia in complex gastrointestinal endoscopy: a joint position statement endorsed by the British Society of Gastroenterology (BSG), joint advisory group (JAG) and Royal College of Anaesthetists (RCoA). Frontline Gastroenterol. 2019;10:141–7.
4. Riphaus A, Wehrmann T, Weber B, et al. S3-Leitlinie "Sedierung in der gastrointestinalen Endoskopie" 2008 (AWMF-Register-Nr. 021 / 014). Z Gastroenterol. 2008;46:1298–330.
5. Early DS, Lightdale JR, Vargo JJ, et al. Guidelines for sedation and anesthesia in GI endoscopy. Gastrointest Endosc. 2018;87:327–37.
6. Rong Q-H, Zhao G-L, Xie J-P, Wang L-X. Feasibility and safety of endoscopic submucosal dissection of esophageal or gastric carcinomas under general anesthesia. Med Princ Pract. 2013;22:280–4.
7. Song BG, Min YW, Cha RR, et al. Endoscopic submucosal dissection under general anesthesia for superficial esophageal squamous cell carcinoma is associated with better clinical outcomes. BMC Gastroenterol. 2018;18:80.
8. Yurtlu DA, Aslan F, Ayvat P, et al. Propofol-based sedation versus general anesthesia for endoscopic submucosal dissection. Medicine (Baltimore). 2016;95:e3680.
9. Brimacombe J, Keller C. The ProSeal laryngeal mask airway: a randomized, crossover study with the standard laryngeal mask airway in paralyzed, anesthetized patients. Anesthesiology. 2000;93:104–9.
10. Agrò F, Brimacombe J, Keller C, Petruzziello L, Barzoi G. Gastroscopy in awake and anaesthetized patients using a modified laryngeal mask. Eur J Anaesthesiol. 2000;17:652–3.
11. Fabbri C, Luigiano C, Cennamo V, et al. The gastro-laryngeal tube for interventional endoscopic biliopancreatic procedures in anesthetized patients. Endoscopy. 2012;44:1051–4.
12. Terblanche NCS, Middleton C, Choi-Lundberg DL, Skinner M. Efficacy of a new dual channel laryngeal mask airway, the LMA®gastro™ airway, for upper gastrointestinal endoscopy: a prospective observational study. Br J Anaesth. 2018;120:353–60.
13. Sorbello M, Pulvirenti GS, Pluchino D, Skinner M. State of the art in airway management during GI endoscopy: the missing pieces. Dig Dis Sci. 2017;62:1385–7.
14. Sorbello M. Evolution of supraglottic airway devices: the Darwinian perspective. Minerva Anestesiol. 2018;84:297–300.
15. von Elm E, Altman DG, Egger M, Pocock SJ, Gøtzsche PC, Vandenbroucke JP. The strengthening the reporting of observational studies in epidemiology (STROBE) statement: guidelines for reporting observational studies. Ann Intern Med. 2007;147:573–7.
16. American Society of Anesthesiologists. ASA Physical Status Classification System. Available from https://www.asahq.org/standards-and-guidelines/asa-physical-status-classification-system. (Accessed 17 May 2019).
17. Sorbello M, Petrini F. Supraglottic airway devices: the search for the best insertion technique or the time to change our point of view? Turk J Anaesthesiol Reanim. 2017;45:76–82.
18. Church NI, Seward EW, Pereira SP, Hatfield AR, Webster GJ. Success of repeat ERCP following initial therapeutic failure. Gastrointest Endosc. 2006;63:AB293.
19. Patel S, Vargo JJ, Khandwala F, et al. Deep sedation occurs frequently during elective endoscopy with meperidine and midazolam. Am J Gastroenterol. 2005;100:2689–95.
20. Sorser SA, Fan DS, Tommolino EE, et al. Complications of ERCP in patients undergoing general anesthesia versus MAC. Dig Dis Sci. 2014;59:696–7.
21. Raymondos K, Panning B, Bachem I, Manns MP, Piepenbrock S, Meier PN. Evaluation of endoscopic retrograde cholangiopancreatography under conscious sedation and general anesthesia. Endoscopy. 2002;34:721–6.
22. Osborn IP, Cohen J, Soper RJ, Roth LA. Laryngeal mask airway--a novel method of airway protection during ERCP: comparison with endotracheal intubation. Gastrointest Endosc. 2002;56:122–8.
23. Orfei P, Ferri F, Panella I, Meloncelli S, Patrizio AP, Pinto G. L'impiego della maschera laringea nelle esofagogastroduodenoscopie in età pediatrica. Minerva Anestesiol. 2002;68:77–82.
24. Löser B, Werner YB, Punke MA, et al. Considérations anesthésiques pour la prise en charge des patients atteints d'achalasie de l'œsophage subissant une myotomie per-orale endoscopique: Compte rendu rétrospectif d'une série de cas. Can J Anaesth. 2017;64:480–8.
25. Tanaka E, Murata H, Minami H, Sumikawa K. Anesthetic management of peroral endoscopic myotomy for esophageal achalasia: a retrospective case series. J Anesth. 2014;28:456–9.
26. Inoue H, Shiwaku H, Iwakiri K, et al. Clinical practice guidelines for peroral endoscopic myotomy. Dig Endosc. 2018;30:563–79.

2

The Clarus Video System (Trachway) and direct laryngoscope for endotracheal intubation with cricoid pressure in simulated rapid sequence induction intubation

Yen-Chu Lin[1], An-Hsun Cho[1,4], Jr-Rung Lin[1,2,3,4] and Yung-Tai Chung[1*] ⓘ

Abstract

Background: During an emergency endotracheal intubation, rapid sequence induction intubation (RSII) with cricoid pressure (CP) is frequently implemented to prevent aspiration pneumonia. We evaluated the CVS in endotracheal intubation in RSII with CP, in comparison with a direct laryngoscope (DL).

Methods: One hundred fifty patients were randomly assigned to one of three groups: the CVS as a video stylet (CVS-V) group, the CVS as a lightwand (CVS-L) group and DL group. Primary outcomes were to assess the power of the CVS, compared with DL, regarding the first attempt success rate and intubation time in simulated RSII with CP. Secondary outcomes were to examine hemodynamic stress response and the incidence of complications.

Results: The first attempt success rates within 30 s and within 60 s were higher in CVS-V and DL group than those in CVS-L group ($p = 0.006$ and 0.037, respectively). The intergroup difference for intubation success rate within 30 s was nonsignificant and almost all the patients were successfully intubated within 60 s (98% for CVS-L and DL group, 96% for CVS-L group). Kaplan-Meier estimator demonstrated the median intubation time was 10.6 s [95% CI, 7.5 to 13.7] in CVS-V group, 14.6 s [95% CI, 11.1 to 18.0] in CVS-L group and 16.5 s [95% CI, 15.7 to 17.3] in DL group ($p = 0.023$ by the log-rank test). However, the difference was nonsignificant after Sidak's adjustment. The intergroup differences for hemodynamic stress response, sore throat and mucosa injury incidence were also nonsignificant.

Conclusions: The CVS-D and DL provide a higher first attempt intubation success rate within 30 and 60 s in intubation with CP; the intubation time for the CVS-V was nonsignificantly shorter than that for the other two intubation methods. Almost all the patients can be successfully intubated with any of the three intubation methods within 60 s.

Keywords: Rapid sequence induction intubation, Cricoid pressure, The Clarus Video System, Direct laryngoscope

* Correspondence: oj8600chung@gmail.com
[1]Department of Anesthesiology, Chang Gung Memorial Hospital, No.5, Fuxing St., Guishan Dist., Taoyuan City 333, Taiwan

Background

Although there has been no scientific evidence to prove that cricoid pressure (CP) will prevent aspiration pneumonia [1, 2], the majority of anesthesiologists (92%) in a national survey in the UK still use CP in rapid sequence induction intubation (RSII) [3]. Therefore, skillfully using a proper intubation device is obligatory for those anesthesiologists to ensure the successful endotracheal intubation with CP.

When properly applied, CP may not affect glottic view during endotracheal intubation with either a direct laryngoscope (DL) or a video laryngoscope [4–6]. However, the application of CP is likely to prolong the intubation time [5, 6]. Limited mouth opening or vulnerable teeth, which often accompany the patients requiring emergency intubation, are the two common factors to deter the intubators from using a laryngoscopic device. Besides, the blade of a laryngoscopic device is often too bulky for a narrow mouth opening, and the blade always bears a level force on upper incisors while the intubator is lifting epiglottis during intubation, which is liable to tooth fracture.

Intubating stylets with a slim handle have been proved to be superior to laryngoscopic devices for the endotracheal intubation in terms of ease of movement [7, 8] and prevention of dental injury [8]. The Clarus Video System (Trachway®, CVS) intubating stylet (Biotronic Instrument Enterprise Ltd., Tai-Chung, Taiwan), a video stylet, has been proved to be a comparable but faster solution to successful intubation than DL [9–11] in intubation without CP. Moreover, the CVS can also be operated as a lightwand when its red light is turned on. This alternative function is practically advantageous when the video image is blurred by mist, secretions or blood in the oral cavity or the intubators just lose their way in locating the glottis. The endotracheal tube will be initially guided into larynx in the dimly lit operating room by a bright glow moving in the anterior soft tissue of the neck and finally by the image of the trachea rings on the video screen. In addition, the CVS barely applies force on the teeth while an endotracheal intubation is being performed. As a result, dental trauma can be avoided.

How the CVS performs in endotracheal intubation with CP has not yet been evaluated in literature, so the study is the first to examine the capability of the CVS in intubation with CP. A lightwand (Surch-Lite; Aaron Medical, St Petersburg, FL), an intubation stylet without video assistance, was not recommended by Hodgson et al. as the first choice of endotracheal intubation with CP because of longer intubation time and higher failure rate for the first attempt [12]. Nevertheless, we hypothesized that the CVS could yield positive results in a study examining the capability of the CVS in endotracheal intubation with CP. In this prospective randomized study, we compare the use of the CVS and that of DL (Macintosh Laryngoscope) in patients undergoing endotracheal intubation in simulated RSII for the primary goals of the first attempt success rate and intubation time.

Methods

This study was approved by Chang Gung Medical Foundation Institutional Review Board and a written informed consent was obtained from each patient. The patients participating in this clinical trial were older than 20 years of age and scheduled for elective surgery under general anesthesia. Patients were excluded if they had BMI (Body Mass Index) > 35 kg/m^2, interincisor distance < 3 cm, poor dentition, upper airway tumor, limited neck mobility, pregnancy or history of difficult tracheal intubation.

One hundred fifty patients were enrolled and, based on computer-generated random numbers, were assigned to one of three groups: the CVS as a video stylet (CVS-V) group, the CVS as a lightwand (CVS-L) group and DL group. All intubations were executed by two anesthesiologists who are experienced in the use of the designated devices, Lin for CVS-V as well as DL group and Chung for CVS-L group. Both Chung and Lin have used the CVS in more than 200 cases, and Chung also has more than 10 years' practice with lighted stylet [13].

After the intravenous line was checked and monitors, including electrocardiography, pulse oximetry and non-invasive blood pressure measurement, were correctively positioned, the patients breathed 100% oxygen for 3 min. Anesthesia was induced with fentanyl (2 μg/kg), lidocaine (20 mg), propofol (2 mg/kg) and rocuronium (1.2 mg/kg) intravenously. No assistant breathing was offered to all the patients before endotracheal intubation. Sixty seconds following the injection of rocuronium, each patient was intubated with the assigned device and an endotracheal tube of proper size while 30-40 N pressure was being applied on the cricoid cartilage by an assistant standing on a weighing scale [14]. Following checking the position and tapping of the tube, sevoflurane 4% in 50% oxygen with a fresh gas flow 4 L/min was initially provided from the circle system of the anesthesia machine and then the concentration of the inhalation anesthetic was adjusted in accordance with the patient's need.

In this trial, successful intubation was defined as the intubation was completed within 30 s. Intubation time was counted from the inserting the device into the patient's mouth to viewing the endotracheal tube into the trachea. The intubation time for patients who required more than one attempt was the sum of the times of all the intubation attempts. The following data were also collected: (1) airway parameters (Mallampati classification, thyromental distance, interincisor distance and neck circumference); (2) hemodynamic stress response; (3) sore throat and mucosa injury (documented by a blinded observer on the next day).

Statistical analyses were conducted using SPSS version 17.0 (SPSS Inc., Chicago, IL, U.S.) and SAS version 9.4 (SAS Institute Inc., Cary, NC, U.S.). The study was designed to allow the intergroup difference of 20% for first attempt success rate to detect at 5% level of significance with a power of 80%. Categorical data were analyzed by the chi-square test and continuous data by one-way analysis of variance. Hemodynamic changes responsive to endotracheal intubation were tested by analysis of covariance, using preinduction variables as the covariates. Bonferroni post hoc tests were performed where appropriate. The log-rank test with Sidak correction was used to compare the intergroup difference for the Kaplan-Meier curves that were obtained from the time to successful intubation with one attempt for each patient. A p value less than or equal to 0.05 was considered to be statistically significant.

Results

A total of 214 patients undergoing elective surgery were screened between November 2016 and April 2018, of which 64 were excluded because they refused to participate or did not meet one or more of the inclusion criteria. The others were randomly allocated into three groups (Fig. 1). Demographics and airway characteristics of the patients in three groups were similar (Table 1).

The first attempt success rate (in either within 30 s or within 60 s) of CVS-V and DL group was significantly higher than that of CVS-L group ($p = 0.006$ and 0.037, respectively) (Table 2). Forty-seven patients (94%) in CVS-V group, 47 in DL group (94%) and 38 in CVS-L group (76%) had their intubation completed within 30 s at the first attempt. Of the ten patients requiring time between 30 and 60 s to be intubated at the first attempt, 2 were from CVS-V group, 6 from CVS-L group and 2 from DL group, respectively. Eight patients required two attempts to be intubated, 1 patient in CVS-V group by the CVS-V, 6 in CVS-L group by the CVS-L and 1 in DL group by the CVS-V (due to unseen glottis with DL at the first attempt). However, the intergroup difference for intubation success rate (including patients who had 2 attempts of intubation) within 30 s was nonsignificant (94% for CVS-L and DL group, 82% for CVS-L group). Almost all the patients were intubated within 60 s (98% for CVS-L and DL group, 96% for CVS-L group).

If the patients with failed intubation at the first attempt were treated as censored observations, Kaplan-Meier estimator (Fig. 2) demonstrates that more patients in CVS-V group than in the other two groups have their intubation completed in shorter time. The median time of successful intubation at the first attempt was faster in

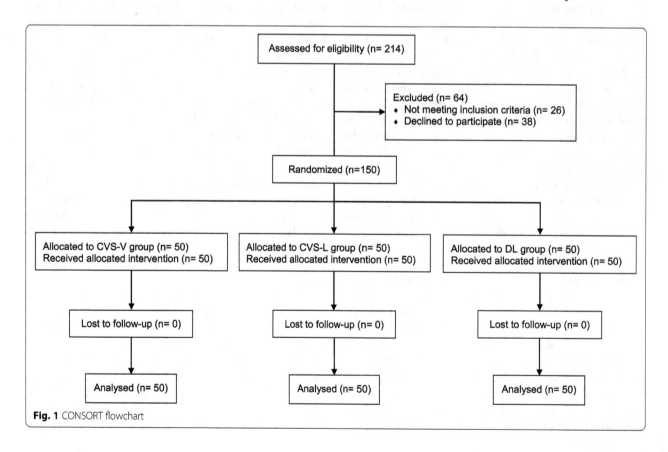

Fig. 1 CONSORT flowchart

Table 1 Demographic data, airway characteristics, complications and hemodynamic responses

	CVS-V group (n = 50)	CVS-L group (n = 50)	DL group (n = 50)	p value
Demographic data				
Age (years)	46 ± 12	47 ± 14	48 ± 12	0.575
ASA class (I/II/III)	16/31/3	15/33/2	10/36/4	0.634
Gender (M/F)	23/27	29/21	24/26	0.437
Body height (cm)	163 ± 8	165 ± 8	163 ± 8	0.313
Body weight (kg)	66 ± 11	68 ± 12	65 ± 13	0.478
BMI (kg/m^2)	25 ± 3	25 ± 3	24 ± 4	0.878
Airway characteristics				
Mallampati classification (1/2/3/4)	8/16/20/6	12/17/12/9	12/11/19/8	0.512
Thyromental distance (cm)	6.5 ± 0.7	6.4 ± 0.7	6.6 ± 0.8	0.360[b]
Interincisor distance (cm)	4.5 ± 0.8	4.6 ± 0.6	4.7 ± 0.6	0.304
Neck circumference (cm)	38 ± 5	39 ± 5	38 ± 4	0.431
Complications				
Sore throat in the next day[a] (n; none/mild/moderate/severe)	37/10/2/1	34/11/5/0	28/17/4/1	0.445
Mucosa injury	2	1	0	0.360
Hemodynamic response[b]				
Patients successfully intubated at the first attempt	49	44	49	
Mean arterial pressure (mmHg)				
Preinduction	98 ± 12	101 ± 15	98 ± 12	0.321
1 min after intubation	98 ± 23[c]	107 ± 21	104 ± 22	0.164
5 min after intubation	74 ± 14	78 ± 16	77 ± 17	0.575
Heart rate (bpm)				
Preinduction	74 ± 14	77 ± 12	70 ± 11	0.149
1 min after intubation	89 ± 15	94 ± 17	88 ± 14	0.571
5 min after intubation	84 ± 15	86 ± 16	81 ± 14	0.926

Values are shown as mean ± standard deviation or number
[a] Sore throat was graded according to numerical rating scale (NRS): none, NRS = 0; mild, NRS = 1–3; moderate, NRS = 4–6; severe, NRS = 7–10
[b] Analysis of hemodynamic response excluded patients who need second attempt. Preinduction variables are referred to as covariate of 1 min or 5 min after intubation variables in the analysis of covariance (ANCOVA). No significant hemodynamic response to endotracheal intubation was seen in any of the three groups
[c] No statistical difference versus preinduction value within the group

Table 2 Data of endotracheal intubations

	CVS-V group (n = 50)	CVS-L group (n = 50)	DL group (n = 50)	p value
Patients successfully intubated				
At the first attempt within 30 s	47 (94)	38 (76)	47 (94)	0.006
At the first attempt within 60 s[a]	49 (98)	44 (88)	49 (98)	0.037
Success within 30 s (including two attempts)	47 (94)	41 (82)	47 (94)	0.069
Success within 60 s (including two attempts)	49 (98)	48 (96)	49 (98)	0.773
Median time to successful intubation at the first attempt (s)	10.6 (7.5 to 13.7)	14.6 (11.1 to 18.0)	16.5 (15.7 to 17.3)	0.023[b]

Values are shown as number (%) or median (95% CI)
[a] Intubation tools at the second attempt were the same in both CVS-V and CVS-L group. In the DL group, CVS-V was used in this case due to unseen glottis at the first attempt
[b] Data from Kaplan-Meier estimator with p value of log-rank test. However, after Sidak's adjustment for multiple comparisons for the log-rank test, the p values were all more than 0.05 in three comparisons (p = 0.0566 between CVS-V group and CVS-L group, p = 0.0762 between CVS-V group and DL group, and p = 0.9998 between CVS-V group and CVS-L group)

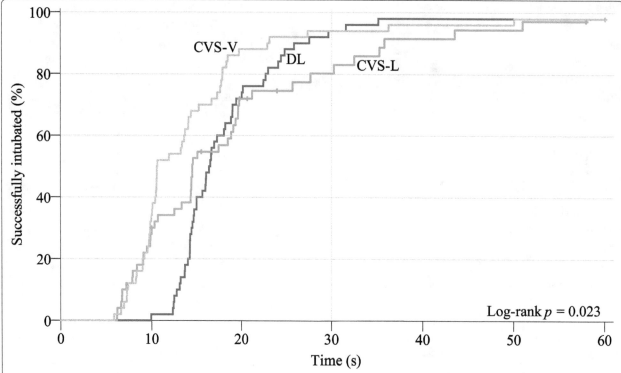

Fig. 2 Duration of the successful intubation at the first attempt demonstrated by Kaplan-Meier estimator. Vertical ticks mark the time point when the first intubation attempt failed (censored observation). Kaplan-Meier estimator demonstrates that the intubation time in CVS-V group is consistently shorter than that in the other two groups. And the intubation time in CVS-L is the most inconsistent. The p value was 0.023 by the log-rank test. However, after Sidak's adjustment for multiple comparisons for the log-rank test, the p values were more than 0.05 between the groups

CVS-V (10.6 s [95% CI, 7.5 to 13.7]) than in CVS-L group (14.6 s [95% CI, 11.1 to 18.0]) or in DL group (16.5 s [95% CI, 15.7 to 17.3]) (Table 2). The p value was 0.023 by the log-rank test, but the intergroup difference was nonsignificant after Sidak's adjustment ($p = 0.0566$ between CVS-V group and CVS-L group, $p = 0.0762$ between CVS-V group and DL group, and $p = 0.9998$ between CVS-V group and CVS-L group).

Although mean blood pressures in CVS-V group appeared the least responsive to intubation, the intergroup difference was nonsignificant (Table 1). There was no patient who had oxygen saturation below 90% during intubation. Sore throat and mucosa injury occurred with a similar frequency in the three groups (Table 1).

Discussion
In a large randomized clinical trial (3472 cases) conducted in urban academic centers, intubation with CP failed to show an advantage over intubation without CP in RSII in terms of preventing pulmonary aspiration [2]. However, the authors also mentioned that the results of the study may not be applied to emergency cases outside operating rooms where there are supposed to be more manpower and equipment, and patients probably has more adequate muscle relaxation for endotracheal

intubation. Aspiration pneumonia is still a major concern to many anesthesiologists, so they will not hesitate to apply CP while intubating patients with risks of the complication [3].

As compared to DL, the video laryngoscopes during endotracheal intubation are associated with less neck manipulation, a better glottic view and a higher success rate of intubation in normal or difficult airways [15], but they don't usually guarantee shorter intubation time [16, 17]. Moreover, like DL with a bulky blade, they are not usually chosen for patients presenting with limited mouth opening or fragile incisors. On the contrary, the CVS can be a tool of choice in such patients thanks to its slim stylet and video screen. The CVS has also been proved to provide faster endotracheal intubation than DL [10] and the Airway Scope (Pentax, Tokyo, Japan) in a simulated difficult airway [18]. Therefore, we assumed that the CVS is a preferable tool of intubation over laryngoscopic devices in intubation with CP.

Regarding the learning curve of the CVS, an inexperienced trainee can be proficient in using it after a few practices. Ten times of practice is sufficient for the inexperienced to learn the proper use of the CVS and after practicing on 20 patients, they are likely to accomplish intubation with the CVS at the first attempt in a mean intubation time less than 20 s [19]. As compared with the studies of intubation with the CVS without CP [10, 11], the median intubation time and success rate at the first attempt of intubation for CVS-V group in our study (50 cases) is 10.6 s [95% CI, 7.5 to 13.7] and 94%, 15 s [IQR, 12 to 19] and 89.9% in Yang et al's study (200 cases) [10] and 9 s (mean) [SD, 4] seconds and 100% in Hsu et al's study (30 cases) [11] (all the data calculated based on same definition of intubation time). Thus, CP does not appear to significantly affect the intubation time in CVS-V group in our study. When it comes to endotracheal intubation with CP, the intubation time in any of the three groups of our study is much shorter than that (78.8 s [SD, 41.2]) in the study by Hodgson et al. [12]. Therefore, with video assistance, the CVS-V as a video stylet is a handy device for endotracheal intubation with CP.

During intubation in CVS-L group, the application of CP may displace the larynx and cause difficulty for the operator to move the tube into the larynx, and under downward direction of the force the esophagus gets closer to anterior neck skin, so the false positive transillumination on the anterior neck tissue becomes more frequent. Nevertheless, the intubation still can be facilitated by checking the position of the tube on the video screen. Endotracheal intubation with the CVS-L may not be as straightforward as that with the CVS-V, but it can be accomplished sooner than that with a lightwand per se [12].

This study was conducted in simulated RSII while patients' muscle power was not being monitored during anesthesia. Instead, we provided rocuronium 1.2 mg/Kg, which is proved by Magolian et al. to allow onset time (55 ± 14 s) [20]. The patients were intubated 1 min after injection of rocuronium and all the intubation conditions in the study were acceptable.

Thirty seconds was set as a cutoff point for the successful intubation time based on the research team's experience and literature [7, 10, 11] where an intubation is usually completed in less than 30 s with either DL or the CVS. This study showed that the median time to successful intubation is within expected 30 s in all of the three groups.

There are three limitations in the study. Firstly, Lin did all the intubations in both CVS-V and DL group, so personal bias was possibly involved in the results. However, the results regarding our primary goals do not deviate from those in previous studies where the intubation using the CVS without CP [10, 11], so the personal bias should be minimal. Secondly, this was a randomized controlled study about how the CVS and DL perform in endotracheal intubation with CP, so ethically we need to conduct a study on patients whose airway conditions meet the indications to the use of the CVS and DL alike. Thirdly, the results revealed that the intubation time in

CVS-V group was shorter than those in the other groups, but the intergroup difference was nonsignificant. It seems that the intergroup difference for intubation time is less than we expected and we should have had a larger sample size of patients to prove our hypothesis. Nevertheless, it is still worthwhile to further study how powerful the CVS-V can be in intubation in RSII when patients present with limited mouth opening or fragile incisors, which are two specific indications where an intubation stylet may be more advantageous over a laryngoscopic device.

Conclusions
Both of the CVS-V and DL can provide comparably higher first attempt intubation success rate within 30 s as well as within 60 s in endotracheal intubation with CP. Intubation time with the CVS-V was nonsignificantly shorter than that with the other two intubation methods. Almost all the patients can be successfully intubated with any of the three intubation methods within 60 s.

Abbreviations
ANCOVA: Analysis of covariance; ASA: American Society of Anesthesiologists; AWS: Pentax airway scope; BMI: Body mass index; CVS: The Clarus Video System; CVS-L: The Clarus Video System as a lightwand; CVS-V: The Clarus Video System as a video stylet; DL: Direct laryngoscope; NRS: Numerical rating scale; RSII: Rapid sequence induction intubation

Acknowledgements
The authors would like to express appreciation to the nurses, Wei-Ching Cheng and Chia-Fang Cheng. They were the blinded observers who documented sore throat and mucosa injury on the next day.

Authors' contributions
YCL designed and conducted the study, collected and analyzed the data, and wrote the manuscript. AHC helped to conduct the study. JRL helped to design the study and to analyze the data. YTC designed and conducted the study, wrote the manuscript, and revised it critically for important intellectual content. All authors read and approved the final manuscript.

Author details
[1]Department of Anesthesiology, Chang Gung Memorial Hospital, No.5, Fuxing St., Guishan Dist., Taoyuan City 333, Taiwan. [2]Clinical Informatics and Medical Statistics Research Center, Chang Gung University, Taoyuan City, Taiwan. [3]Graduate Institute of Clinical Medical Sciences (Joint Appointment), Chang Gung University, Taoyuan City, Taiwan. [4]College of Medicine, Chang Gung University, Taoyuan City, Taiwan.

References
1. Algie CM, Mahar RK, Tan HB, Wilson G, Mahar PD, Wasiak J. Effectiveness and risks of cricoid pressure during rapid sequence induction for endotracheal intubation. Cochrane Database Syst Rev. 2015;11:CD011656.
2. Birenbaum A, Hajage D, Roche S, Ntouba A, Eurin M, Cuvillon P, et al. Effect of cricoid pressure compared with a sham procedure in the rapid sequence induction of anesthesia: the IRIS randomized clinical trial. JAMA Surg. 2018:1–10.
3. Sajayan A, Wicker J, Ungureanu N, Mendonca C, Kimani PK. Current practice of rapid sequence induction of anaesthesia in the UK - a national survey. Br J Anaesth. 2016;117:i69–74.
4. Vanner RG, Clarke P, Moore WJ, Raftery S. The effect of cricoid pressure and neck support on the view at laryngoscopy. Anaesthesia. 1997;52:896–900.

5. Turgeon AF, Nicole PC, Trépanier CA, Marcoux S, Lessard MR. Cricoid pressure does not increase the rate of failed intubation by direct laryngoscopy in adults. Anesthesiology. 2005;102(2):315–9.
6. Komasawa N, Kido H, Miyazaki Y, Tatsumi S, Minami T, Asai T. Cricoid pressure impedes tracheal intubation with the Pentax-AWS Airwayscope®: a prospective randomized trial. Br J Anaesth. 2016;116:413–6. https://doi.org/10.1093/bja/aev438.
7. Byhahn C, Nemetz S, Breitkreutz R, Zwissler B, Kaufmann M, Meininger D. Brief report: tracheal intubation using the Bonfils intubation fibrescope or direct laryngoscopy for patients with a simulated difficult airway. Can J Anesth. 2008;55:232–7.
8. Hung OR, Pytka S, Morris I, Murphy M, Launcelott G, Stevens S, et al. Clinical trial of a new lightwand device (trachlight) to intubate the trachea. Anesthesiology. 1995;83:509–14.
9. Cooney DR, Beaudette C, Clemency BM, Tanski C, Wojcik S. Endotracheal intubation with a video-assisted semi-rigid fiberoptic stylet by prehospital providers. Int J Emerg Med. 2014;7:1–5.
10. Yang M, Kim JA, Ahn HJ, Choi JW, Kim DK, Cho EA. Double-lumen tube tracheal intubation using a rigid video-stylet: a randomized controlled comparison with the macintosh laryngoscope. Br J Anaesth. 2013;111:990–5. https://doi.org/10.1093/bja/aet281.
11. Hsu HT, Chou SH, Chen CL, Tseng KY, Kuo YW, Chen MK, et al. Left endobronchial intubation with a double-lumen tube using direct laryngoscopy or the Trachway® video stylet. Anaesthesia. 2013;68:851–5.
12. Hodgson RE, Gopalan PD, Burrows RC, Zuma K. Effect of cricoid pressure on the success of endotracheal intubation with a lightwand. Anesthesiology. 2001;94:259–62.
13. Huang WT, Huang CY, Chung YT. Clinical comparisons between GlideScope® video laryngoscope and Trachlight® in simulated cervical spine instability. J Clin Anesth. 2007;19:110–4.
14. Clayton TJ, Vanner RG. A novel method of measuring cricoid force. Anaesthesia. 2002;57:326–9.
15. Healy DW, Maties O, Hovord D, Kheterpal S. A systematic review of the role of videolaryngoscopy in successful orotracheal intubation. BMC Anesthesiol. 2012;12(1). https://doi.org/10.1186/1471-2253-12-32.
16. Aziz MF, Dillman D, Fu R, Brambrink AM. Comparative effectiveness of the C-MAC video laryngoscope versus direct laryngoscopy in the setting of the predicted difficult airway. Anesthesiology. 2012;116:629–36. https://doi.org/10.1097/ALN.0b013e318246ea34.
17. Fiadjoe JE, Gurnaney H, Dalesio N, Sussman E, Zhao H, Zhang X, et al. A prospective randomized equivalence trial of the GlideScope Cobalt® video laryngoscope to traditional direct laryngoscopy in neonates and infants. Anesthesiology. 2012;116:622–8.
18. Kim JK, Kim JA, Kim CS, Ahn HJ, Yang MK, Choi SJ. Comparison of tracheal intubation with the airway scope or Clarus Video System in patients with cervical collars. Anaesthesia. 2011;66:694–8.
19. Moon Y-J, Kim J, Seo D-W, Kim J-W, Jung H-W, Suk E-H, et al. Endotracheal intubation by inexperienced trainees using the Clarus video system: learning curve and orodental trauma perspectives. J Dent Anesth Pain Med. 2015;15:207. https://doi.org/10.17245/jdapm.2015.15.4.207.
20. Magorian T, Flannery KB, Miller RD. Comparison of rocuronium, succinylcholine, and vecuronium for rapid-sequence induction of anesthesia in adult patients. Anesthesiology. 1993;79:913–8.

3

Effects of the anesthesiologist's experience on postoperative hoarseness after double-lumen endotracheal tube intubation: A single-center propensity score-matched analysis

Yuji Kamimura[1]* (iD), Toshiyuki Nakanishi[1], Aiji Boku Sato[2], Satoshi Osaga[3], Eisuke Kako[1] and Kazuya Sobue[1]

Abstract

Background: Postoperative hoarseness after general anesthesia is associated with patient discomfort and dissatisfaction. A recent large retrospective study showed that single-lumen endotracheal tube intubation by a trainee did not alter the incidence of postoperative pharyngeal symptoms compared with intubation by a senior anesthesiologist. However, there is limited information about the relationship between the anesthesiologist's experience and hoarseness after double-lumen endotracheal tube intubation. We tested the hypothesis that double-lumen endotracheal tube intubation performed by a trainee increases the incidence of postoperative hoarseness compared to intubation by a senior anesthesiologist.

Methods: This retrospective observational study included patients who underwent lung resection between April 2015 and March 2018 at a university hospital. Double-lumen endotracheal tube intubation was carried out with a Macintosh laryngoscope. We divided the patients into 2 groups - one group comprised of patients who were intubated by a trainee anesthesiologist with < 2 years of experience, and the other group comprised of those who underwent intubation by a senior anesthesiologist with ≥2 years of experience. The primary outcome was the incidence of postoperative hoarseness 24 h after surgery and we collected data on postoperative hoarseness using a checklist of postanesthetic adverse events. One-to-one propensity score matching was conducted and P values < 0.05 were considered statistically significant.

Results: There was a total of 256 eligible patients, of which 153 underwent intubation by trainee anesthesiologists, and the remaining 103 patients were intubated by a senior anesthesiologist. The one-to-one propensity score matching resulted in 96 pairs of patients for the groups. The incidence of postoperative hoarseness 24 h after surgery was significantly higher in patients who were intubated by a trainee anesthesiologist than in patients who were intubated by a senior anesthesiologist (9.4% vs. 2.1%, respectively; $P = 0.03$).

(Continued on next page)

* Correspondence: ez4pixy1118@gmail.com
[1]Department of Anesthesiology and Intensive Care Medicine, Nagoya City University Graduate School of Medical Sciences, 1 Kawasumi, Mizuho-cho, Mizuho-ku, Nagoya 467-8601, Japan

(Continued from previous page)

Conclusions: Double-lumen endotracheal tube intubation by trainee anesthesiologists with < 2 years of experience increased the incidence of postoperative hoarseness 24 h after surgery compared to intubation by senior anesthesiologists with ≥2 years of experience.

Keywords: Tracheal intubation, Double-lumen endotracheal tube, Throat complication, Hoarseness, Trainee

Background

There is a correlation between postoperative hoarseness after general anesthesia and patient discomfort and dissatisfaction. Several risk factors, such as patient demographic factors, quality of intubation, and perioperative management, are reportedly associated with postoperative hoarseness [1–3].

Double-lumen endotracheal tube (DLT) intubation had been the gold-standard for surgical lung separation. However, the use of bronchial blockers is also an effective method for lung separation and has a lower incidence of postoperative hoarseness. This has led to an on-going debate regarding the best device for lung separation. A systematic review evaluating 307 patients from 4 studies showed that the use of DLTs was related to a higher risk of postoperative hoarseness than the use of a combination of single-lumen endotracheal tubes (SLTs) and endobronchial blockers [4]. The reported incidence of postoperative hoarseness after insertion of a DLT is 5 to 50% [4–6]. A high frequency of hoarseness may be caused by the thickness of the DLTs and the skills required for intubation.

The results of a recent large retrospective study including over 20,000 patients suggested that endotracheal intubation by a trainee did not increase postoperative throat symptoms compared to intubation by a senior anesthesiologist [7]. However, the study only included patients who underwent SLT intubation. Therefore, there is limited knowledge of the relationship between the anesthesiologist's experience and hoarseness after DLT intubation.

In this study, we tested the hypothesis that DLT intubation by a trainee increases the incidence of postoperative hoarseness compared to DLT intubation by a senior anesthesiologist.

Methods

The protocol for this study was approved by the Nagoya City University Graduate School of Medical Sciences and Nagoya City University Hospital Institutional Review Boards (Nagoya, Japan, approval number: 60-18-0073). According to our institutional review board's code of ethics, we used an opt-out method and posted a description of the research protocol on the website of the Nagoya City University Graduate School of Medical

Sciences on July 30, 2018, and the patients could withdraw from the study.

Data source and study population

The present retrospective observational study included patients who underwent lung resection between April of 2015 and March of 2018. We included patients who underwent DLT intubation with a Macintosh laryngoscope and a neuromuscular blocking drug, who were ≥ 15 years of age, and who had an American Society of Anesthesiologists physical status classification (ASA-PS) of 1 or 2. Patients with preoperative hoarseness, those who were intubated with a video laryngoscope, those who required emergency surgery, and those with missing data were excluded from this study.

Study variables

The exposure of interest was DLT intubation performed by a trainee or senior anesthesiologist. We divided patients into 2 groups: one group comprising patients who were intubated by a trainee anesthesiologist and the other comprising those who were intubated by a senior anesthesiologist. Anesthesiologists in Japan can only be certified as Qualified Anesthesiologists according to the Japanese Society of Anesthesiologists after completing a 2-year training program. Therefore, we defined trainee anesthesiologists as "anesthesiologists with less than 2 years of anesthesia experience" and senior anesthesiologists as "those with more than 2 years of anesthesia experience". These definitions were the same as those used in a previous study [7]. We collected the following clinical variables: age, gender, height, weight, body mass index (BMI), ASA-PS, duration of anesthesia, intraoperative fluid balance, DLT size, intubation depth, number of intubation attempts, intracuff pressure of the DLT, Mallampati score, and Cormack–Lehane grade.

Outcome measures

The primary outcome was incidence of postoperative hoarseness 24 h after surgery. Anesthesiologists in charge of postanesthetic rounds at our hospital must use a checklist of postanesthetic adverse events and determine the presence of hoarseness 24 h after surgery. The investigator (YK), who did not perform DLT intubation or manage anesthesia, collected data on postoperative hoarseness from electronic medical records using a checklist of postanesthetic adverse events. We defined postoperative hoarseness as "a patient-assessed change in voice quality". We did not qualitatively or objectively evaluate postoperative hoarseness. We investigated whether the anesthesiologist who assessed postoperative hoarseness was the same one who provided anesthesia for the patient and whether he or she was a trainee or senior anesthesiologist.

Perioperative patient treatment

There are no standardized methods for induction or maintenance of anesthesia. Electrocardiography, pulse oximetry, and invasive blood pressure monitoring were performed after patients arrived at the operating room. Patients received a combination of general and epidural anesthesia. General anesthesia was induced with propofol (a bolus dose of 1–2 mg/kg or a target-controlled infusion at 3–3.5 µg/ml), fentanyl (1–4 µg/kg) and remifentanil (0–0.3 µg/kg/min) following placement of a thoracic epidural catheter. An attending trainee or senior anesthesiologist performed DLT intubation with a Macintosh laryngoscope after bolus administration of rocuronium (0.6–1 mg/kg). Neuromuscular monitoring was not performed during tracheal intubation. Blade size (3 or 4) was chosen based on anesthesiologist preference and the patient's physique. Portex® Blue Line® Endobronchial Tubes-left (Smiths Medical, Minneapolis, MN, USA) with a stylet were used in all procedures and a water-soluble lubricant without lidocaine was applied to the tube. We used a 37-Fr DLT for men and a 35-Fr DLT for women, but tube size was determined by the attending anesthesiologist based on the patient's height [8]. The attending anesthesiologist guided the DLT into position via a flexible bronchoscope and assessed tube placement after changing patient to the lateral decubitus position. Anesthesia was maintained with 1–2.5% sevoflurane or propofol (target-controlled infusion at 2–3.5 µg/mL) and the Bispectral Index® value was kept between 40 and 60 throughout the entire procedure. Residual neuromuscular blockade was reversed with sugammadex (2–4 mg/kg), postoperatively, and the DLT was removed in the operating room.

Statistical analysis

For sample size calculation, we assumed that the incidence of postoperative hoarseness 24 h after surgery in patients who underwent intubation by a trainee or senior anesthesiologist would be 20 and 5%, respectively, based on previous reports [4–6]. Thus, 89 patients in each group were required to provide 80% power to detect a statistical difference between groups using Fisher's exact test with a two-sided significance level of 5%.

We conducted propensity score analyses to account for differences in baseline characteristics between the 2 groups. The c-statistic for evaluating goodness of fit was calculated and we performed one-to-one propensity score matching by nearest neighbor matching without replacement. Caliper width was set to 25% of the standard deviation of the propensity scores. Furthermore, the confounding factors used in the propensity score model were age, gender, height, weight, BMI, ASA-PS, duration of anesthesia, intraoperative fluid balance, tube size, tube depth, number of intubation attempts, intracuff pressure, Mallampati score, and Cormack–Lehane grade. We assessed the differences between the 2 groups before and after propensity score matching with standardized differences. Standardized differences of < 10% were considered negligible imbalances in the baseline characteristics between the 2 groups. We compared the incidence of hoarseness 24 h after surgery between the 2 groups using Fisher's exact test for before matching and the McNemar test for after matching. A P value < 0.05 was considered statistically significant. All statistical analyses were performed using the R software package (version 3.5.0, R Foundation for Statistical Computing, Vienna, Austria).

Results

Figure 1 shows a flow diagram for cohort identification. We identified 413 lung cancer patients who underwent lung resection during the study period. Out of these patients, 256 were included in the full study cohort based on predetermined inclusion and exclusion criteria. These 256 patients included 153 patients who were intubated by a trainee anesthesiologist and 103 patients who were intubated by a senior anesthesiologist. Overall, 32 anesthesiologists (10 trainee anesthesiologists (listed in Supplementary Table S1) and 22 senior anesthesiologists) participated in this study. Median (interquartile range) length of experience was 1 year (1–2 years) for trainee anesthesiologists and 10 years (7–14 years) for senior anesthesiologists.

Table 1 shows patient characteristics prior to propensity score matching between the 2 groups. There was no significant difference between the 2 groups regarding the number of intubation attempts. Some characteristics, including age, weight, BMI, ASA-PS, intraoperative fluid balance, tube size, tube depth, intracuff pressure, Mallampati score, and Cormack–Lehane grade, had standardized differences of > 10%.

Table 2 shows patient characteristics after propensity score matching between the 2 groups. The established model for estimating propensity scores had a c-statistic of 0.635. A total of 96 patients from each group were matched through propensity score matching. Patient characteristics were well balanced between the 2 groups after matching and.

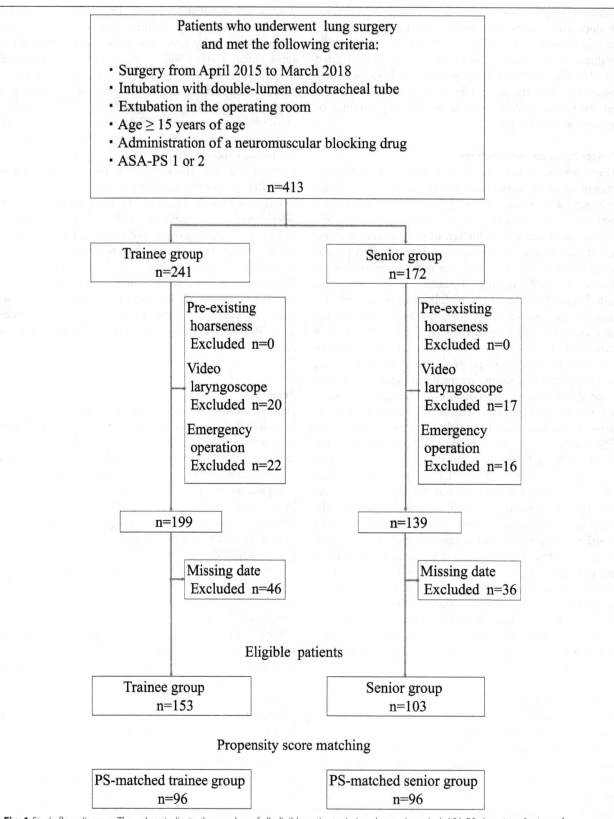

Fig. 1 Study flow diagram. The values indicate the number of all eligible patients during the study period. ASA-PS, American Society of Anesthesiologists physical status classification; PS, propensity score

Table 1 Clinical characteristics prior to propensity score matching

	Prior to propensity score matching		
	Trainee *n* = 153	Senior *n* = 103	Standardized difference (%)
Age (median [IQR]; years)	69 [57, 75]	68 [61, 75]	15.5
Gender (male/female) (%)	90/63 (58.8/41.2)	62/41 (60.2/39.8)	2.8
Height (median [IQR]; cm)	161.4 [155.0, 168.4]	162.2 [155.6, 168.0]	0.6
Weight (median [IQR]; kg)	59.6 [52.6, 66.3]	58.0 [50.7, 64.3]	15
BMI (median [IQR]; kg/m^2)	22.8 [20.5, 25.0]	22.3 [20.1, 24.2]	17.1
ASA-PS (%)			23.3
1	27 (17.6)	10 (9.7)	
2	126 (82.4)	93 (90.3)	
Duration of anesthesia (median [IQR]; h)	4.0 [3.1, 5.0]	4.0 [2.9, 5.0]	1.4
Intraoperative fluid balance (median [IQR]; ml)	1299 [995, 1733]	1232 [926, 1630]	14.8
Tube size (%)			14.6
32 Fr	12 (7.8)	6 (5.8)	
35 Fr	64 (41.8)	45 (43.7)	
37 Fr	69 (45.1)	49 (47.6)	
39 Fr	8 (5.2)	3 (2.9)	
Tube depth (median [IQR]; cm)	28 [27, 30]	29 [27, 30]	15.8
Intubation attempts (%)			4.1
1	147 (96.1)	99 (96.1)	
2	5 (3.3)	3 (2.9)	
3	0 (0.0)	0 (0.0)	
4	1 (0.6)	1 (1.0)	
Cuff pressure (median [IQR]; cmH$_2$O)	20 [20, 20]	20 [20, 20]	10.4
Mallampati score (%)			17.1
1	109 (71.2)	81 (78.6)	
2	44 (28.8)	22 (21.4)	
3	0 (0.0)	0 (0.0)	
4	0 (0.0)	0 (0.0)	
Cormack–Lehane grade (%)			16.3
1	120 (78.4)	82 (79.6)	
2	31 (20.3)	21 (20.4)	
3	2 (1.3)	0 (0.0)	
4	0 (0.0)	0 (0.0)	

Data are described as frequency (%) or median [interquartile range, IQR]

BMI Body mass index; *ASA-PS* American Society of Anesthesiologists physical status classification

the incidence of postoperative hoarseness 24 h after surgery was significantly higher for intubation by a trainee anesthesiologist than for intubation by a senior anesthesiologist (9.4% vs. 2.1%, *P* = 0.03; Table 3). There were no patients with surgical recurrent nerve injury or continuous hoarseness who required referral to an otolaryngologist in either group. Postoperative hoarseness was determined by the anesthesia provider in 85% of trainee intubations and 80% of senior anesthesiologist

intubations. There were no patients who could not be evaluated because they had a Glasgow Coma Scale < 15 or Numerical Rating Scale > 5.

We also compared the incidence of postoperative hoarseness between the first 1–5 cases and after the sixth and subsequent cases for each trainee anesthesiologist. There was no significant difference between the 2 groups (Supplementary Table S1). We also compared the incidence of postoperative hoarseness

Table 2 Clinical characteristics after propensity score matching

	After propensity score matching		
	Trainee n = 96	Senior n = 96	Standardized difference (%)
Age (median [IQR]; years)	71 [63, 76]	68 [61, 75]	1.8
Gender (male/female) (%)	57/39 (59.4/40.6)	56/40 (58.3/41.7)	2.1
Height (median [IQR]; cm)	161.3 [154.6, 166.7]	162.1 [154.7, 167.9]	0.4
Weight (median [IQR]; kg)	57.5 [52.1, 61.97]	58.3[50.5, 64.2]	5.8
BMI (median [IQR]; kg/m^2)	22.1 [20.1, 24.1]	22.4 [20.1, 24.3]	7.1
ASA-PS (%)			3.3
1	11 (11.5)	10 (10.4)	
2	85 (88.5)	86 (89.6)	
Duration of anesthesia (median [IQR]; h)	3.88 [2.75, 4.86]	3.95 [2.96, 5.04]	1.9
Intraoperative fluid balance (median [IQR]; ml)	1222 [931, 1518]	1224 [926, 1630]	3.1
Tube size (%)			7.8
32 Fr	5 (5.2)	6 (6.2)	
35 Fr	43 (44.8)	43 (44.8)	
37 Fr	45 (46.9)	45 (46.9)	
39 Fr	3 (3.1)	2 (2.1)	
Tube depth (median [IQR]; cm)	28 [27, 30]	28 [27, 30]	4.6
Intubation attempts (%)			14.5
1	93 (96.9)	92 (95.8)	
2	3 (3.1)	3 (3.1)	
3	0 (0.0)	0 (0.0)	
4	0 (0.0)	1 (1.0)	
Cuff pressure (median [IQR]; cmH$_2$O)	20 [20, 22]	20 [20, 20]	6.5
Mallampati score (%)			2.5
1	74 (77.1)	75 (78.1)	
2	22 (22.9)	21 (21.9)	
3	0 (0.0)	0 (0.0)	
4	0 (0.0)	0 (0.0)	
Cormack–Lehane grade (%)			< 0.1
1	76 (79.2)	76 (79.2)	
2	20 (20.8)	20 (20.8)	
3	0 (0.0)	0 (0.0)	
4	0 (0.0)	0 (0.0)	

Data are described as frequency (%) or median [interquartile range, IQR]
BMI Body mass index; *ASA-PS* American Society of Anesthesiologists physical status classification

Table 3 Incidence of postoperative hoarseness 24 h after surgery

	Full cohort			Propensity score-matched cohort		
Outcome, n (%)	Trainee n = 153	Senior n = 103	P	Trainee n = 96	Senior n = 96	P
Hoarseness	18 (11.8)	2 (1.9)	0.004	9 (9.4)	2 (2.1)	0.03

Data are described as frequency (%)

between Cormack–Lehane grade 1 and 2, but found no significant difference (Supplementary Table S2).

Discussion

Patients who underwent DLT intubation by a trainee anesthesiologist with < 2 years of experience had a higher incidence of postoperative hoarseness than those who underwent DLT intubation by a senior anesthesiologist with ≥2 years of experience in lung surgery. This result suggests that lack of experience could be a risk factor for postoperative hoarseness in patients undergoing DLT intubation.

The increased incidence of postoperative hoarseness observed in our patients who were intubated by a trainee anesthesiologist differed from the results of a previous study using SLTs [7]. One possible explanation for this difference may be that DLT intubation requires more technical skills than SLT intubation for the following reasons. First, the thicker diameter of DLTs may have made it difficult for trainee anesthesiologists to pass them through the glottis. The incidence of postoperative hoarseness was reported to directly correlate with endotracheal tube size [3]. Second, a DLT has a solid curved body, which can easily come into contact with the vocal cords [9]. During DLT intubation by a trainee anesthesiologist, therefore, the tube may more easily and frequently come into contact with the vocal cords than in intubations by senior anesthesiologists. There was no difference in the number of intubation attempts between trainee and senior anesthesiologists, but there might have been more strain on the vocal cords when trainee anesthesiologists used DLTs. The difference in the incidence of postoperative hoarseness between trainee and senior anesthesiologists, despite adjustments for the number of intubation attempts and tube size, suggests that an unseen skill level may account for the incidence of postoperative hoarseness.

The incidence of postoperative hoarseness 24 h after surgery was lower in both groups in the present study (9.4% for trainee anesthesiologists and 2.1% for senior anesthesiologists) than that in previous studies (5 to 50%) [4–6]. Only patients who subjectively complained were considered to have postoperative hoarseness, and therefore the incidence of postoperative hoarseness may have been underestimated. Thus, it is not easy to compare the results of this study to those of previous studies because of the different definitions of hoarseness. It is essential to know patient comfort level bcause postoperative hoarseness is a subjective patient complaint. Therefore, we believe that the outcome assessed in our study is clinically meaningful. A validated outcome measure, such as voice handicap index [10], may be a more reliable assessment in future studies.

Secondary analyses showed that the first 1–5 intubations for each trainee anesthesiologist, and Cormack–Lehane grade, were not associated with a significant increased risk of postoperative hoarseness 24 h after surgery in patients who underwent DLT intubation. However, postoperative hoarseness tended to be higher in the first 1–5 cases and in Cormack–Lehane grade 2 patients. Since the relatively small sample size of our study cannot provide adequate power for these comparisons, further study is needed to confirm these results.

We acknowledge that this study had some limitations. First, it was a single-center, retrospective observational study with relatively small sample size. Prospective randomized controlled trials are required to validate our results in the future. Second, a significant number of patients were excluded from this study, which may have led to selection bias. Third, we defined trainee anesthesiologists as "anesthesiologists with less than 2 years of anesthesia experience" and senior anesthesiologists as "those with more than 2 years of anesthesia experience". It may be difficult to apply our results directly to other countries even though these definitions were equivalent to those used in a previous study [7]. Fourth, neuromuscular monitoring was not performed during tracheal intubation. The difference between trainee and senior anesthesiologists regarding the depth of muscle relaxation might have affected the incidence of hoarseness. Fifth, 80–85% of the evaluators were anesthesia providers, who were not blinded and may have caused observer bias and ascertainment bias. Moreover, it cannot be ruled out that trainee anesthesiologists may have more aggressively assessed the patient's hoarseness. However, this study has the advantage that neither the evaluators nor the patients were aware of the study's purpose due to the study's retrospective nature. Therefore, evaluator influence on the results of this study, which were analyzed in real-world clinical practice, is likely minimal. Finally, although we attempted to limit selection bias using propensity score matching, the multifactorial etiologies of postoperative hoarseness that affect the outcomes may not have been removed.

Conclusions

DLT intubation by trainee anesthesiologists with < 2 years of experience increased the incidence of postoperative hoarseness 24 h after surgery compared with DLT intubation by senior anesthesiologists with ≥2 years of experience.

Supplementary Information

Additional file 1: Table S1. Details of intubations performed by trainees and incidence of postoperative hoarseness. Table S2. Incidence of postoperative hoarseness in patients with Cormack–Lehane grade 1 and 2.

Abbreviations
ASA-PS: American Society of Anesthesiologists physical status classification; BMI: Body mass index; DLT: Double-lumen endotracheal tube; SLT: Single-lumen endotracheal tube

Acknowledgments
We would like to thank Tadashi Sakane and Ryoichi Nakanishi from Nagoya City University Hospital of Department of Thoracic Surgery for assistance with the data collection.

Authors' contributions
YK, SO and KS designed the study. YK, AS and EK wrote the protocol. YK collected the data. YK, TN and SO analyzed the data. TN, AS and EK made substantial contribution to the interpretation of the data. YK wrote this manuscript under the supervision of TN, AS, EK and KS. All authors have read and approved the final version of the manuscript.

Author details
[1]Department of Anesthesiology and Intensive Care Medicine, Nagoya City University Graduate School of Medical Sciences, 1 Kawasumi, Mizuho-cho, Mizuho-ku, Nagoya 467-8601, Japan. [2]Department of Anesthesiology, Aichi Gakuin University School of Dentistry, 2-11 Suemori-dori, Chikusa-ku, Nagoya 464-8651, Japan. [3]Clinical Research Management Center, Nagoya City University Hospital, 1 Kawasumi, Mizuho-cho, Mizuho-ku, Nagoya 467-8601, Japan.

References
1. Jones MW, Catling S, Evans E, Green DH, Green JR. Hoarseness after tracheal intubation. Anaesthesia. 1992;47:213–6.
2. Mencke T, Echternach M, Kleinschmidt S, Lux P, Barth V, Plinkert PK, Fuchs-Buder T. Laryngeal morbidity and quality of tracheal intubation: a randomized controlled trial. Anesthesiology. 2003;98:1049–56.
3. Hu B, Bao R, Wang X, Liu S, Tao T, Xie Q, Yu X, Li J, Bo L, Deng X. The size of endotracheal tube and sore throat after surgery: a systematic review and meta-analysis. PLoS One. 2013;8:e74467.
4. Clayton-Smith A, Bennett K, Alston RP, Adams G, Brown G, Hawthorne T, Hu M, Sinclair A, Tan J. A comparison of the efficacy and adverse effects of double-lumen endobronchial tubes and bronchial blockers in thoracic surgery: a systematic review and meta-analysis of randomized controlled trials. J Cardiothorac Vasc Anesth. 2015;29:955–66.
5. Knoll H, Ziegeler S, Schreiber JU, Buchinger H, Bialas P, Semyonov K, Graeter T, Mencke T. Airway injuries after one-lung ventilation: a comparison between double-lumen tube and endobronchial blocker: a randomized, prospective, controlled trial. Anesthesiology. 2006;105:471–7.
6. Chang JE, Min SW, Kim CS, Han SH, Kwon YS, Hwang JY. Effect of prophylactic benzydamine hydrochloride on postoperative sore throat and hoarseness after tracheal intubation using a double-lumen endobronchial tube: a randomized controlled trial. Can J Anaesth. 2015;62:1097–103.
7. Inoue S, Abe R, Tanaka Y, Kawaguchi M. Tracheal intubation by trainees does not alter the incidence or duration of postoperative sore throat and hoarseness: a teaching hospital-based propensity score analysis. Br J Anaesth. 2015;115:463–9.
8. Campos JH. Current techniques for perioperative lung isolation in adults. Anesthesiology. 2002;97:1295–301.
9. Seo JH, Kwon TK, Jeon Y, Hong DM, Kim HJ, Bahk JH. Comparison of techniques for double-lumen endobronchial intubation: 90° or 180° rotation during advancement through the glottis. Br J Anaesth. 2013;111:812–7.
10. Mendels EJ, Brunings JW, Hamaekers AE, Stokroos RJ, Kremer B, Baijens LW. Adverse laryngeal effects following short-term general anesthesia: a systematic review. Arch Otolaryngol Head Neck Surg. 2012;138:257–64.

4

Correlation between clinical risk factors and tracheal intubation difficulty in infants with Pierre-Robin syndrome

Yanli Liu[1†], Jiashuo Wang[2†] and Shan Zhong[3*]

Abstract

Background: Difficult tracheal intubation is a common problem encountered by anesthesiologists in the clinic. This study was conducted to assess the difficulty of tracheal intubation in infants with Pierre Robin syndrome (PRS) by incorporating computed tomography (CT) to guide airway management for anesthesia.

Methods: In this retrospective study, we analyzed case-level clinical data and CT images of 96 infants with PRS. First, a clinically experienced physician labeled CT images, after which the color space conversion, binarization, contour acquisition, and area calculation processing were performed on the annotated files. Finally, the correlation coefficient between the seven clinical factors and tracheal intubation difficulty, as well as the differences in each risk factor under tracheal intubation difficulty were calculated.

Results: The absolute value of the correlation coefficient between the throat area and tracheal intubation difficulty was 0.54; the observed difference was statistically significant. Body surface area, weight, and gender also showed significant difference under tracheal intubation difficulty.

Conclusions: There is a significant correlation between throat area and tracheal intubation difficulty in infants with PRS. Body surface area, weight and gender may have an impact on tracheal intubation difficulty in infants with PRS.

Keywords: Tracheal intubation anesthesia, OpenCV, Pierre-Robin syndrome

Background

Difficult tracheal intubation is common in clinical practice, and it mostly refers to tracheal intubation that cannot be successfully completed by an ordinary indirect laryngoscope [1]. It represents the most difficult problem encountered by anesthesiologists in their daily work and is mainly caused by anatomical deformities, restricted back tilting activities, obesity and limited mouth opening [2]. These factors have an adverse effect on treatment. In practice, the level of difficulty is evaluated before the formal implementation of tracheal intubation. For patients with different levels of difficulty, preparations should be done in advance to avoid local mucosal damage caused by multiple intubation or complications such as dislocation of the circular cartilage [3].

In 2016, Münster et al [4] have reported that the position of vocal cords is related to laryngeal exposure and that difficult laryngoscopy is more likely to occur when vocal cords are closer to the head. From 2016 to 2018, many studies have utilized ultrasound for the clinical diagnosis of difficult tracheal intubation [5–10]

* Correspondence: tintin0211@163.com
†Yanli Liu and Jiashuo Wang contributed equally to this work.
3Department of Anesthesiology, Children's Hospital of Nanjing Medical University, No. 72, Guangzhou Road, Gulou District, Nanjing 210008, People's Republic of China

Table 1 Clinical information for children with PRS

Gender	Male: Female	48: 48
Height (Unit: m)	Median (1st Qu., 3rd Qu)	0.5000 (0.5000, 0.5300)
Weight (Unit: kg)	Median (1st Qu., 3rd Qu)	3.400 (3.000, 3.800)
BSA (Unit: m^2)	Median (1st Qu., 3rd Qu)	0.2190 (0.2050, 0.2330)
Throat area (Unit: pixel)	Median (1st Qu., 3rd Qu)	1440.5 (1237.2, 2034.4)
Age (Unit: day)	Median (1st Qu., 3rd Qu)	33.00 (13.67, 50.00)
Pneumonia	Yes: No	32: 64

Descriptive statistics of the seven clinical risk factors for 96 infants enrolled in the study. For categorical variables, the frequency of each category is listed. For numerical variables, the first quartile, median, and third quartiles are calculated

Ultrasound provides not only real-time images but also reveals dynamic structural changes of the airway. In 2019, Lee et al [11] found that the distance from the mandibular groove to the hyoid bone and the distance from the inner edge of the mandible to the hyoid bone on X-ray images of the lateral neck were important for predicting difficult tracheal intubation in patients with acromegaly. However, there are only a few available methods for infant airway assessment and their accuracy is relatively poor [12].

Pierre Robin syndrome [13, 14] is the triad of micrognathia, glossoptosis, and cleft palate. These conditions could easily lead to difficult tracheal intubation which is the most significant risk factor for intubation anesthesia. Accurate preoperative prediction of intubation difficulty and adequate preparations are essential for ensuring successful airway management in infants with PRS. There are many methods for assessing the difficulty of tracheal intubation [3]; yet, no existing method is suitable for infants, especially infants with PRS. Moreover, few reports

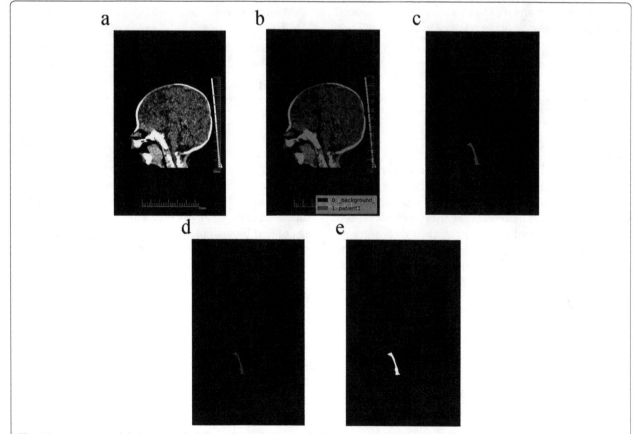

Fig. 1 Images generated during area calculation. **a** Original CT image. **b** The image after labeling by labelme. **c** The *.png* image obtained by single-channel conversion. **d** The grayscale image obtained by color space conversion. **e** The binary image obtained after thresholding is performed

have focused on the application of CT on tracheal intubation difficulty assessment in infants with PRS [15, 16]. Therefore, this study was conducted to assess the difficulty of tracheal intubation in infants with PRS by incorporating CT to guide airway management for anesthesia [17].

Methods

Dataset

This retrospective study was approved by the Institutional Ethics Committee of Children's Hospital of Nanjing Medical University and was conducted using the data obtained from Picture Archiving and Communication System (PACS) database and Operation Anesthesia Information System (OAIS) database. Informed patient consent was waived by our IEC. Clinical information and CT images were collected from infants with PRS who underwent intubation anesthesia in 2018 at Children's Hospital of Nanjing Medical University.

Seven clinical risk factors [18] that may have an impact on tracheal intubation difficulty were provided by experienced clinicians, including gender, height, weight, body surface area (BSA), throat area, age, and pneumonia (Table 1). The calculation of the throat area was elaborated below, and the remaining indicators could be directly obtained or simply calculated. Tracheal intubation difficulty is divided into three levels based on whether glottis can be completely observed under visual laryngoscope, where level I refers to complete observation, level II refers to partial observation, and level III refers to the case when the only epiglottis can be observed.

Labeling criteria

To assess the impact of the throat area on tracheal intubation difficulty, the collected CT images (Fig. 1a) were labeled according to the irregularity of the area being labeled using Labelme, an annotation tool which is based on the Python language and allows for irregular area annotation [19]. A radiologist with 20 years of clinical experience, who was blinded to the infants' difficulty level, was responsible for labeling. Through a three-dimensional reconstruction technique, the median sagittal image of the upper airway of the infants was obtained, after which then the area of the oropharyngeal cavity (ie, the pharyngeal area between the plane of the tongue and the glottis) was labeled.

Annotation file processing and area calculation

The overall workflow is shown in Fig. 2. The annotation file generated by Labelme is in the format of .json (Fig. 1b) [20]. To calculate the throat area, the annotation file was first converted to a single-channel image in .png format (Fig. 1c).

OpenCV performed subsequent processing in the Python environment. First, the single-channel image that was obtained during the previous step underwent color space conversion using the cvtColor function of

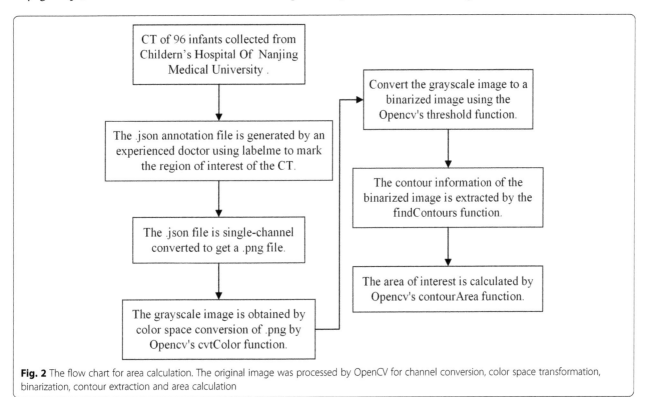

Fig. 2 The flow chart for area calculation. The original image was processed by OpenCV for channel conversion, color space transformation, binarization, contour extraction and area calculation

OpenCV and was converted into a grayscale image (Fig. 1d) [21, 22]. The grayscale image was then thresholded (the threshold was set to 1) using the threshold function and becoming a binary image (Fig. 1e) [22, 23]. The throat contour information of the marker was then obtained by the findContours function, with pixel position difference between two adjacent points in all contour points no larger than 1 [22, 24]. Finally, the contour information obtained in the previous step in the form of a point set was input into the contourArea function of OpenCV to calculate the area [22, 25].

Correlation analysis
Correlation coefficients were used to assess the impact of each risk factor on tracheal intubation difficulty. Clinical risk factors highly correlated with difficulty level had better predicative effects in the clinic.

Statistical analysis
Since clinical risk factors include numerical and categorical variables and tracheal intubation difficulty is categorical, the correlation was measured by the Spearman rank correlation coefficient. Besides, to analyze whether there is a significant difference in each clinical risk factor under tracheal intubation difficulty, the Kruskal-Wallis test was used for numerical factors, and Pearson's Chi-squared test was used for categorical factors.

Results
The flow chart of the study is shown in Fig. 2. Eight infants were excluded due to censored data (4 cases of censored pneumonia data and 4 cases of censored throat area data). Finally, 96 infants were included in the study, among whom 29 were level I difficulty, 43 were level II difficulty, and 24 were level III difficulty of tracheal intubation. Additional data with sufficient clinical information were collected.

The correlation coefficients are integrated in Fig. 3, where darker color indicates stronger correlations, while the lighter color represents weaker correlations. The correlation was strongest between the throat area and

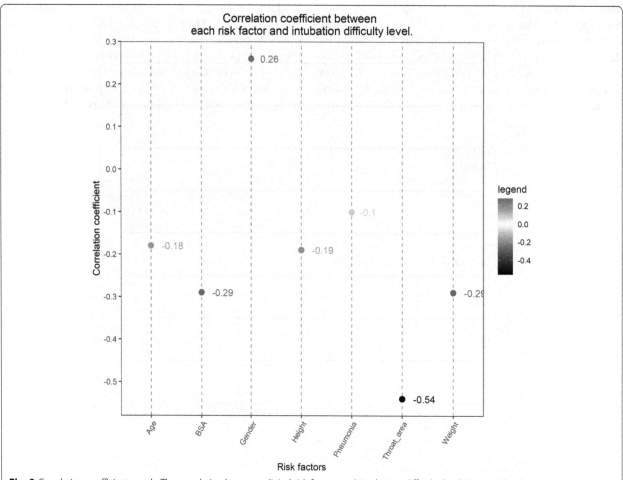

Fig. 3 Correlation coefficient graph. The correlation between clinical risk factors and intubation difficulty level denoted by the Spearman rank correlation coefficient

tracheal intubation difficulty with the correlation coefficient of -0.54. Risk factors that were moderately correlated with tracheal intubation difficulty were BSA, weight, and gender with correlation coefficients of -0.29, -0.29 and 0.26, respectively. All numerical risk factors were negatively correlated with tracheal intubation difficulty. Among categorical risk factors, males were more difficult to intubate than females, and infants with pneumonia had a lower level of difficulty in intubation than infants without pneumonia.

The results of the internal difference analysis of risk factors are shown in Table 2. The difference in throat area under tracheal intubation difficulty was significant, with $P < 0.0001$ (Level I vs. II: $P = 0.0022$, Level II vs. III: $P = 0.0002$, Level I vs.III: $P < 0.0001$). The differences in BSA, weight, and gender under tracheal intubation difficulty were also significant, and their corresponding P values were 0.0117, 0.0117 and 0.0043, respectively. BSA, weight, and gender were significantly different when comparing level II to level III and level I to level III. Height, age, and pneumonia showed no significant difference under tracheal intubation difficulty.

Discussion

In this study, we used clinical data from 96 PRS infants who underwent intubation anesthesia to perform correlation analysis, which demonstrated that the throat area had a significant effect on tracheal intubation difficulty. Our results revealed that a larger throat area was associated with a lower level of tracheal intubation difficulty, which is consistent with the clinician's subjective perception. Besides, we found that high BSA and weight corresponded to low tracheal intubation difficulty, which may be related to the better physical development of these infants. Moreover, male infants had a higher tracheal intubation difficulty than females. Pneumonia, age, and height were slightly correlated with the difficulty of

tracheal intubation, which may be due to the small amount of collected data and thus needs to be further analyzed.

After further P-value analysis, we found that four factors, namely throat area, gender, weight, and BSA, were internally different under the difficulty of tracheal intubation. Among them, the difference in the throat area was significant between all levels of tracheal intubation difficulty. Gender, weight, and BSA were only significantly different between level II and level III, level I, and level III. We speculate that it may be because the sample size of the level I tracheal intubation difficulty is too small. In addition height, age, and pneumonia under tracheal intubation difficulty were not statistically significant, which may be related to the small sample size.

Attention should be paid to some of the limitations of our research. First, we studied the correlation between risk factors and tracheal intubation difficulty without building a predictive model, because the limited number of cases obtained in this study could not meet the requirements for modelling. Second, in order to facilitate the drawing of the correlation coefficient map, the correlation measure was based on the Spearman rank correlation coefficient. In addition, this was a single-center study. Finally, the annotation of the region of interest in the throat was done by one experienced doctor, which may be subjectively biased.

This study has few limitations: first, future studies should expand the number of cases collected and construct a predictive model of intubation difficulty. Secondly, the regional annotation should be performed by multiple physicians, and artificial intelligence annotation tools should be constructed. Finally, the integration of labeling and difficulty prediction should be performed.

Conclusion

The throat area may be helpful for predicting the difficulty of tracheal intubation in infants with PRS. Besides, gender, weight and BSA may also affect the prediction of the difficulty of airway intubation to some extent.

Table 2 Difference analysis results of various factors

	Level 1 vs. 2	Level 2 vs. 3	Level 1 vs. 3	Total
Gender	1	0.0042**	0.0125*	0.0043**
Height	0.2473	0.4621	0.0526	0.1772
Weight	0.476	0.0264*	0.0025**	0.0117*
BSA	0.476	0.0264*	0.0025**	0.0117*
Throat area	0.0022**	0.0002***	< 0.0001***	< 0.0001***
Age	0.4694	0.2924	0.0503	0.1949
Pneumonia	0.4703	1	0.5253	0.5438

P-values for each risk factor under tracheal intubation difficulty. Among them, P values for a numerical variable were calculated by the Kruskal-Wallis test and for the categorical variable by Pearson's Chi-squared test
*$P < 0.05$
**$P < 0.01$
***$P < 0.001$

Abbreviations
PRS: Pierre Robin Syndrome; CT: Computed Tomography; BSA: Body Surface Area

Acknowledgements
Not applicable.

Authors' contributions
YIL is the main contributor in writing the manuscript. SZ is responsible for the collection and annotation of CT images. JSW processes the image and calculates the area, and performs statistical analysis. All authors read and approved the final manuscript.

Author details
[1]Science and technology department, China Pharmaceutical University, Nanjing, People's Republic of China. [2]Research Center of Biostatistics and Computational Pharmacy, China Pharmaceutical University, Nanjing, People's Republic of China. [3]Department of Anesthesiology, Children's Hospital of Nanjing Medical University, No. 72, Guangzhou Road, Gulou District, Nanjing 210008, People's Republic of China.

References

1. Xu Z, Ma W, Hester DL, et al. Anticipated and unanticipated difficult airway management. Curr Opin Anaesthesiol. 2018;31(1):96–103.
2. Cook TM, Woodall N, Frerk C. Major complications of airway management in the UK: results of the fourth National Audit Project of the Royal College of Anaesthetists and the difficult airway society. Part 1: anaesthesia. Br J Anaesth. 2011;106(5):617–31.
3. Rosenblatt WH. Preoperative planning of airway management in critical carepatients. Crit Care Med. 2004;32(4):186–92.
4. Münster T, Hoffmann M, Schlaffer S, et al. Anatomical location of the vocal cords in relation to cervical vertebrae. Eur J Anaesthesiol. 2016;33(4):257–62.
5. Guttman J, Nelson BP. Diagnostic emergency ultrasound: assessment techniques inthe pediatric patient. Pediatr Emerg Med Pract. 2016;13(1):1–27.
6. Erer OF, Erol S, Anar C, et al. Contribution of cell block obtained by endobronchial ultrasound-guided transbronchial needle aspiration in the diagnosis of malignant diseases and sarcoidosis. Endosc Ultrasound. 2017;6(4):265–8.
7. Leversedge FJ, Cotterell IH, Nickel B, et al. Ultrasonography guided de Quervain injection: accuracy and anatomic considerations in a cadaver model. J Am Acad Orthop Surg. 2016;24(6):399–404.
8. Li Y, Wang W, Yang T, et al. Incorporating uterine artery embolization in the treatment of cesarean scar pregnancy following diagnostic ultrasonography. Int J Gynaecol Obstet. 2016;134(2):202–7.
9. Osman A, Sum KM. Role of upper airway ultrasound in airway management. J Intensive Care. 2016;4(1):52.
10. Falcetta S, Cavallo S, Gabbanelli V, Pelaia P, Sorbello M, Zdravkovic I, Donati A. (2018). Evaluation of two neck ultrasound measurements as predictors of difficult direct laryngoscopy: a prospective study. Eur J Anaesthesiol. 2018;35:605–12.
11. Lee HC, Kim MK, Kim YH, et al. Radiographic predictors of difficult laryngoscopy in acromegaly patients. J Neurosurg Anesthesiol. 2019;31(1):50–6.
12. Karišik M, Janjević D, Sorbello M. Fiberoptic bronchoscopy versus video laryngoscopy in pediatric airway management. Acta Clinica Croatica. 2016;55:51–4.
13. Benko S, Fantes JA, Amiel J, et al. Highly conserved non-coding elements on either side of SOX9 associated with Pierre Robin sequence. Nat Genet. 2009;41(3):359–64.
14. Evans KN, Sie KC, Hopper RA, et al. Robin sequence: from diagnosis to development of an effective management plan. Pediatrics. 2011;127(5):936–48.
15. Plaza AM, Valadés RF, López AE, et al. Changes in airway dimensions after mandibular distraction in patients with Pierre-Robin sequence associated with malformation syndromes. Revista Española De Cirugía Oral Y Maxilofacial. 2015;37(2):71–9.
16. Frova G, Guarino A, Petrini F, et al. Recommendations for airway control and difficult airway management in paediatric patients. Minerva Anestesiol. 2006;72(9):723–48.
17. Ondik MP, Kimatian S, et al. Management of the difficult airway in the pediatric patient. J Pediatr Intensive Care. 2007;18(2):121–6.
18. Loftus PA, Ow TJ, Siegel B, et al. Risk factors for perioperative airway difficulty and evaluation of intubation approaches among patients with benign goiter. Ann Otol Rhinol Laryngol. 2014;123(4):279–85.
19. Xue FS, Yuan YJ, Wang Q, et al. Difficulties and possible solutions for tracheal intubation with the airway scope. Am J Emerg Med. 2011;29(1):123–4.
20. Hong L, Jin Q, Li X, et al. Image and medical annotations using non-homogeneous 2D ruler learning models. Comput Electrical Eng. 2016;50:102–10.
21. Domínguez C, Heras J, Pascual V. IJ-OpenCV: combining ImageJ and OpenCV for processing images in biomedicine. Comput Biol Med. 2017;84:189–94.
22. Culjak I, Abram D, Pribanic T, et al. A brief introduction to OpenCV [C]// MIPRO, 2012 proceedings of the 35th international convention. IEEE, 2012.
23. Chernov V, Alander J, Bochko V. Integer-based accurate conversion between RGB and HSV color spaces. Comput Electrical Eng. 2015;46:328–37.
24. Shin JW. High-accuracy skin lesion segmentation and size determination. Dissertations & Theses - Gradworks, 2011.
25. Raymond WH, Garder A. A spatial filter for use in finite area calculations. Mon Weather Rev. 2009;116(1):209–22.

Conditions for laryngeal mask airway placement in terms of oropharyngeal leak pressure: A comparison between blind insertion and laryngoscope-guided insertion

Go Wun Kim[1], Jong Yeop Kim[1], Soo Jin Kim[2], Yeo Rae Moon[2], Eun Jeong Park[1] and Sung Yong Park[1]*

Abstract

Background: Insertion under laryngoscopic guidance has been used to achieve ideal positioning of the laryngeal mask airway (LMA). However, to date, the efficacy of this technique has been evaluated only using fiberoptic evaluation, and the results have been conflicting. Other reliable tests to evaluate the efficacy of this technique have not been established. Recently, it has been suggested that the accuracy of LMA placement can be determined by clinical signs such as oropharyngeal leak pressure (OPLP). The aim of this study was to assess the efficacy of LMA insertion under laryngoscopic guidance using OPLP as an indicator.

Methods: After approved by the institutional ethics committee, a prospective comparison of 100 patients divided into 2 groups (50 with blind technique and 50 with the laryngoscope technique) were evaluated. An LMA (LarySeal™, Flexicare medical Ltd., UK) was inserted using the blind approach in the blind insertion group and using laryngoscopy in the laryngoscope-guided insertion group. The OPLP, fiberoptic position score, whether the first attempt at LMA insertion was successful, time taken for insertion, ease of LMA insertion, and adverse airway events were recorded.

Results: Data were presented as mean ± standard deviation. The OPLP was higher in the laryngoscope-guided insertion group than in the blind insertion group (21.4 ± 8.6 cmH₂O vs. 18.1 ± 6.1 cmH₂O, $p = 0.031$). The fiberoptic position score, rate of success in the first attempt, ease of insertion, and pharyngolaryngeal adverse events were similar between both groups. The time taken for insertion of the LMA was significantly longer in the laryngoscope-guided insertion group, compared to blind insertion group (35.9 ± 9.5 s vs. 28.7 ± 9.5 s, $p < 0.0001$).

Conclusion: Laryngoscope-guided insertion of LMA improves the airway seal pressure compared to blind insertion. Our result suggests that it may be a useful technique for LMA insertion.

Keywords: Laryngeal masks, Blind insertion, Laryngoscopy, Equipment and supplies

* Correspondence: anepark@hanmail.net
[1]Department of Anaesthesiology and Pain Medicine, Ajou University School of Medicine, 164, World Cup-ro, Yeongtong-gu, Suwon 16499, Republic of Korea

Background

The laryngeal mask airway (LMA) has been used routinely during general anaesthesia replacing endotracheal intubation, or has served as a bridge between endotracheal intubation and the facemask in emergent airway management [1, 2]. The blind insertion technique described by Brain is most widely used [3], but insertion of the LMA is not always smooth and anaesthetic gas leakage and gastric insufflation may occur [1, 4]. For achieving the ideal anatomical position of the LMA, various techniques, including insertion with the use of a laryngoscope, have been described [5, 6]. This technique was designed to control the tongue and displace the epiglottis superiorly so that the LMA can be placed over the tongue at a position below the epiglottis, with minimal resistance from the oral soft tissues [5]. However, except fiberoptic assessment which was based on the anatomic position of epiglottis and vocal cords [5, 6], reliable tests for efficacy of this technique have not been established.

In addition, to assess the airway seal and adequate ventilation of LMA, the value of the fiberoptic scoring system has been questioned [4, 7]. Alternative assessment modalities are needed. Recently, it has been suggested that the accuracy of LMA placement can be determined from clinical signs such as oropharyngeal leak pressure (OPLP). OPLP is commonly measured during LMA insertion to evaluate the degree of airway protection. High OPLPs are desirable as they indicate the feasibility of positive pressure ventilation and the likelihood of successful supraglottic airway placement [1, 7–12]. However, so far, no study has evaluated the efficacy of laryngoscope-guided LMA insertion techniques using OPLP as an indicator.

The aim of this randomised prospective study was to assess and compare the efficacy of blind LMA insertion with that of laryngoscope-guided LMA insertion. We considered that OPLP indicates clinical performance or function of the LMA better than fiberoptic score system does. The primary outcome of this study was the OPLP. The secondary outcomes were the fiberoptic position score, rate of success of first attempt at insertion, time taken for insertion of the LMA, ease of insertion, and the occurrence of any pharyngeal adverse event.

Methods

This prospective, randomised controlled trial was performed at Ajou University Hospital, Suwon, Republic of Korea, and was approved by the Institutional Ethics Committee (AJIRB-MED-DEO-16-072). After obtaining written informed consent for participation in the study, we enrolled 100 patients (American Society of Anesthesiologists physical status I or II, Age 19–70 years) scheduled to receive general anaesthesia with LMA insertion for elective minor surgery or ambulatory surgery. The exclusion criteria were as follows: (1) a recent history of upper respiratory tract infection, and (2) contraindication to the use of the LMA,

such as a body mass index (BMI) $\geq 40 \, \text{kg/m}^2$, symptomatic hiatal hernia, or severe oesophageal reflux disease. The trial is registered in a public trial register (Clinical Research Information Service, CRIS) under the identification number KCT0001945.

The patients were randomly divided into two groups with 50 patients in each, using a random group generator: the blind insertion group (Group 1) and the laryngoscope-guided insertion group (Group 2). Preoperative assessment included Mallampati airway classification. After the patient's arrival in the operating room, routine monitoring was applied, including electrocardiography, pulse oximetry, and noninvasive blood pressure measurement. Bispectral index (BIS) was monitored using a commercial device (A-2000™, Aspect medical systems, USA). Without premedication, anaesthesia was induced using a standard anaesthetic protocol without the use of muscle relaxant. Induction of anaesthesia was achieved with intravenous propofol (1.5–2.0 mg/kg) and remifentanil continuous infusion. Remifentanil infusion was started and maintained at effect-site concentration 2.0 ng/ml. For effect-site target-controlled infusion (TCI) of remifentanil, a commercial TCI pump (Orchestra Base Primea, Fresinus Vial, France) was used. After the patient lost consciousness, with continuous infusion of remifentanil, 2 vol% sevoflurane was administered and mask ventilation was performed for approximately 5 min for adequate depth of anaesthesia and muscle relaxation [13]. When an appropriate depth of anaesthesia was achieved (relaxation of the jaw, BIS < 60), the head was placed in the dorsiflexion sniffing position and a lubricated LMA (LarySeal™, Flexicare medical Ltd., UK) was inserted using the blind technique in Group 1 and under laryngoscopic guidance in Group 2. Selection of the LMA size was based on the body weight of the patient, usually size 3 for women and size 4 for men. Laryngoscopy was performed as described by Campbell et al. [5]; a MacIntosh #3 laryngoscope blade was placed in the vallecula and the epiglottis was identified; then, both the tongue and epiglottis were lifted anteriorly. It was not necessary to visualize the tracheal opening or vocal cords. To ensure optimal inflation of LMA cuff, the LMA cuff was inflated with air and the pressure was stabilized at 60 cmH$_2$O using a handheld manometer. Anaesthesiologists who had experience of at least more than 100 insertions of each technique performed the LMA insertion.

The time taken for LMA insertion, ease of LMA insertion, whether the first attempt was successful, OPLP, and fiberoptic position score were recorded. The time taken for LMA insertion was defined as the duration from the time the anaesthesiologist picked up the LMA till the capnography tracing was obtained. A failed attempt was defined as failed passage of the LMA into the pharynx or ineffective ventilation (expiratory tidal volume < 5 mg/kg or absence of a capnography tracing). The second attempt was performed without sniffing position, and if the second attempt failed endotracheal intubation was done. The patients in whom the first insertion was not successful were excluded from the analysis. Following successful LMA placement and ventilation, OPLP was measured by closing the expiratory valve of the circuit at a fixed gas flow rate of 6 L/min and noting the airway pressure at which the gas leaked into the mouth [8]. To ensure safety, the maximal allowable OPLP was fixed at 40 cmH$_2$O. Because position of head can impact the OPLP [11], the head and neck were kept in the sniffing position during the study. A fiberoptic scope was passed through the LMA tube to a position 1 cm proximal to the end of the tube, and the fiberoptic position was evaluated using the fiberoptic scoring system [5, 14]: 4, only the vocal cords seen; 3, vocal cords plus posterior epiglottis seen; 2, vocal cords plus anterior epiglottis seen; 1, vocal cords not seen, but function adequate; and 0, functional failure with the vocal cords invisible. The OPLP and fiberoptic position score were documented by an independent researcher, who was blinded to the insertion technique. Upon completion of the study protocol, the anaesthesiologist who performed the LMA insertion provided a subjective assessment of the insertion procedure by grading it as easy, fair, or difficult. Haemodynamic parameters and BIS were recorded at baseline, 1 min after anaesthesia induction, before insertion of the LMA, and 1 min after insertion of the LMA. During the procedures, anaesthesia was maintained with 2 vol% sevoflurane and effect-site TCI of remifentanil at 2.0 ng/ml.

At the end of the surgery, the independent researcher who was blinded to the group allocation removed the LMA after the patient gained consciousness, and collected data on the following adverse events: The presence of blood (none/trace/moderate/severe) after removal of the LMA. The presence or absence of sore throat and dysphonia was assessed at 1 h postoperatively.

Statistical analysis

The sample size of this study was determined based on previous studies [1, 10]. If the true difference in OPLP between the two groups was 20%, 44 participants would be required in each group to be able to reject the null hypothesis that the population means of the two groups were equal with a probability of 0.8. A total of 100 patients were enrolled considering a 10% dropout rate ($\alpha = 0.05$, $\beta = 0.8$).

We analyzed the data with R software package (R version 3.4.3) and SAS software version 9.4 (2002–2012, SAS Institute Inc., USA). Continuous data were analyzed using Student's t-test. Nonparametric data were analyzed using the Mann-Whitney test for two independent samples. Nominal data were analyzed using the chi-square test. Haemodynamic data were analyzed using the linear mixed effect model. Data were presented as mean ± standard deviation (SD), or numbers. A p value < 0.05 was considered significant.

Results

A total of 100 patients consented to participate in the study. The CONSORT flow diagram is shown in Fig. 1. The patient characteristics are shown in Table 1. There were no differences between the two groups in terms of demographic characteristics and Mallampati airway classification. The types of surgery were excision of breast tumor (11), knee arthroscopy (8), removal of fixation device (6), inguinal herniorrhaphy (6), open reduction of fracture (5), debridement (3), others (11) in Group 1, and excision of breast tumor (12), knee arthroscopy (12), removal of fixation device (6), anal surgery (4), ligation of saphneous vein (3), others (13) in Group 2.

Data on the primary and secondary variables are presented in Table 2. Values were presented as mean ± SD or numbers. The OPLP was higher in the laryngoscope-guided insertion group than in the blind insertion group (21.4 ± 8.6 cmH$_2$O vs. 18.1 ± 6.1 cmH$_2$O, $p = 0.031$). The fiberoptic position score ($p = 0.053$) and ease of insertion ($p = 0.405$) were not significantly different between the two groups. Rate of success at the first insertion attempt was not significantly different between the two groups (88% in Group 1, 90% in Group 2, $p = 0.749$). In all the patients in whom the first insertion attempt was not successful, success was achieved in the second attempt. The time taken for insertion of the LMA was significantly longer in Group 2 (28.7 ± 9.5 s in Group 1 vs 35.9 ± 9.5 s in Group 2, $p < 0.0001$). There was no difference between groups with respect to adverse events (Table 3). During anaesthesia induction and insertion of the LMA, haemodynamic parameters (mean arterial pressure, heart rate, oxygen saturation) and BIS were not significantly different between the two groups (Table 4). There were no episodes of teeth damage or hypoxia (SaO$_2$ < 95%) during the procedures. Anaesthesia was uncomplicated in all patients.

Discussion

In this study, we demonstrate that laryngoscope-guided insertion of LMA offers an advantage in terms of the OPLP compared with blind insertion. The main finding of our study is that laryngoscope-guided insertion results in a higher OPLP than blind insertion. This suggests that laryngoscope-guided insertion of LMA significantly improves the airway seal pressure. The reason that OPLP was higher in the laryngoscope-guided insertion group is probably because use of direct visual laryngoscopy to facilitate insertion the cuff of LMA plugs more firmly into the periglottic tissue. Direct laryngoscope compresses

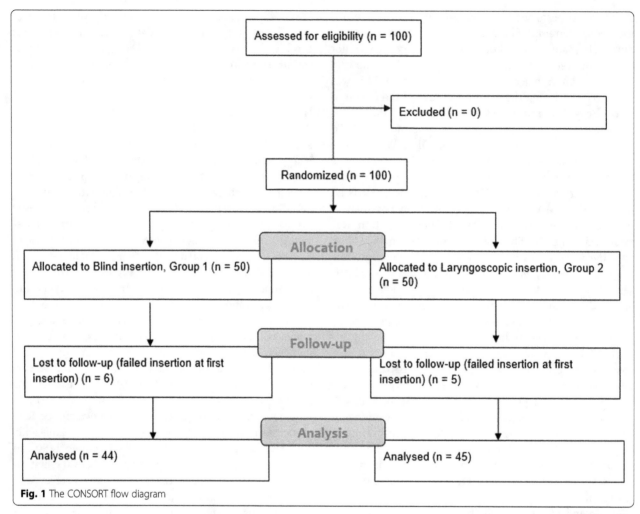

Fig. 1 The CONSORT flow diagram

the tongue to the left so the LMA can be inserted straightforward, minimizing lateral deviation. Under guidance of direct laryngoscope, the LMA can be possibly in alignment with laryngeal skeleton. However, our results indicate that laryngoscope-guided insertion is not superior to blind insertion in terms of achieving proper anatomical placement of the LMA, since the fiberoptic position scores were similar for both techniques.

Table 1 Patient characteristics

	Group 1 (n = 50)	Group 2 (n = 50)	p
Age (yr)	45.7 ± 12.1	44.9 ± 11.9	.740
Height (cm)	164.4 ± 8.2	164.3 ± 8.8	.981
Weight (kg)	62.7 ± 9.7	63.1 ± 10.7	.847
M/F (n)	24/26	23/27	.841
ASA physical status (I/II, n)	41/9	44/6	.400
Mallampati class (I/II/III/IV, n)	21/20/9/0	23/18/9/0	.907
Surgical time (min)	42.0 ± 23.8	48.3 ± 27.7	.235

Values are presented as mean ± SD or numbers
Group 1 = Blind insertion group; Group 2 = Laryngoscope-guided insertion group; M Male; F Female; ASA American Society of Anesthesiologists

It is very important to position the LMA correctly in order to ensure proper ventilation and minimize airway adverse events during the LMA insertion. To achieve this, several techniques of LMA insertion have been proposed [5, 6, 15–18], and laryngoscope-guided insertion is one of them [5, 6]. The proposed aim of this technique is to prevent the occlusion of the epiglottis due to insertion of the LMA by lifting the epiglottis upward using the laryngoscope directly during the insertion, so that the epiglottis does not block the vocal cord [5]. To date, the efficacy of this technique has been evaluated using only fiberoptic evaluation, and the results have been conflicting [5, 6]. Campbell et al. [5] used fiberoptic examination to compare the traditional blind insertion technique with direct visual placement using a laryngoscope. They reported that appropriate positioning of the LMA had been achieved in 91.5% of patients in the direct visual placement group, compared with 42% in the blind insertion group; the difference was significant. Chandan et al. [6], however, reported contradictory findings. They reported that there was no statistically significant difference between the blind insertion group and

Table 2 Safety, efficacy and utility data

	Group 1	Group 2	p
Oropharyngeal leak pressure (cmH$_2$O)	18.1 ± 6.1	21.4 ± 8.6	.031*
First attempt success rate (n, [%])	44/50 (88%)	45/50 (90%)	.749
Time taken for insertion (s)	28.7 ± 9.5	35.9 ± 9.5	< .0001*
Fiberoptic position score (4/3/2/1/0, n)	15/5/16/7/1	20/10/12/3/0	.053
Easy of insertion (easy/fair/difficult, n)	40/4/6	33/12/5	.405

Values are presented as mean ± SD or numbers
Group 1 = Blind insertion group; Group 2 = Laryngoscope-guided insertion group
* P < .05 refers to the statistical difference

the laryngoscope-guided insertion group using the fiberoptic position scoring proposed by Campbell et al. [5], which is similar to our finding. Because of these conflicting reports, the efficacy of laryngoscope-guided LMA placement, assessed using fiberoptic evaluation, seems to be controversial.

Although the most convenient method to assess the accuracy of anatomic placement of the LMA for clinical studies is fiberoptic examination, the value of the fiberoptic scoring system as a means of assessing proper positioning and airway seal function of the LMA has been debatable [4, 11, 19, 20]. Some studies demonstrated that there was no correlation between position and tightness of the LMA, and no prediction of tightness was possible [7, 20]. In Füllekrug et al.'s study [4], the epiglottis was observed to be in various positions obstructing the glottis opening, but clinical signs of improper placement were rarely observed. The airway can be functionally patent and clinically acceptable even when anatomic placement is less than optimal since the accessory vent allows good airflow to continue. Some researchers have suggested that fiberoptic scoring of the cuff position is not an accurate test to assess the airway seal and ventilation function of the LMA [4, 7, 20]. We speculated that the efficacy of the seal or tightness may vary depending on the individual patient's laryngopharyngeal anatomy, in addition to the anatomical placement of the LMA.

In contrast to previous studies that evaluated the efficacy of this technique, we measured the OPLP to judge the appropriateness of the airway maintenance and protection, and the correct mounting of the LMA. Recently,

it was suggested that the actual tightness of the inserted LMA, rather than fiberoptic view, is an important parameter of adequate airway management [1]. As a mean of this evaluation, an airway sealing pressure or OPLP is commonly performed with the supraglottic airway to quantify the seal with the airway and judge the appropriateness of ventilation [1, 7–12]. OPLP values have been widely used as a reference for feasibility of positive pressure ventilation and the degree of airway protection and is regarded as the most important value when testing the stability of a LMA [9]. Studies to date have not achieved a consensus regarding leak pressure of LMA inserted by laryngoscope-guided technique. To our knowledge, it is the first study that evaluate the usefulness of this technique in terms of OPLP.

Someone might state that the reason to use the blind technique is to avoid the sympathetic stimulation and pharyngolaryngeal adverse events from instrumentation of the oropharyngeal soft tissues during laryngoscopy [5, 6]. Although these haemodynamic changes are short-lived, they are undesirable in patients with pre-existing myocardial or cerebral disease [21]. LMA placement without laryngoscopy avoids airway trauma with fewer changes in haemodynamic parameters [6]. In our study, there were no differences between two groups in haemodynamic parameters and incidence of pharyngolaryngeal adverse events. The reason for these findings was probably secondary to the applied laryngoscopy technique in this study – just gently lift the epiglottis and not necessary to visualize the tracheal opening or vocal cords [5]. It also indicated that the depth of anaesthesia was adequate after 5 min of 2 vol% sevoflurane inhalational induction and remifentanil infusion (effect-site concentration 2.0 ng/ml).

Mean insertion time in laryngoscope-guided insertion group tended to be longer than in blind insertion group (35.9 s vs 28.7 s). Possible reason for longer insertion time in the laryngoscope-guided insertion group was the additional time need for laryngoscopy manipulation procedure. But, we do not consider this to be a clinical problem since it is unlike that the magnitude of this differences have clinical significance.

Table 3 Incidence of adverse events

	Group 1 (n = 44)	Group 2 (n = 45)	p
Bleeding (none/trace/moderate, n)	43/1/0	39/5/1	.053
Pharyngolaryngeal adverse event (none/sore throat/dysphonia)	37/6/1	33/12/0	.189

Values are presented as numbers
Group 1 = Blind insertion group; Group 2 = Laryngoscope-guided insertion group

Table 4 Haemodynamic profiles and bispectral indices during laryngeal mask airway insertion

		Baseline	1 min after induction	Pre-insertion	1 min after LMA insertion
MBP (mmHg)	Group 1	96.2 ± 15.0	77.4 ± 12.6	67.2 ± 11.9	71.5 ± 14.0
	Group 2	94.5 ± 12.7	75.4 ± 11.2	65.7 ± 10.8	75.2 ± 12.4
HR (beats/min)	Group 1	72.5 ± 12.7	66.2 ± 11.3	63.5 ± 11.2	63.5 ± 12.3
	Group 2	74.6 ± 11.9	69.2 ± 12.0	65.0 ± 11.5	65.3 ± 12.4
SpO$_2$ (%)	Group 1	99.0 ± 1.3	99.9 ± 0.3	99.8 ± 0.6	99.8 ± 0.4
	Group 2	99.0 ± 1.3	99.9 ± 0.4	99.9 ± 0.4	99.8 ± 0.7
BIS	Group 1	96.7 ± 2.4	42.2 ± 10.7	43.2 ± 8.2	48.0 ± 10.9
	Group 2	96.9 ± 1.6	41.3 ± 11.3	44.1 ± 9.9	48.8 ± 11.4

Values are mean ± SD
LMA laryngeal mask airway, Group 1 = Blind insertion group; Group 2 = Laryngoscope-guided insertion group; *MAP* mean arterial pressure; *HR* heart rate; *SpO$_2$* peripheral oxygen saturation; *BIS* bispectral index

Our study had some limitations. First, assessment of easy of insertion was not blinded; therefore, this is a possible source of bias. Second, the present study was performed by board-certified anaesthesiologists trained in the use of LMA to minimize the bias due to familiarity with each technique. Therefore, we cannot comment on results obtained by naïve users. Thirdly, our data cannot be applied to the all kinds of supraglottic airway. The type of supraglottic airway (e.g. bulky designed i-gel™ or pre-curved LMA) might also play a very important role if laryngoscopic guidance is better than blind insertion. The variety of cuff's properties and shapes of supraglottic airway should be considered. Fourthly, we did not use muscle relaxants before insertion of the LMA, because the LMA can be inserted easily without muscle relaxants if an adequate depth of anaesthesia is reached [9, 12]. Because there is some evidence suggesting that the use of neuromuscular blocker can alter the OPLP [22], this should be considered. Finally, the difference between the groups might be statistical different, but 3 cmH$_2$O may not make a clinically relevant difference. Some clinicians would argue that OPLP of 18 cmH$_2$O is sufficient for most patient in most clinical situations. Although the included number of patients were determined based on previous studies [1, 10], this trial might be underpowered to answer the question of this trial.

Conclusion
When compared to the blind insertion, laryngoscope-guided insertion of LMA improve the airway seal pressure. Our result suggests that it may be a useful technique for LMA insertion.

Abbreviations
BIS: Bispectral index; BMI: Body mass index; LMA: Laryngeal mask airway; OPLP: Oropharyngeal leak pressure; TCI: Target-controlled infusion

Acknowledgements
None.

Authors' contributions
GWK was responsible for study execution and manuscript writing. JYK was resposible for conceived and designed this study. SJK and YRM were responsible for data analysis and interpretation of results. EJP collected the data. SYP was responsible for study execution, supervising of data management and manuscript writing. All authors have read and approved the final version of the manuscript.

Author details
[1]Department of Anaesthesiology and Pain Medicine, Ajou University School of Medicine, 164, World Cup-ro, Yeongtong-gu, Suwon 16499, Republic of Korea. [2]Office of Biostatistics, Ajou University School of Medicine, Suwon, Republic of Korea.

References
1. Seet E, Rajeev S, Firoz T, Yousaf F, Wong J, Wong DT, et al. Safety and efficacy of laryngeal mask airway supreme versus laryngeal mask airway ProSeal: a randomized controlled trial. Eur J Anaesthesiol. 2010;27:602–7.
2. Francksen H, Bein B, Cavus E, Renner J, Scholz J, Steinfath M, et al. Comparison of LMA unique, Ambu laryngeal mask and soft seal laryngeal mask during routine surgical procedures. Eur J Anaesthesiol. 2007;24:134–40.
3. Brain AI. The laryngeal mask-a new concept in airway management. Br J Anaesth. 1983;55:801–5.
4. Füllekrug B, Pothmann W, Werner C, Schulte am Esch J. The laryngeal mask airway: anesthetic gas leakage and fiberoptic control of positioning. J Clin Anesth. 1993;5:357–63.
5. Campbell RL, Biddle C, Assudmi N, Campbell JR, Hotchkiss M. Fiberoptic assessment of laryngeal mask airway placement: blind insertion versus direct visual epiglottoscopy. J Oral Maxillofac Surg. 2004;62:1108–13.
6. Chandan SN, Sharma SM, Raveendra US, Rajendra Prasad B. Fiberoptic assessment of laryngeal mask airway placement: a comparison of blind insertion and insertion with the use of a laryngoscope. J Maxillofac Oral Surg. 2009;8:95–8.
7. Brimacombe J, Keller C. Stability of the LMA-ProSeal and standard laryngeal mask airway in different head and neck positions: a randomized crossover study. Eur J Anaesthesiol. 2003;20:65–9.
8. Keller C, Brimacombe JR, Keller K, Morris R. Comparison of four methods for assessing airway sealing pressure with the laryngeal mask airway in adult patients. Br J Anaesth. 1999;82:286–7.
9. Beleña JM, Núñez M, Anta D, Carnero M, Gracia JL, Ayala JL, et al. Comparison of laryngeal mask airway supreme and laryngeal mask airway Proseal with respect to oropharyngeal leak pressure during laparoscopic cholecystectomy: a randomised controlled trial. Eur J Anaesthesiol. 2013;30:119–23.

10. Eschertzhuber S, Brimacombe J, Hohlrieder M, Keller C. The laryngeal mask airway supreme-a single use laryngeal mask airway with an oesophageal vent. A randomised, cross-over study with the laryngeal mask airway ProSeal in paralysed, anaesthetised patients. Anaesthesia. 2009;64:79–83.

11. Kim HJ, Lee K, Bai S, Kim MH, Oh E, Yoo YC. Influence of head and neck position on ventilation using the air-Q® SP airway in anaesthetized paralysed patients: a prospective randomized crossover study. Br J Anaesth. 2017;118:452–7.

12. Gasteiger L, Ofner S, Stögermüller B, Ziegler B, Brimacombe J, Keller C. Randomized crossover study assessing oropharyngeal leak pressure and fiber optic positioning: laryngeal mask airway supreme™ versus laryngeal tube LTS II™ size 2 in non-paralyzed anesthetized children. Anaesthesist. 2016;65:585–9.

13. Joe HB, Kim JY, Kwak HJ, Oh SE, Lee SY, Park SY. Effect of sex differences in remifentanil requirements for the insertion of a laryngeal mask airway during propofol anesthesia: a prospective randomized trial. Medicine. 2016; 95:e5032.

14. Brimacombe J. Berry a. a proposed fiber-optic scoring system to standardize the assessment of laryngeal mask airway position. Anesth Analg. 1993;76:457.

15. Brimacombe J, Berry A. Insertion of the laryngeal mask airway-a prospective study of four techniques. Anaesth Intensive Care. 1993;21:89–92.

16. Park JH, Lee JS, Nam SB, Ju JW, Kim MS. Standard versus rotation technique for insertion of Supraglottic airway devices: systematic review and meta-analysis. Yonsei Med J. 2016;57:987–97.

17. Jeon YT, Na HS, Park SH, Oh AY, Park HP, Yun MJ, et al. Insertion of the ProSeal laryngeal mask airway is more successful with the 90 degrees rotation technique. Can J Anaesth. 2010;57:211–5.

18. Ghai B, Wig J. Comparison of different techniques of laryngeal mask placement in children. Curr Opin Anaesthesiol. 2009;22:400–4.

19. Joshi S, Sciacca RR, Solanki DR, Young WL, Mathru MM. A prospective evaluation of clinical tests for placement of laryngeal mask airways. Anesthesiology. 1998;89:1141–6.

20. Xue FS, Mao P, Liu HP, Yang QY, Li CW, He N, et al. The effects of head flexion on airway seal, quality of ventilation and orogastric tube placement using the ProSeal laryngeal mask airway. Anaesthesia. 2008;63:979–85.

21. Gupta K, Rastogi B, Gupta PK, Singh I, Singh VP, Jain M. Dexmedetomidine infusion as an anesthetic adjuvant to general anesthesia for appropriate surgical field visibility during modified radical mastectomy with i-gel®: a randomized control study. Korean J Anesthesiol. 2016;69:573–8.

22. Goldmann K, Hoch N, Wulf H. Influence of neuromuscular blockade on the airway leak pressure of the ProSeal laryngeal mask airway. Anasthesiol Intensivmed Notfallmed Schmerzther. 2006;41:228–32.

A clinical prediction rule to identify difficult intubation in children with Robin sequence requiring mandibular distraction osteogenesis based on craniofacial CT measures

Zhe Mao, Na Zhang and Yingqiu Cui[*] [iD]

Abstract

Background: Airway management is challenging in children with Robin sequence (RS) requiring mandibular distraction osteogenesis (MDO). We derived and validated a prediction rule to identify difficult intubation before MDO for children with RS based on craniofacial computed tomography (CT) images.

Method: This was a retrospective study of 69 children with RS requiring MDO from November 2016 to June 2018. Multiple CT imaging parameters and baseline characteristic (sex, age, gestational age, body mass index [BMI]) were compared between children with normal and difficult intubation according to Cormack–Lehane classification. A clinical prediction rule was established to identify difficult intubation using group differences in CT parameters (eleven distances, six angles, one section cross-sectional area, and three segment volumes) and clinicodemographic characteristics. Predictive accuracy was evaluated by receiver operating characteristic (ROC) curve analysis.

Results: The overall incidence of difficult intubation was 56.52%, and there was no significant difference in sex ratio, age, weight, height, BMI, or gestational age between groups. The distance between the root of the tongue and posterior pharyngeal wall was significantly shorter, the bilateral mandibular angle shallower, and the cross-sectional area at the epiglottis tip smaller in the difficult intubation group. A clinical prediction rule based on airway cross-sectional area at the tip of the epiglottis was established. Area > 36.97 mm^2 predicted difficult intubation while area < 36.97 mm^2 predicted normal intubation with 100% sensitivity, 62.5% specificity, 78.6% positive predictive value, and 100% negative predictive value (area under the ROC curve = 0.8125).

Conclusion: Computed tomography measures can objectively evaluate upper airway morphology in patients with RS for prediction of difficult intubation. If validated in a larger series, the measures identified could be incorporated into airway assessment tools to guide treatment decisions.

This was a retrospective study and was granted permission to access and use these medical records by the ethics committee of Guangzhou Women and Children's Medical Center.

Keywords: Difficult intubation, Mandibular micrognathia, Robin sequence

* Correspondence: gzhtwang@163.com
Guangzhou Women and Children's Medical Center, No 9, Jinsui Road,
Guangzhou 510623, Guangdong, China

Background

Robin sequence (RS) is a congenital craniofacial abnormality usually defined by a triad of micrognathia, glossoptosis, and U-shaped cleft palate that collectively result in frequent tongue-based airway obstruction (TBAO). The condition affects 1 in 8500 to 20,000 neonates, and may be associated with several other syndromes [1, 2]. Most RS patients are either asymptomatic or can be treated conservatively [3]. However, patients with severe TBAO may require surgical intervention [4]. Tracheostomy is a direct and effective method to relieve upper airwway obstruction [5]. However, long-term reliance on tracheotomy can lead to bleeding, speech and swallowing difficulties, tracheal stenosis, and even death [6]. In recent years, mandibular distraction osteogenesis (MDO) has become one of the most popular surgical alternatives to tracheostomy. By gradual lengthening the mandible, thereby simultaneously advancing the soft tissues and tongue, MDO can increase upper airway size and relieve airway obstruction safely and effectively [7].

However, MDO surgery requires tracheal intubation for general anesthesia, which may be challenging in RS due to upper airway deformity. Indeed, Denise et al. reported difficult laryngoscopy exposure in 42.7% of children with RS [8] and Yin et al. reported difficult intubation in 71% of children with RS [9]. The need for more than two direct laryngoscopy attempts in children with difficult tracheal intubation is associated with high failure rate and increased incidence of severe complications, including subglottic narrowing, aspiration, and death [10, 11]. Therefore, it is critical to assess the possibility of difficult intubation before MDO.

At present, mouth opening degree, head and neck activity, thyromental distance, ratio of thyromental height to distance, and Mallampati classification are used to assess the possibility of difficult intubation among the general surgical population [12, 13]. However, these prediction methods often lack standard data for children, especially for infants, so at present there is no prediction method that can be reliably applied to RS patients. A new method to predict intubation difficulty before MDO for RS could reduce perioperative complications and improve clinical outcome.

Cone-beam computed tomography (CBCT) allows for extensive anatomic characterization while avoiding excessive radiation exposure [14, 15]. At present, craniofacial CBCT is routinely used to determine the location of upper airway obstruction and depict the mandibular anatomy of infants with RS under consideration for surgical intervention [16–19]. In this retrospective study, we identified quantitative parameters derived from CBCT images that differed between RS patients with normal or difficult intubation and tested their predictive efficacies by receiving operating characteristic (ROC)

analyses. These analyses identified three such parameters that distinguish normal from difficult intubation prior to MDO for RS patients with high sensitivity and predictive value.

Methods

This was a retrospective study and was granted permission to access and use these medical records by the ethics committee of Guangzhou Women and Children's Medical Center .

Our multidisciplinary team followed a comprehensive algorithm using physical examination, laboratory, endoscopic, and polysomnography findings to assess the

Table 1 Definition of all CT Measurements

CT Measurements	Definition of all CT Measurements
D1	Distance between the upper central alveolar ridge and root of the epiglottis
D2	Distance between the root of the epiglottis and glottis midpoint
D3	Distance between the end of the mandible and glottis midpoint
D4	Height of the mandible
D5	Distance between the uvula and posterior pharyngeal wall
D6	Distance between the root of the tongue and posterior pharyngeal wall
D7	Distance between the epiglottis and posterior pharyngeal wall
D8	Length of the epiglottis
D9	Length of the mandibular ramus
D10	Length of the mandible body
D11	Length of the mandible
A1	Angle between lines D1 and D2
A2	The angle between line D2 and the lower edge of the upper central alveolar ridge to the glottis midpoint
A3	The angle of lines D3 and D4
A4	The angle of the point of the lower edge of the upper central alveolar ridge to the trailing edge of the hard palate and then to the root of epiglottis
A5	The angle of the mandible
A6	The angle of the gonion to the angle of the mandible
Airway section area at the tip of epiglottis	The airway section area at the tip of epiglottis
Oral volume	Mouth volume from upper and lower alveolar ridge to the posterior edge of the hard palate
Palatine pharyngeal volume	Palatine pharyngeal volume from the posterior border of the hard palate to the edge of the soft palate
Glossopharyngeal volume	Glossopharyngeal volume from soft palate palatal cusp to epiglottis upper edge.

D Distance, *A* Angle

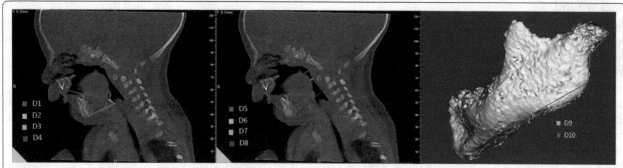

Fig. 1 Upper airway distances D1–D11 derived from 3D reconstructions of craniofacial CBCT images acquired prior to mandibular distention osteogenesis for treatment of Robin sequence. Distances D1 to D10 are shown while D11 is the sum of D9 plus D10

severity of airway obstruction. Exclusion criteria were (1) severe cardiopulmonary disease, (2) head and neck tumors or trauma leading to local anatomical structure changes, (3) laryngomalacia, brain-induced central apnea, or mixed apnea, and (4) other anomalies unrelated to RS causing airway obstruction.

All patients underwent intubation by the same experienced anesthesiologist. Patients were divided into two groups according to the Cormack–Lehane classification recorded in the anesthesia record. The degree of difficult intubation was graded as follows: grade I, glottis was completely exposed; grade II, glottis was partially exposed; grade III, epiglottis only was exposed; grade IV, glottis and epiglottis were not seen by endoscopy. Patients of grade I/II were defined as the normal intubation group (group A), while those of grade III/IV were defined as the difficult intubation group (group B). Among infants in the two groups, baseline characteristics collected were sex, age, gestational age, and body mass index (BMI).

CBCT measurements.

Cone-beam CT scans were obtained as part of clinical management using standard institutional protocols. All images were acquired with patients in the left-lateral position at slice thickness between 0.625 mm and 1.25 mm. Axial images were reformatted parallel to the Frankfort horizontal plane and sagittal images were

subsequently generated, providing a standardized reference plane. Two experienced raters performed CT analysis for all patients. All CT reformatting and analyses were conducted using MIMICS 17.0 image processing software (Materialise NV, Leuven, Belgium). Airway volumes for each division were calculated on axial images using region of interest (ROI) analysis set at a threshold for air density and the MIMICS ROI volume calculator. Volumes occupied by the radio-opaque border of an artificial airway were not included in the reported palatine pharyngeal volume and glossopharyngeal volume. Craniocaudal lengths for each division were calculated on the reformatted sagittal images. Mandible measures were performed using 3D reconstructed views. A total of 21 parameters (Table 1) were measured as potential predictors of difficult tracheal intubation by a special surveyor. Each index was measured three times by an experienced rater and the average value was taken as the final result. An additional rater performed a second reading to evaluate inter-rater reliability. These parameters included eleven distances (D1 – D11) (Fig. 1), six angles (A1 – A6) (Fig. 2), one airway cross-sectional area, and three volumes (Fig. 3).

Statistical analyses.

All statistical analyses were performed using SPSS21.0 (IBM, Armonk, NY, USA). To control for differences in

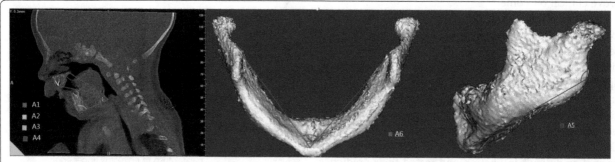

Fig. 2 Measurements of upper airway angles A1 to A6

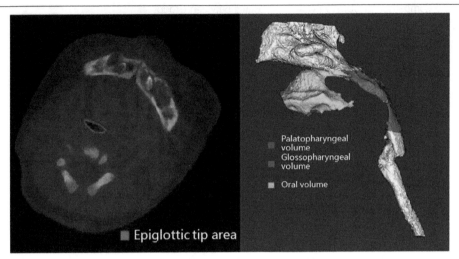

Fig. 3 Measurements of upper airway cross-sectional area and segment volumes

skeletal distance among patients of various sizes and ages, all distances were normalized to each patient's nasion to sella turcica center distance according to the formula $y^{(norm)} = y/y^{NB}$, where y is the raw measure and y^{NB} is the nasion to sella turcica center distance. Baseline clinicodemographic characteristics of the two RS patient groups were compared by t test, while CT measurements were compared by the Mann-Whitney rank sum test. A $P < 0.05$ (two-tailed) was considered significant for all tests. Spearman's rank correlation coefficient (ρ) was used to evaluate inter-rater reliability respectively, with $\rho > 0.9$ indicating high reliability. According to the test results, a clinical prediction rule was established. Thirty-two individual patient datasets were randomly selected as training sets to build the decision tree model, and the remaining 37 datasets were used as a prediction set to verify the prediction rule. A receiving operating characteristic (ROC) curve was constructed to evaluate predictive efficacy.

Results

Baseline characteristics of normal and difficult intubation groups of RS patients.

Of the 69 patients enrolled, 30 were classified as normal intubation cases (group A) and 39 as difficult intubation cases (group B), for an overall difficult intubation incidence of 56.52% (Group B/total). There was no significant difference in sex ratio, weight, height, BMI, or gestational age between groups ($P > 0.05$) (Table 2).

Comparison of CBCT measures between groups.

The inter-rater reliability of CBCT parameters met the requirement of $\rho > 0.9$. The distance between the root of the tongue and posterior pharyngeal wall (D6) was significantly shorter, the bilateral mandibular angle (A5) shallower, and the cross-sectional area at the epiglottis tip smaller in the difficult intubation group (all $P < 0.05$) (Table 3).

Construction of a clinical prediction rule

According to the test results, D6, A5, and cross-sectional area at the epiglottis tip differed significantly between normal and difficult intubation groups. However, the measurement of D6 is based on soft tissue images and so can be influenced by tongue movement, which is not conducive to clinical application. At the

Table 2 Baseline characteristic of the two groups of RS patients

Variable	Normal intubation group(n = 30)	Difficult intubation group(n = 39)	P Value
Female, No. (%)	12 (40.0)	14 (35.9)	0.922
Birth weight.kg. (mean (sd))	3.01 (0.56)	2.97 (0.58)	0.762
Weight.kg. (mean (sd))	3.70 (0.79)	3.46 (0.58)	0.14
Birth height.cm. (mean (sd))	50.70 (2.25)	49.67 (3.28)	0.232
Height.cm. (mean (sd))	52.03 (3.42)	51.19 (3.44)	0.32
Gestational age. Week. (mean (sd))	38.22 (2.39)	38.48 (1.78)	0.611
BMI (mean (sd))	13.52 (1.87)	12.98 (1.77)	0.233

A comparison of baseline characteristic between these groups can be found in the Table. P<0.05 means a significant difference between the two groups

Table 3 Reliability and Comparison of Upper Airway CT Measures between Groups

Variable	Normal intubation group(n = 30)	Difficult intubation group(n = 39)	ρ Value	P Value
D1 (mean (sd))	40.86 (3.15)	39.84 (2.80)	0.997	0.192
D2 (mean (sd))	6.92 (3.11)	6.28 (2.09)	0.991	0.357
D3 (mean (sd))	25.02 (3.96)	23.44 (4.31)	0.998	0.164
D4 (mean (sd))	15.52 (2.09)	15.63 (3.17)	0.993	0.877
D5 (mean (sd))	3.79 (1.44)	3.69 (1.33)	0.994	0.772
D6 (mean (sd))	2.78 (1.65)	2.00 (1.19)	0.997	0.045*
D7 (mean (sd))	4.87 (2.29)	5.27 (2.18)	0.999	0.511
D8 (mean (sd))	5.66 (1.77)	5.63 (0.99)	0.994	0.942
D9. Left. (mean (sd))	16.54 (2.55)	15.32 (2.49)	0.998	0.068
D9.Right. (mean (sd))	16.41 (2.50)	15.19 (2.67)	0.998	0.078
D10.Left. (mean (sd))	40.32 (3.83)	40.04 (3.05)	0.999	0.762
D10.Right. (mean (sd))	40.54 (4.01)	40.08 (2.95)	0.997	0.613
D11.Left. (mean (sd))	56.91 (5.58)	55.41 (3.77)	0.997	0.227
D11.Right. (mean (sd))	54.96 (11.14)	53.87 (9.58)	0.993	0.686
Area (mean (sd))	40.64 (19.34)	25.61 (11.72)	0.995	0.001*
A1 (mean (sd))	144.29 (14.25)	142.53 (19.61)	0.999	0.705
A2 (mean (sd))	4.82 (2.26)	4.63 (2.35)	0.998	0.758
A3 (mean (sd))	116.71 (11.20)	118.45 (14.62)	0.999	0.622
A4 (mean (sd))	100.05 (12.54)	101.60 (7.18)	0.998	0.554
A5.Left. (mean (sd))	135.46 (4.89)	131.45 (8.12)	0.997	0.012*
A5.Right. (mean (sd))	135.74 (6.18)	130.73 (8.00)	0.998	0.01*
A6 (mean (sd))	87.22 (7.78)	88.08 (8.14)	0.999	0.675
Oral volume (mean (sd))	2000.66 (1389.55)	1948.27 (1192.55)	0.992	0.88
Palatine pharyngeal volume (mean (sd))	652.45 (410.90)	538.90 (267.63)	0.993	0.212
Glossopharyngeal volume (mean (sd))	400.81 (226.37)	321.45 (274.75)	0.992	0.239

Spearman's rank correlation coefficient was used to evaluate the Inter-observer correlation
D Distance, A Angle Area: Airway section area at the tip of epiglottis
*Statistically significant at p < 0.05
P<0.05 means a significant difference between the two groups
ρ>0.9 shows that the measurement results are credible

same time, not all hospitals have the capacity for three-dimensional reconstruction of CT images, so A5 is not widely applicable. Alternatively, it may be possible to use radiation-free methods such as magnetic resonance imaging (MRI) to measure the cross-sectional area at the epiglottis tip. Considering these factors, we constructed a decision tree model by the airway cross-sectional area at the epiglottis tip (Fig. 3) using Classification and Regression Trees (CART) for predicting difficult intubation. When the cross-sectional area was more than 36.97 mm², difficult intubation was more likely, while normal intubation was more likely when the cross-sectional area was less than 36.97 mm².

Evaluation of the decision tree model
Based on CART evaluation, the airway cross-sectional area at the epiglottis tip was subjected to ROC analysis,

which yielded an area under of ROC curve 0.8125 (Fig. 4) and prediction of difficult intubation with 100% sensitivity, 62.5% specificity, 78.6% positive predictive value, and 100% negative predictive value (Table 4).

Discussion
This study compared multiple airway dimensions from CT images between RS patients demonstrating normal or difficult intubation during MDO to identify factors useful for presurgical prediction of difficult airway management. Over half of this patient cohort exhibited difficult intubation, and such patients demonstrated a shorter distance between the root of the tongue and posterior pharyngeal wall (D6), a shallower bilateral mandibular angle (A5), and smaller cross-sectional area at the epiglottis tip (Table 3). Based on these findings, we established a clinical prediction rule and verified its

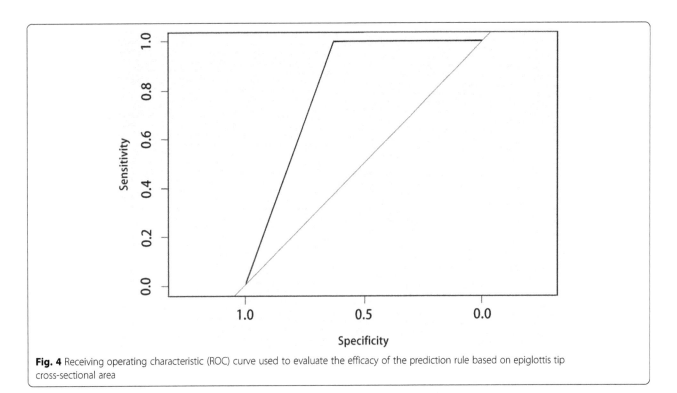

Fig. 4 Receiving operating characteristic (ROC) curve used to evaluate the efficacy of the prediction rule based on epiglottis tip cross-sectional area

efficacy by ROC curve analysis. While tongue root to posterior pharyngeal wall distance (D6) differed significantly between groups, it is also influenced by tongue movement and so may not be reliable for clinical applications. Similarly, many hospitals lack the technology for routine three-dimensional reconstruction of CT images, limiting the use of A5. Therefore, in an attempt to simplify the CT composite score for routine clinical use, we constructed a decision tree model based only one cross-sectional area at the epiglottis tip (Fig. 3) as this metric is not influenced by tongue movement and may be measurable using radiation-free techniques, such as MRI. ROC analysis of this parameter yielded a high AUC (0.8125) using a cut-off cross-sectional area of 36.97 mm^2, indicating that a cross-sectional area above 36.97 mm^2 is predictive of difficult intubation.

Mallampati score, nail–chin spacing, chest–chin spacing, upper and lower incisor spacing, mandibular protrusion, cervical retroversion, and ratio of thyromental height to distance are the most widely used methods to identify laryngoscopic exposure difficulties [20–25]. However, most of these methods were established by screening the general population, and are not applicable for patients with maxillofacial deformities [26]. Robin sequence

patients have unusual and highly heterogeneous jaw and upper airway morphologies, making it difficult to predict difficult intubation. Computed tomography can be used to evaluate infant bony and soft tissue anatomy of the upper airway in 2 and 3 dimensions, which is not possible with cephalometrics [27–29]. While CT scanning does require radiation exposure, maxillofacial CT is a routine preoperative examination for MDO [16–18], so this evaluation method will not require additional exposure. Further, cone-beam delivery can markedly reduce total radiation dose, so there is no additional safety limitation for clinical practice. Surgical treatment is often unavoidable for the treatment of severe RS [19], and early identification of difficult intubation will help reduce complications from multiple intubation attempts.

This is an exploratory study and has several limitations. First, we were unable to observe the effects of mouth opening on glottic exposure in children with oral closure and quiet breathing during CT scan. The small sample size also limits statistical strength, so other factors predictive of difficult intubation may have been missed. However, we did try to minimize the impact of growth, development, and age through normalization of the CT metrics to baseline values. In addition, this study

Table 4 Results of the decision tree model for the prediction set

Sensitivity	Specificity	Accuracy	Positive predictive value	negative predictive value	AUC
(%)	(%)	(%)	(%)	(%)	
1	62.5	78.571	66.667	1	0.8125

was conducted at a single center, which may introduce selection bias. For instance, these CBCT metrics were derived from RS infants with severe airway obstruction, and it is not clear whether they persist in infants with mild airway obstruction. However, only severe RS patients require presurgical intubation, so we believe that patient selection does not limit the clinical applicability of the prediction rule. Severe RS patients who need MDO all have potentially life-threatening breathing difficulties. In order to minimize the risk of airway obstruction, our hospital stipulates no more than two attempts at laryngoscopic visualization and intubation. Therefore, we have no clinical information on patients with three or more unsuccessful intubation attempts. This is why patients were divided into normal and difficult intubation groups according to Cormack–Lehane classification instead of by the number of laryngoscopic visualization and intubation attempts.

This work represents a first step toward development of an evidence-based decision tool for predicting difficult intubation in patients with RS, but prospective validation is needed. To further advance our understanding of factors conferring difficult intubation in children with RS, we plan to compare other airway and bone measurements as well as clinical severity measurements. Future work should also assess the effectiveness of imaging modalities that do not involve ionizing radiation, such as MRI.

Conclusion

Computed tomography was used to quantify morphological parameters of the upper airway predictive of difficult intubation during mandibular distraction osteogenesis for infants with Robin sequence. These measures may help guide RS treatment decisions.

Abbreviations
AUC: Area under curve; BMI: Body mass index; CART: Classification and Regression Tree; CBCT: Cone-beam computed tomography; CT: Computed tomography; MDO: Mandibular distraction osteogenesis; ROC: Receiver operating characteristic; ROI: Region of interest; RS: Robin sequence; TBAO: Tongue-based airway obstruction

Acknowledgements
Not applicable.

Authors' contributions
Authors Z.M, N.Z, and Y.Q.C had full access to study data and take responsibility for data integrity and the accuracy of data analysis. Concept and design:Z.M,YQ.C. Acquisition, analysis, or interpretation of data: N.Z. Drafting of the manuscript: Z.M. Critical revision of the manuscript for important intellectual content: All authors. Statistical analysis:N.Z. Obtained funding: Y.Q.C. All authors have read and approved the manuscript, and ensure that this is the case.

References

1. Evans KN, Sie KC, Hopper RA, Glass RP, Hing AV, Cunningham ML. Robin sequence: from diagnosis to development of an effective management plan. Pediatrics. 2011;127(5):936–48.
2. Bush PG, Williams AJ. Incidence of the Robin Anomalad (Pierre Robin syndrome). Br J Plast Surg. 1983;36(4):434–7.
3. Printzlau A, Andersen M. Pierre Robin sequence in Denmark: a retrospective population-based epidemiological study. Cleft Palate Craniofac J. 2004;41(1):47–52.
4. Ren XC, Gao ZW, Li YF, et al. The effects of clinical factors on airway outcomes of mandibular distraction osteogenesis in children with Pierre Robin sequence. Int J Oral Maxillofac Surg. 2017;46(7):805–10.
5. Tomaski SM, Zalzal GH, Saal HM. Airway obstruction in the Pierre Robin sequence. Laryngoscope. 1995;105:111–4.
6. Bookman LB, Melton KR, Pan BS, et al. Neonates with tongue-based airway obstruction: a systematic review. Otolaryngol Head Neck Surg. 2012;146(1):8–18.
7. Collins B, Powitzky R, Rumbled C, Rose C, Glade R. Airway management in Pierre Robin sequence: patterns of practice. Cleft Palate Craniofac J. 2014;51:283–9.
8. Manica D, Schweiger C, Sekine L. Severity of clinical manifestations and laryngeal exposure difficulty predicted by glossoptosis endoscopic grades in Robin sequence patients. Int J Pediatr Otorhinolaryngol. 2016;28(9):214–9.
9. Yin N, Fang L, Shi X, et al. A comprehensive scoring system in correlation with perioperative airway management for neonatal Pierre Robin sequence. PLoS One. 2017;12(12):e0189052.
10. Fiadjoe JE, Nishisaki A, Jagannathan N, et al. Airway management complications in children with difficult tracheal intubation from the pediatric difficult intubation (PeDI) registry: a prospective cohort analysis. Lancet Respir Med. 2016;4(1):37–48.
11. Manica D, Schweiger C, Sekine L. Severity of clinical manifestations and laryngeal exposure difficulty predicted by glossoptosis endoscopic grades in Robin sequence patients. Int J Pediatr Otorhinolaryngol. 2016;90:214–9.
12. Hekiert AM, Mandel J, Mirza N. Laryngoscopies in the obese: predicting problems and optimizing visualization. Ann Otol Rhinol Laryngol. 2007; 116:312–6.
13. Lundstrom LH, Vester-Andersen M, et al. Poor prognostic value of the modified Mallampati score: a meta-analysis involving 177088 patients. Br J Anaesth. 2011;107(5):659–67.
14. Zeiberg AS, Silverman PM, Sessions RB, et al. Helical (spiral) CT of the upper airway with three-dimensional imaging: technique and clinical assessment. Am J Roentgenol. 1996;166(2):293–9.
15. Loubele M, Bogaerts R, Van Dijck E, et al. Comparison between effective radiation dose of CBCT and MSCT scanners for dentomaxillofacial applications. Eur J Radiol. 2009;71(3):461–8.
16. Lee VS, Evans KN, Perez FA, Oron AP, Perkins JA. Upper airway computed tomography measures and receipt of tracheotomy in infants with Robin sequence. JAMA Otolaryngol Head Neck Surg. 2016;142(8):750–7.
17. Ramieri V, Basile E, Bosco G, Caresta E, Papoff P, Cascone P. Three-dimensional airways volumetric analysis before and after fast and early mandibular osteodistraction. J Craniomaxillofac Surg. 2017;45(3):377–80.
18. Zellner EG, Mhlaba JM, Reid RR, Steinbacher DM. Does mandibular distraction vector influence airway volumes and outcome? J Oral Maxillofac Surg. 2017;75(1):167–77.
19. Gómez OJ, Barón OI, Peñarredonda ML. Pierre Robin sequence: an evidence-based treatment proposal. J Craniomaxillofac Surg. 2018;29(2):332–8.
20. Kheterpal S, Healy D, Aziz MF, et al. Incidence, predictors, and outcome of difficult mask ventilation combined with difficult laryngoscopy. Anesthesiology. 2013;119:1360–9.
21. Law AJ, Broemling N, Cooper RM, et al. The difficult airway with recommendations for management-part 2-the anticipated difficult airway. Can J Anaesth. 2013;60:1119–38 with permission.
22. Heinrich S, Birkholz T, Irouschek A, Ackermann A, Schmidt J. Incidences and predictors of difficult laryngoscopy in adult patients undergoing general anesthesia: a single-center analysis of 102,305 cases. Anesthesiology. 2013; 27:815–21.
23. Ling-shuang Z, Ma X-y, Gao J. Predictive system study of difficult laryngoscopy. J Clin Anesth. 2013;29:789–91.

24. Yu T, Wang B, Jin XJ, et al. Predicting difficult airways: 3-3-2 rule or 3-3 rule? Ir J Med Sci. 2015;184:677–83.
25. Ittichaikulthol W, Chanpradub S, Amnoundetchakorn S, et al. Modified Mallampati test and thyromental distance as a predictor of difficult laryngoscopy in Thai patients. J Med Assoc Thail. 2010;93:84–9.
26. Al Ramadhani S, Mohamed LA, Rocke DA, et al. Sternomental distance as the sole predictor of difficult laryngoscopy in obstetric anaesthesia. Br J Anaesth. 1996;77(3):312–6.
27. Abramson Z, Susarla S, Troulis M, Kaban L. Age-related changes of the upper airway assessed by 3-dimensional computed tomography. J Craniofac Surg. 2009;20(suppl 1):657–63.
28. Li H, Lu X, Shi J, Shi H. Measurements of normal upper airway assessed by 3-dimensional computed tomography in Chinese children and adolescents. Int J Pediatr Otorhinolaryngol. 2011;75(10):1240–6.
29. Mattos CT, Cruz CV, da Matta TC, et al. Reliability of upper airway linear, area, and volumetric measurements in cone-beam computed tomography. Am J Orthod Dentofac Orthop. 2014;145(2):188–97.

Radiological indicators to predict the application of assistant intubation techniques for patients undergoing cervical surgery

Bingchuan Liu[1,2†], Yanan Song[3†], Kaixi Liu[3], Fang Zhou[1,2], Hongquan Ji[1,2], Yun Tian[1,2*] and Yong Zheng Han[3*]

Abstract

Background: We aimed to distinguish the preoperative radiological indicators to predict the application of assistant techniques during intubation for patients undergoing selective cervical surgery.

Methods: A total of 104 patients were enrolled in this study. According to whether intubation was successfully accomplished by simple Macintosh laryngoscopy, patients were divided into Macintosh laryngoscopy group ($n = 78$) and Assistant technique group ($n = 26$). We measured patients' radiographical data via their preoperative X-ray and MRI images, and compared the differences between two groups. Binary logistic regression model was applied to distinguish the meaningful predictors. Receiver operating characteristic (ROC) curve and area under the curve (AUC) were used to describe the discrimination ability of indicators. The highest Youden's index corresponded to an optimal cut-off value.

Results: Ten variables exhibited significant statistical differences between two groups ($P < 0.05$). Based on logistic regression model, four further showed correlation with the application of assistant techniques, namely, perpendicular distance from hard palate to tip of upper incisor (X2), atlanto-occipital gap (X9), angle between a line passing through posterior-superior point of hard palate and the lowest point of the occipital bone and a line passing through the anterior-inferior point and the posterior-inferior point of the second cervical vertebral body (Angle E), and distance from skin to hyoid bone (MRI 7). Angle E owned the largest AUC (0.929), and its optimal cut-off value was 19.9° (sensitivity = 88.5%, specificity = 91.0%). the optimal cut-off value, sensitivity and specificity of other three variables were X2 (30.1 mm, 76.9, 76.9%), MRI7 (16.3 mm, 69.2, 87.2%), and X9 (7.3 mm, 73.1, 56.4%).

Conclusions: Four radiological variables possessed potential ability to predict the application of assistant intubation techniques. Anaesthesiologists are recommended to apply assistant techniques more positively once encountering the mentioned cut-off values.

Keywords: Difficult laryngoscope, Assistant intubation technique, Radiological indicator, Clinical study

* Correspondence: tiany@bjmu.edu.cn; hanyongzheng@163.com
†Bingchuan Liu and Yanan Song are co–first authors.
¹Department of Orthopaedics, Peking University Third Hospital, Beijing, China
³Department of Anesthesiology, Peking University Third Hospital, 49 North Garden Rd, Haidian District, Beijing 100191, China

Background

Airway management is regarded as the most important aspect in clinical anesthesia and a successful intubation remains crucial for surgical procedures [1]. Clinically, there are many factors associated with difficulty of intubation during laryngoscopy, including head-neck trauma [2], airway abnormalities [3], gastroesophageal reflux disease [4], hard to open mouth [5], impaired cervical mobility [6], etc. The incidence of difficulty to undergo laryngoscopy and intubation ranges widely among different studies, and patients with cervical spondylosis have a higher incidence of difficult laryngoscopy (17.1%) [7] than those without cervical spondylosis (7.3%) [8]. This might in turn cause unexpected difficult airways in large proportion of patients, significantly increasing the morbidity and mortality rates [9]. Difficulty during laryngoscopy due to unexpected situations brings huge challenge to anesthesiologists. Under such circumstances, multiple attempts of intubation and application of assistant intubation techniques are considered inevitable.

A pre-planned induction strategy involves consideration of various interventions that are designed to facilitate intubation during difficult airway conditions. The interventions that are intended to manage difficult airway include, but are not limited to [10]: (1) video-assisted laryngoscopy, (2) lighted stylets (e.g., shikani, light wand), (3) fiberoptic-guided intubation, (4) supraglottic airway for ventilation and intubation (e.g., intubating laryngeal mask airway), and (5) invasive airway access (e.g., tracheostomy). However, the clinical application and promotion of these assisted techniques were still associated with some limitations. Firstly, overuse without any specific indications not only causes wastage of medical resources, but reduces the productivity of anesthesiologist. Secondly, the opportunity of optimal intubation might be missed when these techniques are forced to be applied under unexpected situations and multiple attempts of intubation might cause iatrogenic guttural injury. Therefore, before undergoing intubation, an effective predictive strategy that can provide anesthesiologists with information on the necessity and possibility of assistant techniques is required and considered crucial in clinical practice.

Many researchers have attempted to predict difficult of intubation by preoperative radiologic data, but very few studies have specifically targeted at the necessity and possibility of the application of assistant techniques for intubation. Hence, in the present study, this prediction was carried out based on radiological indicators of patients who underwent cervical surgery. Our study findings could provide valuable information for airway management practice, especially for patients with special conditions where traditional assessment methods such as thyromental distance, mouth opening, cervical mobility and Mallampati classification are difficult to be obtained.

Methods

Study design

From June 2019 to December 2019, patients who underwent elective cervical spine surgery under general anesthesia were recruited in this cohort study. Inclusion criteria of patients were as follows: (1) age ranging from 20 to 70 years; (2) with good mental health; and (3) complete radiographic and clinical materials. Exclusion criteria were as follows: patients (1) with airway tumor or foreign body; (2) severe cervical trauma; (3) cervical spine instability; (4) poor physical conditions (ASA IV or V); and (5) anticipated difficult mask ventilation. The clinical and radiological data of patients were acquired by reviewing their medical history and measuring the values on the Picture Archiving and Communication Systems (PACS). This study was approved by Medical Ethics Committee of Peking University Third Hospital, Peking University Health Science Center, Beijing (IRB00006761–2015021). Informed consents were obtained from the patients.

Measurement of radiological indicators

Radiological data were obtained by cervical X-ray examination and neck MRI (MR750; GE Medical Systems, Milwaukee, WI, USA). X-ray examination was performed by informing patients to maintain standing position and MRI scan was completed in the supine position. All X-ray and MRI data were evaluated using radiography information system (Centricity RIS-IC CE V3.0; GE Healthcare, Little Chalfont, UK) of the Peking University Third Hospital. All distance and angle indicators on cervical lateral X-rays were measured in the neutral position (Figs. 1 and 2), which indicated that the cervical spine was maintained its natural curvature without flexion and extension, and sagittal T2-weighted neck MRI indicators were also measured in neutral position (Fig. 3). All imaging indicator measurements were completed by the same orthopedic surgeon for all patients in batches. The detailed measurement methods of all parameters are described in the figure legends. Bias was avoided as orthopedic surgeon was blinded to group allocation, and not involved in the intubation and anesthesia management.

Intubation procedure

Routine preoperative monitoring of non-invasive blood pressure, heart rate, pulse oximetry, and electrocardiography were performed. Anesthesia was induced with sufentanil (0.3 μg/kg) and propofol (2 mg/kg). For patients who lost consciousness, neuromuscular blockade was injected by rocuronium (0.6 mg/kg). The Macintosh laryngoscope was applied by senior anesthesiologists who were not involved in the preoperative radiologic assessment. Patients who were successfully intubated with Macintosh laryngoscope were assigned to the Macintosh group, and those unsuccessfully intubated with Macintosh laryngoscope

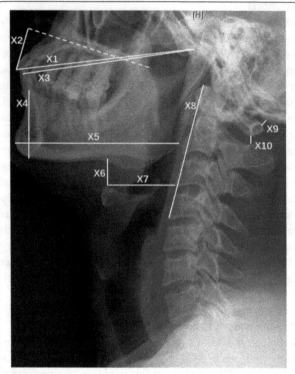

Fig. 1 Distance indicators on the lateral cervical X-ray in the neutral position. X1: distance between temporomandibular joint and the tip of upper incisor; X2: perpendicular distance from hard palate to the tip of upper incisor; X3: distance between temporomandibular joint and the tip of lower incisor; X4: anterior depth of mandible; X5: length of mandibular body; X6: vertical distance from the highest point of hyoid bone to mandibular body; X7: horizontal distance from the highest point of hyoid bone to the border of the nearest cervical vertebra; X8: distance from the anterior-inferior border of the fourth cervical vertebra to the anterior-superior border of the first vertebra; X9: atlanto-occipital gap; X10: distance between the spinous processes of the first and second cervical vertebra

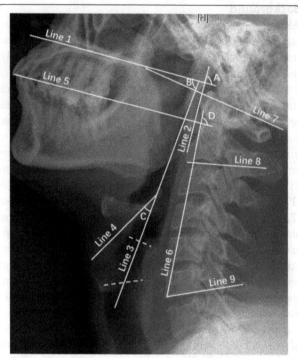

Fig. 2 Angle indicators on the lateral cervical X-ray in the neutral position. Angle A: angle between Line 1 and Line 2; Angle B: angle between Line 1 and Line 3; Angle C: angle between Line 3 and Line 4; Angle D: angle between Line 5 and Line 6; Angle E: angle between Line 7 and Line 8; Angle F: angle between Line 8 and Line 9. (Line 1: a line parallel to hard palate; Line 2: a line passing through the anterior point of the bodies of atlas and axis; Line 3: a line passing through the airway midpoint crossing the cricoid cartilage; Line 4: a line parallel to epiglottis; Line 5: a line along the occlusal surface of maxillary teeth; Line 6: a line passing through anterior-inferior border of the sixth cervical vertebra and the most anterior aspect of the first cervical vertebra; Line 7: a line passing through the posterior-superior point of hard palate and the lowest point of the occipital bone; Line 8: a line passing through the anterior-inferior point and the posterior-inferior point of the second cervical vertebral body; Line 9: a line passing through the anterior-inferior point and the posterior-inferior point of the sixth vertebral body)

were settled according to the Difficult Airway Society 2015 guidelines [11].

Selection of different assistant intubation techniques

Patients who were unsuccessfully intubated with Macintosh laryngoscope were further dealt with assistant techniques in this study. In this study, unsuccessful intubation was defined as the clinical situation in which a conventionally trained anesthesiologist (working more than 5 years) could not successfully complete tracheal intubation less than three attempts with Macintosh laryngoscope. The video-assisted laryngoscopy is the first choice as it is easy to handle, and can be inserted into the patient's mouth. If failed, shikani or fiberoptic-guided intubation was considered as alternative techniques. If the patient has poor oxygenation, then the intubating laryngeal mask airway should be chosen. In emergency situation or those in need for invasive airway access, tracheostomy could also be considered.

Patient and public involvement

No patients were involved in the radiological data measurements nor were they involved in developing plans for design and accomplishment of the present study. No patients were asked to advise on interpretation. The final results will be disseminated to investigators and patients through this publication.

Statistical analysis

SPSS 22.0 software was used to execute statistical analysis. Kolmogorov-Smirnov test assists in determining whether the distribution was normal. Continuous variables that were normally distributed were analyzed by independent-samples T test, while non-normal variables were assessed by Mann-Whitney test. Categorical data were analyzed by Chi-square test. After that, binary

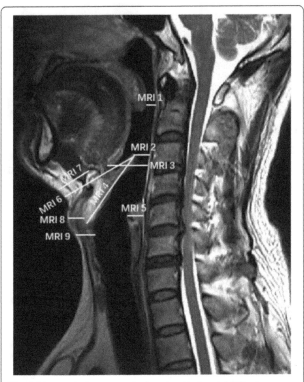

Fig. 3 Distance indicators on the lateral sagittal neck MRI in the neutral position. MRI 1: distance between uvula and the posterior pharyngeal wall; MRI 2: distance between the tip of epiglottis and the posterior pharyngeal wall; MRI 3: distance between the base of tongue and the posterior pharyngeal wall; MRI 4: the length of epiglottis; MRI 5: distance between vocal cord and the posterior pharyngeal wall; MRI 6: distance from skin to the tip of epiglottis; MRI 7: distance from skin to hyoid bone; MRI 8: distance from skin to thyroid cartilage at the level of vocal cord; MRI 9: distance from skin to vocal cord

logistic regression model was applied to distinguish multivariate predictors. Odds ratio (OR) and 95% confidence interval (95% CI) signifies the strength of association. The receiver operating characteristic (ROC) curve was used to describe the discrimination ability of the predictive indicators. Area under the curve (AUC) was used as a quantitative index. Youden's index (= sensitivity + specificity - 1) was calculated and the highest score was considered as an optimal predictive cut-off value. $P < 0.05$ was considered to be statistically significant.

Results

A total of 104 patients were enrolled in this study. Based on whether assistant techniques were applied during intubation, patients were divided into Macintosh laryngoscopy group (78 cases) and Assistant technique group (26 cases). In the Assistant technique group, 4 patients underwent intubation with video-assisted laryngoscope successfully, 4 patients underwent intubation with shikani optical stylet, 15 patients with fiberoptic bronchoscopy, 2

patients with laryngeal mask airway, and 1 patient with tracheostomy tube. The average age of the patients was 51.77 years, and included 92 males and 12 females. Patients' demographics and measurement data were displayed in Table 1. There were no significant differences in the aspects of gender, age, height, weight and BMI between two groups ($P > 0.05$). With regard to radiological measurement, ten indicators that showed significant differences between the two groups were found, namely, X2 ($P < 0.001$), X6 ($P = 0.028$), X7 ($P = 0.001$), X9 ($P = 0.039$), Angle B ($P = 0.037$), Angle E ($P < 0.001$), Angle F ($P = 0.017$), MRI 1 ($P = 0.002$), MRI 4 ($P = 0.013$), and MRI 7 ($P < 0.001$).

Based on the binary logistic regression model (Forward: LR) presented in Table 2, among the ten mentioned indicators with significant differences between the two groups, 4 indicators showed further correlation with the application of assistant techniques during intubation. These included X2 ($P = 0.005$, OR = 0.526), X9 ($P = 0.019$, OR = 3.175), Angle E ($P < 0.003$, OR = 1.723), and MRI 7 ($P = 0.018$, OR = 1.375), and their 95% CI were (0.337 to 0.819), (1.213 to 8.309), (1.206 to 2.463), (1.058 to 1.796), respectively.

The ROC curve and the AUC were used to understand the predictive ability of the 4 radiological predictors established by the logistic regression model. As shown by Table 3 and Fig. 4, Angle E owned the largest AUC (0.929) (95% CI was 0.873 to 0.986), and the AUCs of X2 and MRI 7 were higher than 0.8. According to the highest Youden's index, the optimal cut-off value of Angle E was 19.9° (sensitivity = 88.5%, specificity = 91.0%), and the optimal cut-off value, sensitivity and specificity of other variables were X2 (30.1 mm, 76.9, 76.9%), MRI7 (16.3 mm, 69.2, 87.2%), and X9 (7.3 mm, 73.1, 56.4%).

Discussion

Due to the existence of cervical degeneration, instability or spondylosis, difficult laryngoscopy has a higher incidence in patients undergoing elective cervical spine surgery. To reduce the unnecessary attempts and increase the efficiency and accuracy of the anaesthesiologist during application of assistant techniques during intubation, and based on patients' preoperative cervical X-ray and MRI images, this study was conducted to distinguish radiological predictors that were reported in the previous literature in difficult conditions where assisted techniques should be prepared and applied in a more positive manner and where necessary. To our knowledge, only few studies have focused on the prediction of the application of assisted techniques according to the preoperative radiological measurements. Our findings would hold great value in providing references to clinical anesthesia.

Table 1 Demographics and measurement data between two groups

Items	Macintosh laryngoscopy group (n = 78)	Assistant technique group (n = 26)	Statistic (χ^2/z/t)	P-value
Male (%)	71 (91.0)	21 (80.8)	2.010	0.156
Age (years)	51.2 ± 8.6	53.4 ± 10.4	1.062	0.291
Height (cm)	170.7 ± 5.9	168.3 ± 6.6	−1.349	0.177
Weight (kg)	71.2 ± 8.2	68.2 ± 9.1	−1.524	0.128
BMI (kg/m^2)	24.4 ± 2.7	24.0 ± 2.7	− 0.641	0.534
X1 (mm)	106.0 ± 7.7	108.0 ± 6.8	1.178	0.242
X2 (mm)	28.1 ± 3.5	33.0 ± 4.1	− 4.857	**< 0.001**
X3 (mm)	103.5 ± 7.4	104.1 ± 6.7	− 0.184	0.854
X4 (mm)	40.9 ± 3.8	39.2 ± 5.0	−1.793	0.076
X5 (mm)	98.8 ± 6.9	101.1 ± 7.9	1.396	0.166
X6 (mm)	19.3 ± 6.3	16.3 ± 4.9	− 2.225	**0.028**
X7 (mm)	44.7 ± 6.1	40.0 ± 6.2	−3.323	**0.001**
X8 (mm)	95.0 ± 7.3	93.6 ± 8.2	−0.825	0.411
X9 (mm)	7.9 ± 2.8	6.6 ± 1.7	−2.064	**0.039**
X10 (mm)	6.1 ± 1.8	6.1 ± 2.6	− 0.833	0.405
Angle A (°)	97.1 ± 7.9	95.8 ± 5.9	− 0.748	0.456
Angle B (°)	83.1 ± 7.4	80.2 ± 9.9	− 2.091	**0.037**
Angle C (°)	28.7 ± 3.9	29.4 ± 2.8	− 0.214	0.831
Angle D (°)	99.8 ± 7.7	101.6 ± 9.6	0.155	0.338
Angle E (°)	27.2 ± 6.3	14.8 ± 5.7	−8.866	**< 0.001**
Angle F (°)	15.9 ± 6.1	12.5 ± 6.3	−2.391	**0.017**
MRI 1 (mm)	8.1 ± 1.7	6.9 ± 1.8	−3.125	**0.002**
MRI 2 (mm)	7.4 ± 1.9	7.2 ± 2.4	−0.721	0.471
MRI 3 (mm)	16.7 ± 3.8	15.9 ± 3.7	−0.998	0.321
MRI 4 (mm)	39.5 ± 4.5	42.1 ± 4.2	2.541	**0.013**
MRI 5 (mm)	9.3 ± 1.7	8.7 ± 1.3	−1.653	0.101
MRI 6 (mm)	46.5 ± 5.94	44.8 ± 6.1	−1.263	0.209
MRI 7 (mm)	20.7 ± 4.2	16.1 ± 6.1	−4.212	**< 0.001**
MRI 8 (mm)	11.6 ± 3.6	11.3 ± 6.2	−1.723	0.085
MRI 9 (mm)	8.6 ± 2.1	9.8 ± 4.3	−1.156	0.248

Angle E, which is the angle between a line passing through the posterior-superior point of hard palate and the lowest point of the occipital bone and a line passing through the anterior-inferior point and the posterior-inferior point of the second cervical vertebral body, could reflect the upper cervical spine mobility. Less

Table 2 The binary logistic regression model (Forward: LR) of the enrolled variables

Items	B	SE	P-value	OR	95% CI
X2	−0.643	0.226	0.005	0.526	0.337, 0.819
X9	1.155	0.491	0.019	3.175	1.213, 8.309
Angle E	0.544	0.182	0.003	1.723	1.206, 2.463
MRI 7	0.321	0.135	0.018	1.378	1.058, 1.796

Angle E seen in our study implied the limited flexion of upper cervical spine, which might result in difficult laryngoscopy. The occipitoatlantal junction contributes 23.0°–24.5° of flexion/extension of the skull and the atlantoaxial joint provides an additional 10.1°–22.4° [12] movement. Hence, the upper cervical spine contributes a vast majority of flexion and extension of the cervical spine mobility. Besides, the atlantoaxial joint serves as an important hub structure that connects the skull and spine, where many important vessels and nerves were located [13]. The limitation of flexion and extension might increase the risk of disastrous iatrogenic injuries if laryngoscopy is forced to be applied [14]. In our study, Angle E demonstrated the best ability to predict the necessity of assistant technique application (AUC = 0.929), and the

Table 3 The AUC and the optimal cut-off value based on the highest Youden's index

Items	AUC	Highest Youden's index	Optimal cut-off value	Sensitivity	Specificity
Angle E	0.929	0.795	19.9	0.885	0.910
X2	0.819	0.538	30.1	0.769	0.769
MRI 7	0.805	0.564	16.3	0.692	0.872
X9	0.636	0.295	7.3	0.731	0.564

cut-off value of 19.9° had the highest sensitivity (88.5%) and specificity (91.0%). The results suggested that if the Angle E was less than 19.9° in clinical intubation, higher vigilance and more positive application of assistant techniques are required.

X2, the perpendicular distance from hard palate to the tip of upper incisor, was also an effective radiological indicator in predicting the difficult laryngoscopy in this study (AUC = 0.819). The patients in Assistant technique group were detected with longer X2 distance (33.0 ± 4.1 mm vs. 28.1 ± 3.5 mm, $P < 0.001$). In a sense, longer X2 distance caused by bucktooth and abnormal hard palate indicates shorter inter-incisor gap and smaller oral cavity space anatomically [15, 16]. These two limiting factors further restrict the intraoral operation of laryngoscopy and create difficulty in exposing the glottis [17, 18]. In this study, the optimal cut-off value of X2 was 30.1 mm (sensitivity = 76.9%, specificity = 76.9%), and this indicated that a X2 distance of more than 30.1 mm reminded us the

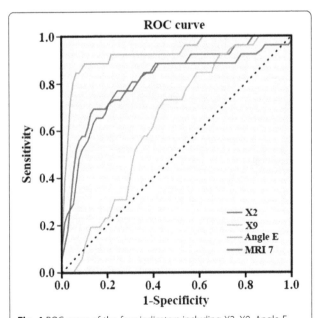

Fig. 4 ROC curve of the four indicators including X2, X9, Angle E, MRI 7. (X2: perpendicular distance from hard palate to the tip of upper incisor; X9: atlanto-occipital gap; Angle E: angle between Line 7 and Line 8; MRI 7: distance from skin to hyoid bone. Line 7: a line passing through the posterior-superior point of hard palate and the lowest point of the occipital bone; Line 8: a line passing through the anterior-inferior point and the posterior-inferior point of the second cervical vertebral body)

application of assisted techniques during intubation more possibly and necessarily.

MRI 7 is the distance from skin to hyoid bone. Adhikari et al. [19] have reported that this distance could be used to distinguish difficult and easy laryngoscopies, and found that it was higher in patients in difficult laryngoscopy group when compared with easy laryngoscopy group (1.69 cm, 95% CI 1.19 to 2.19 vs 1.37 cm, 95% CI 1.27 to 1.46) in a study of 51 American patients who underwent intubation in neutral position without a pillow. Besides, MRI 7 also had higher specificity and sensitivity for predicting difficult airway management, and this is because the hyoid acts as a vital factor of the upper airway, which was connected to tongue by genioglossus muscle and to the larynx via the hyoepiglottic and thyrohyoid [20]. In our study, the shorter distance from skin to hyoid bone indicated difficult laryngoscopy, which was different from the result of Adhikari [19]. The reason for this might be that the shorter MRI 7 could suggest connection of anatomical structures to the hyoid bone that were located more anteriorly and lower, which might in turn influence the exposure of glottis during laryngoscope examination. In our study, the distance from skin to hyoid bone acts as a moderate accuracy predictor with an AUC = 0.805. It was significantly different between the Macintosh laryngoscope and Assistant technique groups (20.7 ± 4.2 mm vs 16.1 ± 6.1 mm, $P < 0.001$). This result was consistent with some previous studies [21, 22], in which the distance from skin to hyoid bone as measured by ultrasound had certain predictive function for difficult laryngoscopy.

X9 is the atlanto-occipital gap, and the distance between the occipital bone and first cervical vertebra in patients undergoing intubation in neutral position. Patients with atlantooccipital distance impairment had a higher prevalence of difficulty laryngoscopy [23, 24]. X9 is related to occipito-atlanto complex, and is associated with mandibular protrusion. Patients with lesions in the occipito-atlanto complex had a higher prevalence of difficult airway than those with disease below the complex [23]. Besides, shorter X9 distance might reflect decreased motion range and slight fusion of atlanto-occipital joint to some extent. In our study, atlanto-occipital gap was significantly different between Macintosh laryngoscopy group and Assistant technique group (7.9 ± 2.8 mm vs. 6.6 ± 1.7 mm, $P = 0.039$). However, the AUC of X9 was 0.636, representing low accuracy and its optimal cut-off value was 7.3 mm with a sensitivity of 73.1% and specificity of 56.4%.

However, there are some limitations in our study. Firstly, the present study included a relatively small number of patients, and larger sample size and a multi-center study might make the results more convincing. Secondly, this was a retrospective study, and a prospective study for predicting the necessity and possibility of assistant technique application during intubation might have the potential to provide more references to clinical anesthesia. Additionally, some measurement errors might exist because the measurements were completed by a single surgeon.

Conclusions

In summary, four radiological parameters were recognized to predict the application of assistant intubation techniques in this study. Based on the optimal cut-off values of each preoperative predictor, the possibility of difficult airway is warned, and the anaesthesiologist should then apply the assistant technique more positively before many attempts during intubation.

Abbreviations
ASA: American Society of Anesthesiologists; PACS: picture archiving and communication systems; MRI: magnetic resonance imaging; ROC: receiver operating characteristic; AUC: area under the curve

Acknowledgements
We thank Xiaoyan Niu for her help in collecting clinical data.

Authors' contributions
BCL and YNS analyzed the data and wrote the manuscript. BCL and KXL collectively reviewed patients' clinical data and accomplished the radiological measurement. FZ, HQJ, YT and YZH designed the study and analyzed the results. All authors read and approved the final manuscript.

Author details
[1]Department of Orthopaedics, Peking University Third Hospital, Beijing, China. [2]Beijing Key Laboratory of Spinal Disease Research, Beijing, China. [3]Department of Anesthesiology, Peking University Third Hospital, 49 North Garden Rd, Haidian District, Beijing 100191, China.

References
1. Schumacher J, Arlidge J, Dudley D, et al. The impact of respiratory protective equipment on difficult airway management: a randomised, crossover, simulation study. Anaesthesia. 2020. https://doi.org/10.1111/anae.15102.
2. Lee J, Kim JS, Kang S, et al. Prediction of difficult airway management in traumatic cervical spine injury: influence of retropharyngeal space extension. Ther Clin Risk Manag. 2019;15:669–75.
3. Hews J, El-Boghdadly K, Ahmad I. Difficult airway management for the anaesthetist. Br J Hosp Med (Lond). 2019;80(8):432–40.
4. Nasr VG, Abdallah C. Gastroesophageal reflux disease causing a difficult airway. J Clin Anesth. 2010;22(5):389–90.
5. Han YZ, Tian Y, Xu M, et al. Neck circumference to inter-incisor gap ratio: a new predictor of difficult laryngoscopy in cervical spondylosis patients. BMC Anesthesiol. 2017;17(1):55.
6. Han Y, Fang J, Zhang H, et al. Anterior neck soft tissue thickness for airway evaluation measured by MRI in patients with cervical spondylosis: prospective cohort study. BMJ Open. 2019;9(5):e029987.
7. Han YZ, Tian Y, Zhang H, et al. Radiologic indicators for prediction of difficult laryngoscopy in patients with cervical spondylosis. Acta Anaesthesiol Scand. 2018;62(4):474–82.
8. Etezadi F, Ahangari A, Shokri H, et al. Thyromental height: a new clinical test for prediction of difficult laryngoscopy. Anesth Analg. 2013;117(6):1347–51.
9. Shiga T, Wajima Z, Inoue T, et al. Predicting difficult intubation in apparently normal patients: a meta-analysis of bedside screening test performance. Anesthesiology. 2005;103(2):429–37.
10. Apfelbaum JL, Hagberg CA, Caplan RA, et al. Practice guidelines for management of the difficult airway: an updated report by the American Society of Anesthesiologists Task Force on management of the difficult airway. Anesthesiology. 2013;118(2):251–70.
11. Frerk C, Mitchell VS, McNarry AF, et al. Difficult Airway Society intubation guidelines working g. Difficult Airway Society 2015 Guidelines for management of unanticipated difficult intubation in adults. Br J Anaesth. 2015;115(6):827–48.
12. Lopez AJ, Scheer JK, Leibl KE, et al. Anatomy and biomechanics of the craniovertebral junction. Neurosurg Focus. 2015;38(4):E2.
13. Ferreira MP, Waisberg CB, Conti PCR, et al. Mobility of the upper cervical spine and muscle performance of the deep flexors in women with temporomandibular disorders. J Oral Rehabil. 2019;46(12):1177–84.
14. Bransford RJ, Alton TB, Patel AR, et al. Upper cervical spine trauma. J Am Acad Orthop Surg. 2014;22(11):718–29.
15. Schieren M, Kleinschmidt J, Schmutz A, et al. Comparison of forces acting on maxillary incisors during tracheal intubation with different laryngoscopy techniques: a blinded manikin study. Anaesthesia. 2019;74(12):1563–71.
16. Wijngaarde CA, Stam M, de Kort FAS, et al. Limited maximal mouth opening in patients with spinal muscular atrophy complicates endotracheal intubation: an observational study. Eur J Anaesthesiol. 2018;35(8):629–31.
17. Khan ZH, Mohammadi M, Rasouli MR, et al. The diagnostic value of the upper lip bite test combined with sternomental distance, thyromental distance, and interincisor distance for prediction of easy laryngoscopy and intubation: a prospective study. Anesth Analg. 2009;109(3):822–4.
18. Jiang LX, Qiu SL, Zhang P, et al. The midline approach for endotracheal intubation using GlideScope video laryngoscopy could provide better glottis exposure in adults: a randomized controlled trial. BMC Anesthesiol. 2019;19(1):200.
19. Adhikari S, Zeger W, Schmier C, et al. Pilot study to determine the utility of point-of-care ultrasound in the assessment of difficult laryngoscopy. Acad Emerg Med. 2011;18(7):754–8.
20. Falcetta S, Cavallo S, Gabbanelli V, et al. Evaluation of two neck ultrasound measurements as predictors of difficult direct laryngoscopy: a prospective observational study. Eur J Anaesthesiol. 2018;35:605–12.
21. Alessandri F, Antenucci G, Piervincenzi E, et al. Ultrasound as a new tool in the assessment of airway difficulties: an observational study. Eur J Anaeshesiol. 2019;36(7):509–15.
22. Wu JH, Dong J, Ding YC, et al. Role of anterior neck soft tissue quantifications by ultrasound in predicting difficult laryngoscopy. Med Sci Monit. 2014;20:2343–50.
23. Calder I, Calder J, Crockard HA. Difficult direct laryngoscopy in patients with cervical spine disease. Anaesthesia. 1995;50(9):756–63.
24. Cook TM, MacDougall-Davis SR. Complications and failure of airway management. Br J Anaesth. 2012;Suppl 1:i68–85.

8

Improving mucosal anesthesia for awake endotracheal intubation with a novel method

Chunji Han[1†], Peng Li[2†], Zhenggang Guo[3], Ying Guo[1], Li Sun[1], Gang Chen[1], Xiaojue Qiu[4], Weidong Mi[1], Changsheng Zhang[1*] (ID) and Lorenzo Berra[5]

Abstract

Background: Topical anesthesia is a crucial step in awake endotracheal intubation for providing favorable intubation conditions. The standard of care technique for awake intubation at our institution, which consists of oropharyngeal tetracaine spray, can result in inadequate mucosal anesthesia. Therefore, we sought to compare the effectiveness of dyclonine hydrochloride mucilage to the standard of care tetracaine in achieving anesthesia of the upper airways for awake endotracheal intubation.

Methods: This is a randomized, assessor-blinded, prospective study. From Jun. 1st, 2019 to Aug. 1st, 2019, patients scheduled for either endoscopic submucosal dissection or peroral endoscopic myotomy were enrolled and randomly allocated into two groups after obtaining written informed consent: patients allocated to novel awake intubation care (Group N-AIC) received a single administration of oral dyclonine hydrochloride mucilage, whereas patients allocated to standard awake intubation care (Group S-AIC) received three oropharyngeal tetracaine sprays before transcricoid tetracaine injection before awake intubation. Mean arterial pressure (MAP), which was the primary outcome of this study, as well as heart rate (HR) were recorded throughout the procedure and compared between the two groups. Feeling of numbness, nausea, and intubation conditions after topical anesthesia were also assessed.

(Continued on next page)

---

* Correspondence: powerzcs@126.com
†Chunji Han and Peng Li contributed equally to this work.
[1]Anesthesia and Operation Center, The First Medical Center of Chinese PLA General Hospital, 28th Fuxing Rd., Haidian District, Beijing 100853, P. R. China

(Continued from previous page)

Results: Sixty patients were enrolled and completed the study. Baseline MAP and HR were similar between the two groups. However, hemodynamic responses to intubation and gastrointestinal endoscopy, especially MAP, were significantly less elevated in Group N-AIC. The degree of numbness of the oropharyngeal mucosa after topical anesthesia did not differ between the two groups, neither did the feeling of nausea during laryngoscopy. The amount of pharyngeal secretions before intubation was less in Group N-AIC. Total intubation time was significantly shorter in Group N-AIC when compared to Group S-AIC (18.4 ± 2.86 vs. 22.3 ± 6.47, $P < 0.05$). Extubation bucking was significantly less frequent in Group N-AIC (13.3% vs. 76.7%). Patients received in Group N-AIC had a lower rate of post-extubation sore throat compared to Group S-AIC (6.7% vs. 43.3%). No adverse side effects attributable to either tetracaine or dyclonine were observed in this study.

Conclusions: In awake endotracheal intubation, novel care using oral dyclonine hydrochloride mucilage can provide more favorable mucosal anesthesia and better intubation conditions compared to standard of care practice using oropharyngeal tetracaine spray.

Keywords: Topical anesthesia, Awake endotracheal intubation, Dyclonine, tetracaine

Key points

Question: Does novel awake intubation care using oral dyclonine hydrochloride mucilage improve mucosal anesthesia for awake endotracheal intubation?

Findings: Novel awake intubation care using 10 ml of oral dyclonine hydrochloride mucilage is associated with fewer pharyngeal secretions, shorter intubation time, minor mean arterial pressure fluctuations, lower extubation bucking and sore throat rate perioperatively than the standard awake intubation care using three oropharyngeal tetracaine sprays (1%).

Meaning: In awake endotracheal intubation, novel care using oral dyclonine hydrochloride mucilage can provide more favorable intubation conditions and more stable hemodynamics than the standard of care using oropharyngeal tetracaine spray.

Background

Awake intubation consists of placing an endotracheal tube in the trachea while a patient continues to breathe spontaneously. This technique can be utilized in many different situations to help control a potentially unstable airway. However, awake intubation can be a difficult, time-consuming maneuver for the anesthesiologist and an unpleasant experience for the patient [1]. Satisfactory execution of awake intubation needs both moderate sedation and sufficient topical anesthesia. Thus, topical anesthesia of the upper airways, including the oropharyngeal and subglottic tracheal mucosa, is a crucial element in providing adequate comfort for the patient throughout the procedure [2].

Traditionally, the standard of care at our institution for topical anesthesia of the oropharyngeal mucosa is with oropharyngeal tetracaine ($0.5 \sim 1\%$) or lidocaine (4%) sprays, while topical anesthesia of the subglottic tracheal mucosa is provided by tetracaine (2%) transcricoid or intratracheal injection [3–6]. Tetracaine is a potent local anesthetic commonly used as the standard of care for awake intubation in many health care institutions. Application of tetracaine can effectively blunt the cough reflex and provide topical anesthesia for procedures requiring mucosal anesthesia, such as bronchoscopy and endotracheal intubation. However, the standard of care for awake intubation is potentially complicated by the undesirable properties of tetracaine sprays, including its narrow safety profile, sialogogic effects, and bitter taste [7].

Dyclonine hydrochloride, a relatively new and different chemical compound with local anesthetic properties, was initially adopted for endoscopic procedures to reduce pain, nausea, patient movements, and to lubricate the gastroscope [8]. Multiple reports have shown that dyclonine is more effective than tetracaine and lidocaine in providing adequate mucosal anesthesia [9, 10]. In daily clinical practice, the oral application of dyclonine hydrochloride mucilage does not involve as many complicated steps as tetracaine sprays do in the current standard of care regimen for awake intubation. Additionally, dyclonine can be safely used in patients with documented allergy to bupivacaine and procaine [11]. However, dyclonine is rarely utilized as a topical anesthetic for patients requiring awake endotracheal intubation. Therefore, it is worth further investigating whether dyclonine could be a potential mucosal anesthetic for use in awake intubation.

In this prospective, assessor-blinded, randomized controlled trial, the authors compared the mucosal anesthetic efficacy of oral dyclonine hydrochloride mucilage to the current standard of care, pharyngeal tetracaine sprays, for performing awake endotracheal intubation.

Methods

This was a prospective, randomized controlled trial performed at the endoscopy center, First Medical Center of

Chinese PLA General Hospital. This study was approved by the Ethical Committee of Chinese PLA General Hospital (#2019–088-01), and written informed consent was obtained from all subjects participating in the trial. The trial was registered prior to patient enrollment at the Chinese Clinical Trial Registry (ChiCTR1900023151, Principal investigator: Changsheng Zhang, Date of registration: May 14th, 2019). This manuscript adheres to the applicable CONSORT guidelines.

Study population

From Jun. 1st, 2019 to Aug. 1st, 2019, 60 patients aged 20–65 years were enrolled in this study. Inclusion criteria included patients meeting criteria for American Society of Anesthesiology (ASA) Class I or II who were scheduled for endoscopic submucosal dissection (ESD) or peroral endoscopic myotomy (POEM) under general anesthesia. Patients were excluded if they had one or more of the following criteria: a history of asthma, known allergy to study drugs, anticipated difficult intubation, history of documented chronic organ failure, hypertension, ischemic heart disease, atrioventricular block, incomplete or partial heart blocks, application of vasoactive drugs perioperatively.

Study procedures

Patients were randomly allocated to the standard awake intubation care group (Group S-AIC) or novel awake intubation care group (Group N-AIC) in an assessor-blinded fashion based on a computer-generated code. The anesthesiologists participating in this study had at least 5 years of experience as attending physicians at our institution. In this study, topical anesthesia administration to the upper airway was performed alone by an anesthesia nurse to ensure that the anesthesiologist, the clinical investigator, and the data analyst were all blinded to the study grouping.

After arriving in the operation room, venous access was obtained with an 18-gauge cannula placed in the left forearm. Electrocardiogram, pulse oximetry, and noninvasive blood pressure (cuff placed on the right upper arm) were continuously monitored. The standard of care for awake intubation at our institution is to perform topical anesthesia using tetracaine sprays of both the oropharyngeal mucosa and the tracheal mucosa after Bispectral index (BIS) has reached 80–85. The patient is then intubated with a video laryngoscope, video stylet, and flexible fiberoptic scope. Thus, in Group S-AIC, moderate sedation of the patient was provided with intravenous midazolam (0.03 mg/kg) and fentanyl (2 μg/kg) boluses. After adequate sedation was achieved, patients received oropharyngeal tetracaine (Chengdu Tiantaishan Pharmaceutical Co., Ltd., China) spray three times every 2 min (9 sprays and 2 intervals of 2 min in

total. See supplemental video). First, the soft palate was sprayed. Then, the radix linguae were sprayed while the patient was instructed to pronounce *ha*. Finally, the epiglottis was sprayed with the guidance of delicate video laryngoscopy. The total volume of tetracaine (1%) used for oropharyngeal spray was 0.5 ml. In Group N-AIC, patients received oral administration of dyclonine hydrochloride mucilage (10 mg/10 ml, Yangtze River Pharmaceutical Co. Ltd., China) for topical anesthesia of the oropharyngeal mucosa using the same sedation index. The first 2 ml were slowly swallowed as a test-dose to rule out possible allergic reaction. After 2 min, the remaining 8 ml were administered and kept in the oropharynx for 3 min before swallowing.

The degree of oropharynx mucosal numbness was evaluated 2 min after both study procedures. After obtaining adequate pharyngeal anesthesia, needle cricothyroidotomy was performed in both groups, and 2 ml of tetracaine (2%) were injected to provide topical anesthesia of the subglottic tracheal mucosa. Three minutes later, all patients were instructed to swallow all the secretions and drug residues in the mouth and were intubated with a video laryngoscope while spontaneously breathing. The total time and number of attempted intubations were recorded.

After tube insertion, a cuff pressure between 24 and 28 cm H_2O was maintained using an aneroid manometer to provide an adequate seal of the airway. Patients were instructed to place themselves in the left lateral position with the tube in place. General anesthesia induction was achieved by initiating target-controlled infusion (TCI) of propofol (Marsh model, target effect-site concentration of 2–4 μg/kg·min) and remifentanil (Minto model, target effect-site concentration of 3–4 ng/kg·min). The propofol and remifentanil targets were adjusted to maintain target BIS values between 40 and 60 during the entire procedure. All patients were mechanically ventilated to maintain end-tidal CO_2 ($EtCO_2$) between 32 and 36 mmHg during the surgery.

Patients' hemodynamic parameters, mean arterial pressure (MAP) and heart rate (HR), were recorded at the following time points: 10 min after arriving in the endoscope room (T0), before the needle cricothyroidotomy (T1), immediately after intubation (T2), 5 min after intubation (T3), 3 min after left lateral positioning (T4), and immediately after extubation (T5). The degree of oropharyngeal mucosal numbness was defined as invalid, slight numbness, numbness, or significant numbness. The severity of nausea during laryngoscopy was assessed using a verbal numerical rating scale of 0–10 (0 = no feeling of nausea, 10 = severe nausea). The best view obtained by video laryngoscope in each subject was described as that which visualized the glottis or the epiglottis. The amount of secretions before intubation was classified as few, medium or heavy secretions, and the amount of suctioning required before intubation was recorded. The patient's tolerance of endotracheal tube presence was assessed by the anesthesiologist during the patient self-positioning into left lateral decubitus as good, medium, or bad. Bucking response and presence of sore throat were recorded at extubation. The severity of sore throat at 24 h and 48 h after surgery was assessed using a verbal numerical rating scale of 0–10 (0 = no sore throat, 10 = worst sore throat imaginable).

Statistical analysis

We anticipated enrolling 30 subjects (27 + 10% possible dropouts) in both groups. According to our pilot study, sample size calculations showed that 27 patients were needed in both groups in order to detect a difference in MAP immediately after intubation between the two groups of 7.7 mmHg (standard deviation 9.8 mmHg) with a power of 0.8 and a two-sided p value of less than 0.05.

The statistical analysis was conducted using Statistical Package for Social Sciences (SPSS Inc., Chicago, IL, Version 17.0 for Windows). Results are expressed as means and standard deviations, medians and ranges, or numbers and percentages. The comparison of normally distributed continuous variables between the groups was performed using t-test. For time-dependent changes, repeated measures analysis of variance was applied. Normality of data was checked by measures of skewness and Kolmogorov Smirnov tests of normality. Nominal categorical data between the groups were compared using the chi-squared test or Fisher's exact test as appropriate.

Ordinal categorical variables and non-normal distribution of continuous variables were compared using the Mann-Whitney U-test. A p value of less than 0.05 was considered statistically significant.

Results

A total of 60 patients who underwent ESD or POEM were enrolled in this study. No patients were excluded from further analysis (Fig. 1). No adverse side effects of either method for awake intubation care was observed in this study. The demographic data did not differ between the two groups with regard to age and body mass index (BMI). The distribution as per sex, ASA status, and surgery type was similar in both groups, and the mean duration of surgery was comparable in both groups and statistically non-significant (Table 1).

Perioperative mean arterial pressure is more stable in patients who underwent novel awake intubation care

MAP and HR measurements of the six perioperative time points are summarized in Figs. 2 and 3. The baseline (T0 and T1) MAP and HR were comparable between the two groups. However, there was an overall statistically significant differences among the two groups regarding MAP immediately after intubation (T2) and subsequent time points T3 and T4 ($P < 0.0083$, Bonferroni corrected significance level). The novel awake intubation care using dyclonine was found to significantly reduce MAP at intubation and left lateral positioning when compared to standard awake intubation care. However, although the mean HR in the N-AIC group was slightly lower at T2, T3, T4, and T5 as compared

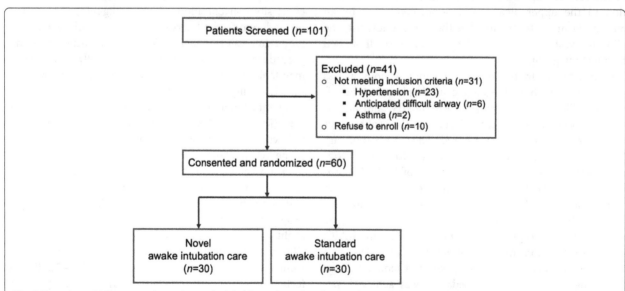

Fig. 1 Flow chart of 101 consecutive patients scheduled for endoscopic submucosal dissection (ESD) or peroral endoscopic myotomy (POEM) under general anesthesia during the study period. After 41 patients were excluded for reasons stated above, 30 patients were randomized to novel awake intubation care, and 30 patients were randomized to standard awake intubation care

Table 1 Patient characteristics

Characteristic	Group N-AIC	Group S-AIC	P value
Age, Median (Quartile)	55 (48–61)	54.5 (44–60)	0.51[a]
BMI, mean (SD)	24.02 (2.94)	23.78 (3.54)	0.77[b]
Sex, Male (%)	16 (53.3)	17 (56.67)	
ASA (I/II)	6/24	6/24	
Surgical procedure			
ESD (%)	25 (83.33)	25 (83.33)	
POEM (%)	5 (16.67)	5 (16.67)	
Duration of surgery (min), Median (Quartile)	63.5 (40–86)	62 (45–106)	
Fluids infused (ml), Median (Quartile)	500 (446–500)	500 (400–500)	

BMI Body mass index, *ASA* American Society of Anesthesiology, *ESD* Endoscopic submucosal dissection, *POEM* Peroral endoscopic myotomy, *N-AIC* Novel awake intubation care, *S-AIC* Standard awake intubation care

[a] Two-sample *t* test. Chi-squared test

[b] chi-squared test

with the S-AIC group, the difference was not statistically significant ($P = 0.124$) (Table 2).

Patients who underwent novel awake intubation care had fewer secretions in the oropharynx and shorter intubation duration

The amount of secretions in patients' oropharynx before intubation was less in the N-AIC group compared to the S-AIC group ($P = 0.01$). Favorable intubation conditions (visualized glottis) were reported in 30 patients in the N-AIC group and 27 patients in the S-AIC group ($P = 0.237$). No patients in the N-AIC group required suctioning before intubation, and only three patients in the S-AIC group required upper airway suctioning before intubation ($P = 0.237$). The total time of intubation was significantly shorter in the N-AIC group (18.4 ± 2.86 vs. 22.3 ± 6.47, $P < 0.05$, Fig. 4). All the patients in the N-

AIC group were successfully intubated at the first attempt, while only one patient in the S-AIC group required two attempts. The endotracheal tube was well tolerated in lateral decubitus in most patients, except for two patients in the S-AIC group whose tolerance was reported as *"medium"*.

Novel awake intubation care did not improve patients' subjective sensation but reduced extubation bucking and sore throat at 24 h after extubation

The degree of numbness of the oropharyngeal mucosa after topical anesthesia and the feeling of nausea during laryngoscopy were not different between the two groups ($P = 0.546$ and $P = 0.317$, respectively). However, only 13.3% of patients who received N-AIC had bucking at extubation, compared to 76.7% with S-AIC ($P < 0.001$). Patients in the N-AIC had a much lower rate of

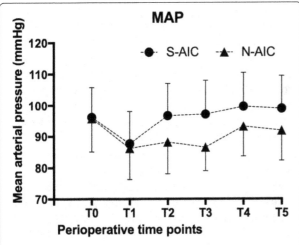

Fig. 2 Results of mean arterial pressure (MAP) of the six perioperative time points. Error bars are +/− standard error of the mean. There were significant differences between groups at the time points of T2, T3, T4, T5 ($P < 0.05$)

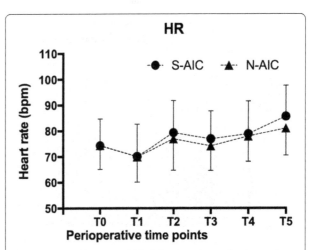

Fig. 3 Results of heart rate (HR) of the six perioperative time points. Error bars are +/− standard error of the mean. No significant differences were found between groups

Table 2 Comparison of MAP and HR between the study groups at various time points

Time points	Parameter	Group N-AIC		Group S-AIC		P Value[a]
		Mean	SD	Mean	SD	
T0	MAP (mmHg)	95.83	10.74	96.17	9.57	0.899
	HR (bpm)	74.43	9.25	74.27	10.46	0.948
T1	MAP (mmHg)	86.23	9.98	87.70	10.39	0.579
	HR (bpm)	69.97	9.78	70.07	12.62	0.630
T2	MAP (mmHg)	88.17	10.11	96.67	10.32	0.002*
	HR (bpm)	76.90	12.16	79.33	12.49	0.448
T3	MAP (mmHg)	86.53	7.49	97.13	10.79	0.000*
	HR (bpm)	74.17	9.51	76.87	10.97	0.312
T4	MAP (mmHg)	93.23	9.50	99.70	10.75	0.000*
	HR (bpm)	77.90	9.77	78.87	12.757	0.743
T5	MAP (mmHg)	91.90	9.54	99.03	10.42	0.008*
	HR (bpm)	81.10	10.58	85.73	11.942	0.120

MAP Mean arterial pressure, *HR* Heart rate, *SD* Standard deviation
* $P < 0.05$ considered statistically significant
[a] Repeated measurement analysis of variance

extubation sore throat than the S-AIC group (6.7% vs. 43.3%, $P < 0.001$). At 24 h after surgery, the severity of sore throat was significantly lower in the N-AIC group than the S-AIC group (0[0–1] vs. 3[0–4], $P = 0.001$). However, this difference in throat soreness between the two groups did not achieve statistical significance at 48 h after surgery (0[0–0] vs. 0[0–0], $P = 0.31$).

Discussion

In this prospective, randomized, controlled trial, we compared the effect of two different types of topical anesthesia for awake intubation care, using oral dyclonine hydrochloride mucilage (10 mg/10 ml) or tetracaine spray (1%, 0.5 ml). We found that awake intubation care

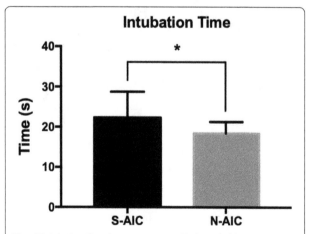

Fig. 4 Intubation time between groups. Each vertical bar represents the mean ± standard error ($n = 30$ in each group). The total time of intubation was significantly shorter in the N-AIC group (*$P < 0.05$)

using oral dyclonine hydrochloride mucilage provides more favorable intubation conditions and better hemodynamics during the perioperative periods than standard awake intubation care.

The reason why awake intubation is a routine method for patients who undergo general anesthesia at our endoscopy center is because it is a relatively safer method for airway management, which could decrease potential aspiration risks and free from muscle relaxants perioperatively. Thus, satisfactory methods for awake intubation are always taken into account. Topical anesthesia of the oropharyngeal mucosa is of crucial importance before awake intubation, and can provide the patient with a relatively comfortable feeling during the laryngoscopic examination. Adequate topical anesthesia of the oropharyngeal mucosa could also result in better cooperation from the patient. Induction of amnesic sedation followed by awake intubation is a common technique at our institution. Given the rapid absorption of tetracaine in the pharynx, tetracaine spray is routinely used to provide topical anesthesia for fiberoptic tracheal intubation and other procedures requiring mucosal anesthesia. In addition, tetracaine frequently provides topical anesthesia for gastrointestinal and ocular procedures. It is reported that the maximum effective concentration of tetracaine is 1%, with a latent period of 1.1 min and a duration of 55.5 min [12].

However, in our experience, topical tetracaine is far from being the ideal mucosal anesthetic due to the following two reasons. First, the bitter taste and feeling of nausea after oropharyngeal application cause patients to regurgitate or swallow the drug, which significantly reduces the amount of drug acting on the mucosa. Additionally, anesthesiologists who are not experienced in administering topical anesthesia of the oropharyngeal mucosa often leave some parts of the mucosa unanesthetized, and thus still sensitive to stimulation. Stevens et al. tested the effects of tetracaine inhalation before intubation. He found that a small dose of nebulized tetracaine may completely coat mucosal surfaces and significantly attenuates the hemodynamic response to tracheal intubation [13]. Therefore, complete coating of mucosal surfaces is a crucial factor of successful topical anesthesia. This may explain why the effects of tetracaine spray used in the S-AIC group is not as good as dyclonine hydrochloride mucilage used in N-AIC in attenuating the hemodynamic response of intubation.

Dyclonine hydrochloride mucilage is a topical anesthetic that reversibly binds to activated sodium channels on the neuronal membrane, thereby decreasing the neuronal membrane's permeability to sodium ions, leading to an increased threshold for excitation [14]. It very effectively produces topical anesthesia and lubricates the mucosal surfaces for gastrointestinal endoscopy and endotracheal intubation [15, 16]. When applied to mucus membranes, the onset of topical anesthesia is 2-10 min and lasts for 20–30 min [12]. Beginning in 1983, the safety and effectiveness of dyclonine were recognized as superior to lidocaine and tetracaine for awake intubation [17]. In 1997, Bacon et al. reported the use of oral and nebulized dyclonine for topical anesthesia of the airway to facilitate awake intubation in a patient with a stated allergy to bupivacaine and procaine [11]. In our study, we found that dyclonine hydrochloride mucilage may have a more prolonged effect than reported because the incidence of extubation bucking and sore throat was significantly lower in the N-AIC group, factors that contributed in providing a better anesthesia and intubation experience to patients.

In this study, we did not find any difference in the subjective sensation of topical anesthesia between the two kinds of awake intubation care, which demonstrate the similar anesthetic effects of both drugs after proper administration. However, patients who received N-AIC had a significantly better hemodynamic profile during and after the procedure, suggesting that dyclonine mucilage significantly attenuates hemodynamic distress induced by laryngoscopy and endotracheal intubation, especially if compared to tetracaine.

Notably, the duration of the intubation process was significantly shorter in patients who received novel awake intubation care. The defoaming effect of dyclonine hydrochloride mucilage, which eliminate the mucous bubbles in the oral-pharyngeal cavity, leads to a better view and fewer visible secretions during the video-laryngoscopic examination [18]. Thus, dyclonine mucilage administration not only provides better mucosal anesthesia (i.e., better attenuates hemodynamic response of laryngoscopy and intubation, is an efficacious anesthetic effect, and leads to excellent patient cooperation), but can also provide better intubation conditions (i.e., fewer visually obstructive secretions and faster intubation).

However, the limitations of our study must be acknowledged. The subjective assessments of the intubation condition by anesthesiologists, and the subjective sensation of the numbness of oropharynx mucosa, nausea and sore throat reported by the patients may lead to subjective bias, which may be the underlying reason for lack of statistically significant differences in some of these parameters. The sedation level prior to intubation was not recorded, which may lead to a difference in subjective sensation during and after topical anesthesia among the patients. Future studies are expected to reveal the effects of dyclonine as a nasal mucosal topical anesthetic during nasotracheal intubation and could provide more comprehensive information for its clinical application.

Conclusion

In awake endotracheal intubation, novel care using oral dyclonine hydrochloride mucilage can provide more favorable mucosal anesthesia and better intubation conditions than standard of care using oropharyngeal tetracaine sprays.

Supplementary Information

Additional file 1: Supplementary Video. The video is a demonstration of the standard awake intubation care in the First medical center of Chinese PLA General Hospital. First, a certain sedation basis was provided by intravenous midazolam (0.03 mg/kg) and fentanyl (2 µg/kg) boluses. Then, the patient received oropharyngeal tetracaine spray (1%) every 2 min for three times. 1. The soft palate was sprayed. 2. The radix linguae was sprayed while the patient was instructed to pronounce *ha*. 3. The epiglottis was sprayed after exposure through delicate video laryngoscopy. Two minutes later, needle cricothyroidotomy was performed, and 2 ml of tetracaine (2%) were injected to provide topical anesthesia of subglottic tracheal mucosa. Three minutes later, the patient was instructed to swallow all the secretions and drug residues in the mouth and intubated with a video laryngoscope. After successful intubation, the patient was instructed to place herself to the left lateral position with the tube in place before the surgery.

Abbreviations

S-AIC: Standard awake intubation care; N-AIC: Novel awake intubation care; ASA: American Society of Anesthesiology; ESD: Endoscopic submucosal dissection; POEM: Peroral endoscopic myotomy; BIS: Bispectral index; TCI: Target-controlled infusion; EtCO$_2$: End-tidal CO$_2$; MAP: Mean arterial pressure; HR: Heart rate

Acknowledgements

The authors thank Dr. Massimiliano Pirrone from the Department of Anesthesia and Critical Care, Fondazione IRCCS Ca' Granda Ospedale Maggiore Policlinico, University of Milan, Italy, and Dr. David AE Imber from the Department of Pediatrics, Boston Children's Hospital, United States, for professional writing services and preparing the manuscript.

Authors' contributions

All authors have read and approved the manuscript. The detailed contribution of each author were listed below. CH: This author helped design the study, collect and analyze data, interpret data, and prepare the manuscript. PL: This author helped design the study, collect and analyze data, interpret data, and prepare the manuscript. ZG: This author helped search the literature, analyze the data, interpret data, and prepare the manuscript. YG: This author helped search the literature, analyze the data, interpret data, and prepare the manuscript. LS: This author helped design the study, collect and analyze data, and interpret data. GC: This author helped collect and analyze data, and interpret data. XQ: This author helped collect and analyze data. WM: This author helped design the study, collect and analyze data, and interpret data. CZ: This author helped search the literature, design the study, collect and analyze data, interpret data, prepare the manuscript, and collect funds. LB: This author helped search the literature, design the study, interpret data, and prepare the manuscript.

Author details

[1] Anesthesia and Operation Center, The First Medical Center of Chinese PLA General Hospital, 28th Fuxing Rd., Haidian District, Beijing 100853, P. R. China. [2] Department of Anesthesia, The Sixth Medical Center of Chinese PLA General Hospital, Beijing, China. [3] Department of Anesthesiology, Peking University Shougang Hospital, Beijing 100144, China. [4] Department of Gastroenterology, The First Medical Center of Chinese PLA General Hospital, Beijing, China. [5] Department of Anesthesia, Critical Care and Pain Medicine, Massachusetts General Hospital, Boston, MA, USA.

References

1. Xue FS, Liu QJ. Tracheal intubation awake or under anesthesia for potential difficult airway: look before you leap. Chin Med J. 2018;131(6):753–6.

2. Simmons ST, Schleich AR. Airway regional anesthesia for awake fiberoptic intubation. Reg Anesth Pain Med. 2002;27(2):180–92.

3. Madineh H, Amani S, Kabiri M, Karimi B. Evaluation of the anesthetic effect of nasal mucosa with tetracaine 0.5% on hemodynamic changes and postoperative pain of septoplasty: a randomized controlled trial. J Adv Pharm Technol Res. 2017;8(4):116–9.

4. Xue FS, Liu HP, He N, Xu YC, Yang QY, Liao X, Xu XZ, Guo XL, Zhang YM. Spray-as-you-go airway topical anesthesia in patients with a difficult airway: a randomized, assessor blinded comparison of 2 and 4% lidocaine. Anesth Analg. 2009;108(2):536–43.

5. Ji M, Tao J, Cheng M, Wang Q. Endotracheal administration of sufentanil and tetracaine during awake fiberoptic Intubation. Am J Ther. 2016;23(1): e92–7.

6. Peng Liang WY, Liu B. Application of tetracaine spray through thyrocricoid puncture before intubation in intensive care unit. Chin J Respir Crit Care Med. 2012;11(1):76–9.

7. Morris MJ, Kwon HP, Zanders TB. Monitoring, sedation, and anesthesia for flexible fiberoptic bronchoscopy. In: Haranath SP, editor. Global perspectives on bronchoscopy. Rijeka: InTech; 2012.

8. Ping RS, White JG, Spear LB. Dyclonine hydrochloride as a topical anesthetic in dentistry; a preliminary report. Oral Surg Oral Med Oral Pathol. 1957;10(6): 623–6.

9. Jichao S, Cuida M, Mingxing C, Yunyun W, Dongdong Z. Oral dyclonine hydrochloride mucilage versus tetracaine spray in electronic flexible laryngoscopy: a prospective, randomized controlled trial. Am J Otolaryngol. 2016;37(2):169–71.

10. Groeben H, Grosswendt T, Silvanus MT, Pavlakovic G, Peters J. Airway anesthesia alone does not explain attenuation of histamine-induced bronchospasm by local anesthetics: a comparison of lidocaine, ropivacaine, and dyclonine. Anesthesiology. 2001;94(3):423–8 discussion 425A-426A.

11. Bacon GS, Lyons TR, Wood SH. Dyclonine hydrochloride for airway anesthesia: awake endotracheal intubation in a patient with suspected local anesthetic allergy. Anesthesiology. 1997;86(5):1206–7.

12. Adriani J, Zepernick R. Clinical effectiveness of drugs used for topical anesthesia. JAMA. 1964;188:711–6.

13. Stevens JB, Vories PA, Walker SC. Nebulized tetracaine attenuates the hemodynamic response to tracheal intubation. Acta Anaesthesiol Scand. 1996;40(6):757–9.

14. Dyclonine Hydrochloride (Code C66875). In. NCIthesaurus. https://ncit.nci. nih.gov/ncitbrowser/ConceptReport.jsp?dictionary=NCI_Thesaurus&ns= ncit&code=C66875.

15. Levine DS, Blount PL, Rudolph RE, Reid BJ. Safety of a systematic endoscopic biopsy protocol in patients with Barrett's esophagus. Am J Gastroenterol. 2000;95(5):1152–7.

16. Groeben H, Schlicht M, Stieglitz S, Pavlakovic G, Peters J. Both local anesthetics and salbutamol pretreatment affect reflex bronchoconstriction in volunteers with asthma undergoing awake fiberoptic intubation. Anesthesiology. 2002;97(6):1445–50.

17. Adriani J, Savoie A, Naraghi M. Scope and limitations of topical anesthetics in anesthesiology prictis. Anesthesiol Rev. 1983;7:10–5.

18. Sun T, Gu X, Lu H, Chen M. Oral preparation of dyclonine hydrochloride. In: United States. Taizhou: Yangtze River Pharmaceutical (Group) Co., Ltd.; 2010.

9

Analysis of pre- and intraoperative clinical factors for successful operating room extubation after living donor liver transplantation

Min Suk Chae[1], Jong-Woan Kim[1], Joon-Yong Jung[2], Ho Joong Choi[3], Hyun Sik Chung[1], Chul Soo Park[1], Jong Ho Choi[1] and Sang Hyun Hong[1*] (ORCID)

Abstract

Background: Early extubation after liver transplantation is safe and accelerates patient recovery. Patients with end-stage liver disease undergo sarcopenic changes, and sarcopenia is associated with postoperative morbidity and mortality. We investigated the impact of core muscle mass on the feasibility of immediate extubation in the operating room (OR) after living donor liver transplantation (LDLT).

Methods: A total of 295 male adult LDLT patients were retrospectively reviewed between January 2011 and December 2017. In total, 40 patients were excluded due to emergency surgery or severe encephalopathy. A total of 255 male LDLT patients were analyzed in this study. According to the OR extubation criteria, the study population was classified into immediate and conventional extubation groups (39.6 vs. 60.4%). Psoas muscle area was estimated using abdominal computed tomography and normalized by height squared (psoas muscle index [PMI]).

Results: There were no significant differences in OR extubation rates among the five attending transplant anesthesiologists. The preoperative PMI correlated with respiratory performance. The preoperative PMI was higher in the immediate extubation group than in the conventional extubation group. Potentially significant perioperative factors in the univariate analysis were entered into a multivariate analysis, in which preoperative PMI and intraoperative factors (i.e., continuous renal replacement therapy, significant post-reperfusion syndrome, and fresh frozen plasma transfusion) were associated with OR extubation. The duration of ventilator support and length of intensive care unit stay were shorter in the immediate extubation group than in the conventional extubation group, and the incidence of pneumonia and early allograft dysfunction were also lower in the immediate extubation group.

Conclusions: Our study could improve the accuracy of predictions concerning immediate post-transplant extubation in the OR by introducing preoperative PMI into predictive models for patients who underwent elective LDLT.

Keywords: Psoas muscles, Liver transplantation, Airway extubation, Operating rooms

* Correspondence: shhong7272@gmail.com
[1]Department of Anesthesiology and Pain medicine, Seoul St. Mary's Hospital, College of Medicine, The Catholic University of Korea, 222, Banpo-daero, Seocho-gu, Seoul 06591, Republic of Korea

Background

Patients with end-stage liver disease (ESLD) frequently suffer from sarcopenia, where sarcopenia before liver transplantation (LT) is one of major risk factors for post-operative morbidity and mortality [1, 2]. A recent study revealed that the degree of perioperative core muscular loss is significantly associated with poor overall patient survival in living donor liver transplantation (LDLT) [3]. Because the model for end-stage liver disease (MELD) score has a limitation in terms of reflecting the physical and nutritional conditions of patients with ESLD, sarcopenia has additional prognostic value for morbidity and mortality in patients with ESLD [4–7]. Particularly, a MELD-Sarcopenia model proved superior to the MELD score in terms of predicting waiting list mortality in LT waiting-list patients with a low MELD score [8].

After LT, prolonged ventilator care with sedation in the intensive care unit (ICU) has been the typical postoperative management strategy [9]. However, studies of other surgeries showed that early tracheal extubation has favorable effects on postoperative patient recovery [10, 11]. Additionally, because the use of ventilator support in the ICU accounts for a large proportion of LT costs, successful early extubation may effectively reduce the financial burden [12]. However, although there is much evidence that early extubation after LT is a safe and feasible practice [12–18], many transplant centers still use routine mechanical ventilation in the ICU after LT. Because LT surgery is one of the most complex procedures currently performed, some transplant clinicians remain concerned regarding the potential risk of cardiopulmonary complications, re-operation, failed extubation, and impaired recovery from surgical stress [13, 19], despite the identification in previous studies of predictors of early extubation in the operating room (OR) after LT [14, 15].

The aim of this study was to investigate the association between pre- and intraoperative factors, including core muscle mass, and immediate extubation in the OR after LDLT. In addition, we compared short-term postoperative complications and outcomes according to OR extubation.

Patients and methods

Ethical considerations

The Institutional Review Board of Seoul St. Mary's Hospital Ethics Committee approved this study for LDLT recipients (KC18RESI0205) on April 13, 2018, and it was performed according to the principles of the Declaration of Helsinki. The requirement for informed consent was waived due to the retrospective study design.

Inclusion and exclusion criteria

The inclusion criteria were 1) male; 2) adult (age ≥ 19 years); and 3) patients who underwent elective LDLT.

The clinical exclusion criteria were 1) emergency LDLT and 2) severe encephalopathy (West-Haven criteria III or IV) [20], because patients with those conditions underwent routine mechanical ventilation after surgery to protect the airway from pulmonary aspiration. Recipients or donors whose electronic medical records contained defective or missing data were also excluded.

Living donor liver transplantation

Surgery and anesthesia were consistently provided by expert transplant surgeons and anesthesiologists with > 5 years' experience in LDLT, respectively. The surgical procedure and anesthetic management were described in detail in our previous studies [3, 21, 22]. Briefly, the piggyback technique was performed using the right liver lobe with reconstruction of the middle hepatic vein. Following the hepatic vessel and bile duct anastomoses, patency of the hepatic vessels was confirmed by Doppler ultrasonography.

Balanced anesthesia was performed under multiple invasive monitoring. The optimal hemodynamic adjustment was made with a mean arterial pressure (MAP) of ≥65 mmHg and a central venous pressure of ≤10 mmHg. According to the Practice Guidelines for Perioperative Blood Management [23], packed red blood cells (PRBCs) were transfused to a hematocrit level of ≥25%, and coagulation factors were replaced as determined by laboratory assessment or thromboelastography (Thromboelastograph Model 5000; Haemoscope Corporation, Niles, IL, USA) [24]. The kidney function of patients who scheduled elective LDLT was regularly monitored by nephrologists, and patients with severely decreased kidney function before surgery (an increase in serum creatinine to ≥4.0 mg.dL^{-1} or to 3-fold baseline level, a urine output of ≤0.3 mL.kg^{-1}.h^{-1} for 24 h, or anuria for 12 h) were intraoperatively given continuous renal replacement therapy (CRRT) (PRISMAFLEX System; Baxter) [25–27]. The expert transplant anesthesiologists classified post-reperfusion syndrome (PRS) as significant, immediately after graft reperfusion, when unstable and persistent vital signs (i.e., hypotension ≥30% in the anhepatic phase or hypotensive duration ≥5 min); fatal arrhythmias (i.e., asystole or ventricular tachycardia); requirement for strong rescue vasopressors (i.e., epinephrine or norepinephrine infusion); continuing or reoccurring fibrinolysis; or a requirement for an anti-fibrinolytic drug were present [28].

An immunosuppression regimen (calcineurin inhibitor, mycophenolate mofetil, and prednisolone) was applied according to the hospital LDLT protocol. Basiliximab was administered before transplant surgery and 4 days after the surgery. The immunosuppressive drugs were progressively discontinued after LDLT.

Criteria for immediate extubation in the operating room

Immediate extubation was defined as tracheal extubation in the OR at the end of surgery, and conventional extubation was defined as tracheal extubation in the ICU. The five attending anesthesiologists (M.S.C.; H.S.C.; C.S.P.; J.H.C.; S.H.H.), who specialized in anesthetic management for LT, decided whether to extubate patients in the OR, immediately after surgery, based on standardized and universally accepted criteria: adequate oxygenation ($SpO_2 \geq 95\%$, with $FiO_2 \leq 0.5$); adequate ventilation (tidal volume ≥ 5 mL.kg^{-1} and spontaneous respiration rate < 25 min^{-1} with normocarbia [$ETCO_2$ 30–40 mmHg]); stable hemodynamic condition or minimal use of a vasopressor (norepinephrine infusion < 0.1 µg.kg^{-1}.min^{-1}); full clinical reversal of muscle relaxation (sustained head lift for 5 s or hand grasp); neurologically intact condition (able to follow simple verbal orders, spontaneous eye opening, and proper cough/ gag reflex); appropriate metabolic status (pH > 7.25, normal electrolytes, and euvolemia); normothermia (≥ 35.5 °C); and no surgical concerns regarding ongoing bleeding or hepatic vascular patency [12, 15, 17]. The surgeon was not consulted unless a surgical issue arose. All patients were transferred to the ICU after surgery.

The patients were classified into two groups: those who were extubated in the OR were classified into the immediate extubation group and those who were not extubated in the OR were classified into the conventional extubation group.

Measurement of psoas muscle area

The abdominal condition of patients who were scheduled for elective LDLT was routinely investigated using computed tomography (CT) within 1 month prior to surgery.

The cross-sectional areas of both PMAs between lumbar vertebrae 3 and 4 were manually evaluated on abdominal CT images (PACS Viewer; INFINITT Healthcare Co., Ltd., Phillipsburg, NJ, USA) using a two-dimensional module, with intramuscular fatty infiltration removed from the PMA images using automated software (AQI; TeraRecon, Foster City, CA, USA). The average of the two PMAs was estimated and normalized to the patient's height squared (PMI = PMA.height^{-2}). The abdominal CT images were analyzed by a radiologist (J.Y.J.) with 10 years' experiences who was blinded to the clinical data.

In this study, the PMI was considered a core muscle index in patients who underwent elective LDLT [3, 29, 30].

Correlations between respiratory performance and preoperative PMI

We studied the correlations between respiratory performance using preoperative spirometry parameters (i.e., forced vital capacity [FVC], the first second of forced expiration [FEV$_1$], and forced expiratory flow [FEF]) and preoperative PMI.

Perioperative recipient and donor-graft factors

Preoperative recipient findings included age, body mass index (BMI), etiology of ESLD, comorbidities (diabetes mellitus [DM], systemic hypertension [HBP], diseases of the heart and kidney, lung disease determined by symptoms of dyspnea with atelectasis, consolidation, or pleural effusion using chest X-ray or CT images, smoking status, history of abdominal surgery, MELD score, complications of ESLD (mild encephalopathy [West-Haven grade I or II] [20], varix, and ascites [>1 L]), transthoracic echocardiography (ejection fraction and diastolic dysfunction), and laboratory findings (hematocrit, creatinine, total bilirubin, sodium, potassium, albumin, ammonia, glucose, international normalized ratio [INR], and platelet count). Intraoperative recipient findings included surgical duration, CRRT, administration of a strong vasopressor (i.e., norepinephrine infusion ≥ 0.1 µg.kg^{-1}.min^{-1}), significant PRS [28], hourly fluid infusion, hourly urine output, total amount of blood product transfused (PRBCs, fresh frozen plasma [FFP], platelet concentrate [PC], single donor platelets [SDPs], and cryoprecipitate), mean laboratory values (lactate, glucose, and brain natriuretic peptide [BNP]), and mean arterial blood gas analysis values (pH, hemoglobin, PaO$_2$, SaO$_2$, and PaCO$_2$). Donor-graft findings included age, sex, BMI, graft-recipient weight ratio (GRWR), steatosis, and total graft ischemic time.

Clinical postoperative outcomes

Clinical postoperative outcomes included duration of ventilator support, and the incidence of re-intubation, pneumonia and early allograft dysfunction (EAD) in the ICU. EAD was defined as the presence of one or more of the following: total bilirubin ≥ 10 mg.dL^{-1} or INR ≥ 1.6 on postoperative day 7; and AST or ALT ≥ 2000 IU.mL^{-1} during the first week [31]. The total lengths of the ICU and hospital stays were compared between the immediate and conventional extubation groups.

Statistical analysis

The perioperative recipient and donor-graft factors were compared between the immediate extubation and conventional groups using the Mann–Whitney U test and the χ^2 test. The normality of the distribution of continuous data was analyzed using the Shapiro–Wilk test. The OR extubation rates were compared among five expert anesthesiologists using the χ^2 test. The correlations of spirometry parameters and preoperative PMI were evaluated using Spearman's method. Perioperative factors affecting immediate extubation in the OR were analyzed using univariate and multivariate logistic regression. Significant factors ($p < 0.1$) in the univariate analysis were entered into the forward and backward multivariate analyses. The most relevant clinical factors were determined when multiple perioperative factors were correlated. The

PMIs were compared between the two groups using the Mann–Whitney U test. In addition, the accuracy of the predictive model was analyzed using the area under the receiver operating characteristic curve (AUC). An optimal cut-off value of preoperative PMI according to OR extubation was determined using the AUC method. Values are expressed as means ± standard deviation (SD), medians and interquartile ranges (IQR), or as numbers and proportions. All tests were two-sided, and a p-value < 0.05 was considered significant. Statistical analyses were conducted using SPSS for Windows (ver. 24.0; SPSS Inc., Chicago, IL, USA) and MedCalc for Windows software (ver. 11.0; MedCalc Software, Ostend, Belgium). The TRIPOD reporting guidelines were followed during the development of the prediction model, and in the validation study [32].

Results
Baseline characteristics of the study population
The initial study population consisted of 295 male adult patients (age ≥ 19 years) who underwent LDLT at our hospital between January 2011 and December 2017. After removing 40 patients based on the exclusion criteria, 255 male patients who underwent elective LDLT remained. The average age of the patients was 52 ± 8 years and the BMI was 24.8 ± 3.6 kg.m^{-2}. The most common etiology was hepatitis B (66.3%), followed by alcohol (20.8%), hepatitis C (5.5%), toxin or drug (3.9%), hepatitis A (1.2%), autoimmune (0.4%), and cryptogenic hepatitis (2.0%). The median (IQR) MELD score was 13 (8–21) points and hepatic decompensation signs were as follows: ascites > 1 L (41.2%), encephalopathy (West-Haven grade I or II) (27.1%), varix (23.5%), and hepatorenal syndrome (12.2%). The average preoperative PMI was 359.4 ± 95.8 mm^2.m^{-2}. In total, 101 of 255 patients (39.6%) were extubated in the OR immediately after surgery. There were no significant differences in OR extubation rate among the attending transplant anesthesiologists (Additional file 1).

Based on OR extubation, the optimal cut-off value of preoperative PMI was 352.2 mm^2.m^{-2} (AUC: 0.862; 95% confidence interval: 0.814–0.902; $p < 0.001$). Thus, 125 patients (49.0%) had non-sarcopenic features and 130 (51.0%) showed sarcopenic features (Additional file 2).

Correlation between respiratory performance and preoperative PMI
Additional file 3 shows that preoperative PMI was weakly correlated with respiratory performance parameters, such as FVC (L), FVC (%), FEV$_1$ (L), FEV$_1$/FVC (%), FEF$_{25-75\%}$ (L.sec^{-1}), and FEF$_{75-85\%}$ (L.sec^{-1}). Only FEV$_1$ (%) was moderately correlated with the PMI.

Comparison of clinical characteristics between the immediate and conventional extubation groups
The preoperative recipient findings differed between the two groups, including with respect to BMI; incidence of lung disease; MELD score; the incidence rates of encephalopathy (West-Haven grade I or II) and ascites (>1 L); and the levels of hematocrit, sodium, albumin, platelets, total bilirubin and INR (Table 1).

The intraoperative recipient findings of the two groups also differed, in terms of surgical duration; frequency of administration of a strong vasopressor; incidence of significant PRS; hourly fluid infusion and urine output; requirement for blood products transfusion (i.e., PRBCs, FFP, PC, SDPs and cryoprecipitates); and the levels of BNP and hemoglobin (Table 2). Although SaO$_2$ was lower in the immediate extubation group than in the conventional extubation group, the range of SaO$_2$ was within normal limits (≥ 94%) in both groups [33]. Despite differences in the donor-graft findings, such as total graft ischemic time and GRWR, all transplant recipients received a graft of sufficient size (GRWR ≥0.8) [34].

Preoperative PMI (median and IQR) was significantly higher in the immediate extubation group than in the conventional extubation group: 309.0 (259.6–352.7) mm^2.m^{-2} vs. 414.9 (367.7–480.0) mm^2.m^{-2} in the immediate extubation group (Fig. 1).

Predictive factors for immediate extubation in the operating room
Table 3 suggests an association between perioperative recipient and donor-graft findings and immediate extubation in the OR among male patients who underwent elective LDLT. After an analysis of the potentially significant preoperative and intraoperative recipient and donor-graft findings in a multivariate logistic regression, the model revealed that preoperative PMI and intraoperative factors (i.e., use of CRRT, development of significant PRS, and FFP transfusion requirement) were independently associated with immediate extubation in the OR (AUC: 0.914; 95% confidence interval: 0.88–0.949; $p < 0.001$ in the predictive model).

Comparison of postoperative outcomes between the immediate and conventional extubation groups
The length of ICU stay and duration of ventilator support were shorter in the immediate extubation group than in the conventional extubation group, and the incidence of pneumonia and EAD were also lower in the immediate extubation group (Table 4). Three patients in the immediate extubation group underwent re-intubation in the ICU. The causes of re-intubation in the immediate extubation group were development of graft dysfunction ($n = 2$ patients) and respiratory distress due to pneumonia

Table 1 Comparison of preoperative recipient findings between the conventional and immediate extubation groups

Group	Conventional extubation	Immediate extubation	p
n	154	101	
Preoperative recipient findings			
Age (year)	53 (47–59)	54 (49–57)	0.983
Body mass index (kg.m^{-2})	23.9 (21.9–26.6)	24.9 (23.2–26.7)	0.016
Etiology of end-stage liver disease			
Alcohol	33 (21.4%)	20 (19.8%)	
Hepatitis A	2 (1.3%)	1 (1.0%)	
Hepatitis B	98 (63.6%)	71 (70.3%)	
Hepatitis C	11 (7.1%)	3 (3.0%)	
Autoimmune	0 (0.0%)	1 (1.0%)	
Toxin & drug	7 (4.5%)	3 (3.0%)	
Cryptogenic	3 (1.9%)	2 (2.0%)	
Comorbidity			
Diabetes mellitus	42 (27.3%)	19 (18.8%)	0.121
Systemic hypertension	32 (20.8%)	17 (16.8%)	0.434
Heart disease	7 (4.5%)	1 (1.0%)	0.152
Lung disease	25 (16.2%)	7 (6.9%)	0.028
Kidney disease	19 (12.3%)	6 (5.9%)	0.093
Current smoker	34 (22.1%)	20 (19.8%)	0.664
History of abdominal surgery	33 (21.4%)	13 (12.9%)	0.082
Model for end-stage liver disease (pts)	16 (10–26)	9 (7–14)	< 0.001
Complications of end-stage liver disease			
Mild encephalopathy	50 (32.5%)	19 (18.8%)	0.016
Varix	40 (26.0%)	20 (19.8%)	0.256
Ascites (> 1 L)	73 (47.4%)	32 (31.7%)	0.013
Transthoracic echocardiography			
Ejection fraction (%)	64.5 (62.0–67.9)	64.8 (62.0–67.0)	0.656
Diastolic dysfunction	52 (33.8%)	28 (27.7%)	0.379
Laboratory findings			
Hematocrit (%)	28.3 (24.4–33.9)	32.7 (26.6–38.2)	< 0.001
Creatinine (mg.dL^{-1})	0.8 (0.7–1.2)	0.8 (0.7–0.9)	0.199
Total bilirubin (mg.dL^{-1})	3.4 (1.0–14.5)	1.6 (0.7–4.2)	0.002
Sodium (mEq.L^{-1})	138.0 (133.8–141.0)	141.0 (138.0–142.0)	< 0.001
Potassium (mEq.L^{-1})	4.0 (3.7–4.3)	4.0 (3.8–4.3)	0.95
Albumin (g.dL^{-1})	2.9 (2.7–3.5)	3.2 (2.7–3.7)	0.015
Ammonia (μg.dL^{-1})	98.0 (65.0–159.0)	121.0 (73.3–178.0)	0.147
Glucose (mg.dL^{-1})	113.5 (93.8–139.0)	101.0 (91.0–129.0)	0.053
International normalized ratio	1.6 (1.3–2.1)	1.4 (1.2–1.7)	0.004
Platelet count (× 10^9.L^{-1})	58.5 (42.0–87.3)	73.0 (48.0–124.0)	0.003

Values are expressed as medians (with interquartile range) or numbers (with % proportion)

($n = 1$ patient). A total of 10 patients in the conventional extubation group had re-intubation due to graft dysfunction ($n = 3$ patients), respiratory distress related to pneumonia ($n = 5$ patients), and miscellaneous reasons ($n = 2$ patients).

Discussion

The main finding of this study was that preoperative PMI was an independent predictor of immediate extubation in the OR after elective LDLT, together with CRRT, significant

Table 2 Comparison of intraoperative recipient and graft-donor findings between the conventional and immediate extubation groups

Group	Conventional extubation	Immediate extubation	p
n	154	101	
Intraoperative recipient finding			
Surgical duration (min)	515 (464–586)	490 (450–556)	0.031
Continuous renal replacement therapy	13 (8.4%)	3 (3.0%)	0.078
[a]Strong vasopressor administration	38 (24.7%)	11 (10.9%)	0.006
Significant postreperfusion syndrome	41 (26.6%)	5 (5.0%)	< 0.001
Hourly fluid infusion ($mL.kg^{-1}.h^{-1}$)	10.9 (7.9–13.7)	9.3 (6.7–11.8)	0.001
Hourly urine output ($mL.kg^{-1}.h^{-1}$)	1.2 (0.6–2.0)	1.6 (0.9–2.3)	0.002
Total amount of blood product transfusion during surgery (unit)			
Packed red blood cell	9 (5–15)	4 (2–8)	< 0.001
Fresh frozen plasma	10 (5–13)	5 (3–7)	< 0.001
Platelet concentrate	0 (0–6)	0 (0–0)	< 0.001
Single donor platelet	0 (0–1)	0 (0–0)	0.003
Cryoprecipitate	0 (0–0)	0 (0–0)	0.001
Average of laboratory factors during entire surgery			
Lactate ($mmol.L^{-1}$)	4.4 (3.2–5.6)	4.2 (3.6–5.4)	0.85
Glucose ($mg.dL^{-1}$)	183 (156–206)	187 (163–206)	0.624
Brain natriuretic peptide ($pg.mL^{-1}$)	83 (40–172)	59 (31–103)	0.027
Average of ABGA factors during entire surgery			
pH	7.32 (7.28–7.37)	7.34 (7.31–7.38)	0.055
Hemoglobin ($g.dL^{-1}$)	9.5 (8.7–10.2)	10.5 (9.7–11.5)	< 0.001
PaO_2 (mmHg)	189.4 (160.8–222.5)	187.0 (163.4–216.4)	0.971
SaO_2 (%)	99.4 (99.0–99.6)	99.2 (98.8–99.5)	0.01
$PaCO_2$ (mmHg)	36.0 (34.9–37.2)	36.0 (34.1–37.4)	0.76
Donor-graft findings			
Age (year)	33 (25–46)	32 (24–43)	0.923
Sex (Male)	89 (57.8%)	66 (65.3%)	0.227
Body mass index ($kg.m^{-2}$)	23.5 (22.1–25.1)	23.4 (21.0–25.0)	0.285
Graft-recipient weight ratio	1.2 (1.0–1.5)	1.1 (1.0–1.3)	0.019
Steatosis (%)	5.0 (0.0–5.0)	3.0 (0.0–5.0)	0.463
Steatosis type			0.264
None	51 (33.1%)	30 (29.7%)	
Microvesicular	13 (8.4%)	3 (3.0%)	
Macrovesicular	81 (52.6%)	62 (61.4%)	
Mixed	9 (5.8%)	6 (5.9%)	
Total graft ischemic time (min)	107 (74–147)	90 (66–113)	0.001

Values are expressed as medians (with interquartile range) or numbers (with % proportion)
Abbreviation: ABGA arterial blood gas analysis
[a]Strong vasopressor administration is defined as norepinephrine infusion ≥ 0.1 $\mu g.kg^{-1}.min^{-1}$

PRS and a large FFP transfusion. The PMI value was higher in the immediate extubation group than in the conventional extubation group. Based on the standardized and universally accepted criteria for endotracheal extubation, the predictive accuracy of our model for OR extubation was high.

In our study, preoperative PMI positively correlated with respiratory performance quantified by spirometry parameters (i.e., FVC, FEV_1, $FEF_{25-75\%}$, and $FEF_{75-85\%}$). This finding was supported by recent studies showing that preoperative muscular quantity and quality parameters (i.e., PMI and intramuscular adipose content

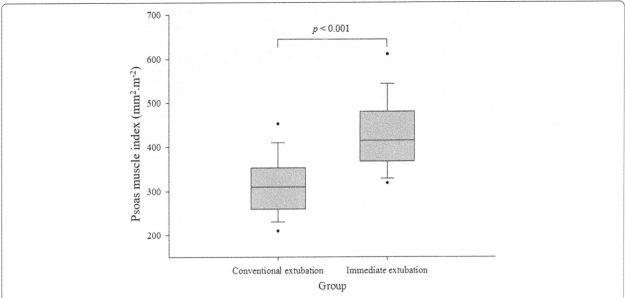

Fig. 1 Comparison of preoperative psoas muscle index between the conventional extubation and immediate extubation groups in male patients who underwent elective living donor liver transplantation (LDLT). The box plots show the median (line in the middle of the box), interquartile range (box), 5th and 9^{5}th percentiles (whiskers), and outliers (dots)

[IMAC]) are associated with preoperative respiratory function parameters (i.e., vital capacity [VC] and FEV$_1$) in patients who underwent hepatectomy for liver cancer [35]. In male patients who underwent LDLT, preoperative levels of PMI and IMAC, as well as grip strength (GS) were associated with preoperative VC and FEV$_1$. In female patients, preoperative levels of IMAC and GS were associated with preoperative VC and FEV$_1$ [29]. These studies suggested that patients with low muscular quantity and quality had poorer respiratory function than those with normal muscular quantity and quality [29, 35].

Our LDLT study suggested that increased preoperative core muscle mass (i.e., PMI) significantly increased the feasibility of OR extubation after elective surgery. Based on the standardized and universally accepted criteria for endotracheal extubation, sufficient core muscle mass before surgery seems to guarantee the recovery and maintenance of patient respiratory capacity immediately after surgery and improves the success rate of OR extubation without fatal complications. LDLT patients who are eligible for successful OR extubation may have sufficient physiological reserves to maintain homeostasis in the presence of external stress (i.e., surgery) whereas a low preoperative core muscle mass may be a marker of an increased risk of failed OR extubation [5, 36, 37]. In a surgical ICU study, muscle weakness in the extremities, measured as the ability to move against gravity and/or resistance, was associated with a higher re-intubation rate following extubation, with the additional consequences of prolonged mechanical support and weaning failure [38]. The MELD score is of limited value in reflecting the

nutritional and functional condition of patients with ESLD, and preoperative core muscle mass measurements may help to identify patients suitable for immediate OR extubation, preventing unnecessary ventilator support after transplantation surgery [1, 5–7, 13, 39].

Many studies have focused on preoperative hepatic decompensation or intraoperative hemodynamic instability for predicting early extubation after LT [14, 15, 18], and our results also show that intraoperative factors related to hemodynamic disturbance (i.e., the use of CRRT, the occurrence of significant PRS, and a requirement for a large FFP transfusion) were negatively associated with immediate extubation in the OR. A prospective study by Biancofiore et al. [14] suggested that patients suitable for immediate postoperative extubation were predominantly male, and that a MELD score of 11 points was the optimal cut-off for immediate postoperative extubation. The immediate postoperative extubation group suffered less severe intraoperative hemorrhage and showed a lower requirement for blood product transfusion than the non-extubation group. Immediately after liver graft reperfusion, patients in the immediate extubation group experienced low blood pressure that required a vasopressor less frequently than those in the non-extubation group. Skurzak et al. [18] devised a prognostic score for early extubation in the OR after LT that consisted of two major factors (intraoperative PRBC transfusion ≥7 units and lactate level ≥ 3.4 mmol.L^{-1} at the end of surgery) and three minor factors (home vs. hospitalized patients before LT; surgical duration ≥5 h; and dopamine ≥5 µg.kg^{-1}.min^{-1} or norepinephrine ≥0.05 µg.kg^{-1}.min^{-1}

Table 3 Association of perioperative recipient and donor-graft factors with early extubation in operating room in male patients undergoing elective living donor liver transplantation

	Univariate logistic regression				Multivariate logistic regression			
	β	OR	95% CI	p	β	OR	95% CI	p
Preoperative recipient findings								
Body mass index (kg.m^{-2})	0.067	1.069	0.997–1.146	0.061				
Psoas muscle index (mm^2.m^{-2})	0.02	1.02	1.015–1.025	< 0.001	0.025	1.025	1.017–1.033	< 0.001
Lung disease	−0.956	0.384	0.16–0.926	0.033				
History of abdominal surgery	−0.613	0.542	0.27–1.089	0.085				
Model for end-stage liver disease (pts)	−0.089	0.915	0.884–0.948	< 0.001				
Complications of end-stage liver disease								
Mild Encephalopathy	−0.73	0.482	0.264–0.88	0.018				
Ascites (> 1 L)	−0.664	0.515	0.304–0.87	0.013				
Laboratory findings								
Hematocrit (%)	0.07	1.072	1.032–1.114	< 0.001				
Total bilirubin (mg.dL^{-1})	−0.047	0.954	0.927–0.983	0.002				
Sodium (mEq.L^{-1})	0.088	1.091	1.035–1.151	0.001				
Ammonia (μg.dL^{-1})	0.003	1.003	0.999–1.006	0.097				
International normalized ratio	−0.762	0.467	0.289–0.754	0.002				
Platelet count (× 10^9.L^{-1})	0.006	1.006	1.002–1.011	0.007				
Intraoperative recipient finding								
Surgical duration (min)	−0.003	0.997	0.995–1.000	0.08				
Continuous renal replacement therapy	−1.103	0.332	0.092–1.196	0.092	−3.781	0.023	0.002–0.301	0.004
Strong vasopressor administration	−0.986	0.373	0.181–0.771	0.008				
Significant postreperfusion syndrome	−1.941	0.144	0.055–0.378	< 0.001	−1.781	0.168	0.043–0.654	0.01
Hourly fluid infusion (mL.kg^{-1}.h^{-1})	−0.105	0.901	0.847–0.958	0.001				
Hourly urine output (mL.kg^{-1}.h^{-1})	0.306	1.358	1.079–1.708	0.009				
Total amount of blood product transfusion during surgery (unit)								
Packed red blood cell	−0.123	0.885	0.841–0.931	< 0.001				
Fresh frozen plasma	−0.224	0.799	0.739–0.864	< 0.001	−0.163	0.85	0.774–0.933	0.001
Platelet concentrate	−0.123	0.884	0.824–0.948	0.001				
Single donor platelet	−0.172	0.842	0.689–1.029	0.093				
Cryoprecipitate	−0.563	0.569	0.372–0.872	0.01				
Average of ABGA factors during entire surgery								
Hemoglobin (g.dL^{-1})	0.609	1.838	1.479–2.285	< 0.001				
SaO$_2$ (%)	−0.313	0.731	0.508–1.051	0.091				
Donor-graft findings								
Graft-recipient weight ratio	−1.028	0.358	0.167–0.766	0.008				
Total graft ischemic time (min)	−0.011	0.989	0.983–0.995	< 0.001				

Abbreviations: CI confidence interval, *ABGA* arterial blood gas analysis

at the end of surgery). Another LT study suggested that the possibility of early extubation (within 3 h after surgery) was affected by intraoperative blood transfusion volume, vital organ function (i.e., kidney, heart, and lung), and hepatic encephalopathy, but early extubation did not correlate with patient age or severity of liver disease (i.e., United Network for Organ Sharing [UNOS] status and Child–Pugh classification) [15].

This study had some limitations. First, we were unable to investigate muscular strength because of the retrospective study design. GS was considered a useful proxy for muscular strength and was related to certain pulmonary

Table 4 Comparison of postoperative outcomes between the conventional and immediate extubation groups

Group	Conventional extubation	Immediate extubation	p
n	154	101	
Hospital stay (day)	23 (21–31)	23 (21–31)	0.53
Intensive care unit stay (day)	7 (6–8)	7 (5–7)	0.008
Ventilator support duration (min)	524 (225–764)	0 (0–0)	< 0.001
Re-intubation	10 (6.5%)	3 (3.0%)	0.211
Pneumonia	26 (16.9%)	4 (4.0%)	0.002
Early allograft dysfunction	26 (16.9%)	2 (2.0%)	< 0.001

Values are expressed as medians (with interquartile range) or numbers (with % proportion)

parameters in previous studies [29, 35]. Second, we only analyzed factors associated with OR extubation in male LDLT patients because there are differences in muscle size and strength between the sexes [6, 40]; therefore, further studies that include female LDLT patients are needed. The effect of sex-specific muscular features on recovery of respiratory ability in patients with ESLD immediately after surgery would be an interesting topic for study [40]. Third, we were unable to investigate the relationship between age-related core muscle loss and the possibility of immediate extubation in the OR, because our cirrhotic patients were in their late 40s and 50s. Because aging influences muscle strength and mass, an age-specific study of cirrhotic patients is required. Fourth, although there were no significant differences in the OR extubation rates among attending transplant anesthesiologists, there may be differences in OR extubation methods, because there is no consensus on the specific OR extubation criteria that should be applied for LDLT patients. Further studies that use a standardized protocol for OR extubation are needed. Finally, there were some differences in preoperative and/ or intraoperative conditions between the two groups, so the possibility of selection bias was not totally excluded. Therefore, further prospective matched studies are required to determine whether OR extubation has positive effects on postoperative outcomes, and whether the PMI can stand as an independent major parameter to determine immediate extubation in the OR after LT surgery.

Conclusions

Immediate tracheal extubation in the OR is safe and beneficial as part of a rapid recovery pathway after elective LDLT. However, as respiratory failure can occur postoperatively, it is important to accurately identify LDLT patients who are eligible for immediate extubation in the OR. Our study could improve the accuracy of prediction of immediate post-transplant extubation in the OR by

introducing preoperative PMI into predictive models of patients who underwent elective LDLT. Eventually, a predictive model of early extubation in the OR, including preoperative levels of PMI and intraoperative hemodynamic factors (i.e., the use of CRRT, the development of significant PRS and a requirement for a large FFP transfusion), may help transplant clinicians to determine which patients are suitable for successful immediate OR extubation, and prevent inadequate ventilator care and unnecessary ICU administration after elective LDLT.

Additional files

Additional file 1: Comparison of OR extubation rates among five anesthesiologists.

Additional file 2: Comparison of PMI between patients with and without sarcopenic features.

Additional file 3: Correlation of preoperative psoas muscle index with spirometry parameters.

Abbreviations
BMI: Body mass index; BNP: Brain natriuretic peptide; CT: Computed tomography; DM: Diabetes mellitus; ESLD: End-stage liver disease; FFP: Fresh frozen plasma; GWRW: Graft-recipient weight ratio; HBP: Systemic hypertension; ICU: Intensive care unit; INR: International normalized ratio; LDLT: Living donor liver transplantation; LT: Liver transplantation; MELD: Model for end-stage liver disease; OR: Operating room; PC: Platelet count; PMA: Psoas muscle area; PMI: Psoas muscle index; PRBCs: Packed red blood cells; PRS: Post-reperfusion syndrome; SDP: Single donor platelet

Acknowledgments
The authors wish to acknowledge the financial support of the Catholic Medical Center Research Foundation made in the program year of 2013.

Authors' contributions
MSC and SHH designed the study, wrote the manuscript, and analyzed and interpreted the data. JWK collected the data. JYJ, HJC, HSC, CSP and JHC collected the data and provided critical comments. All authors revised the manuscript critically for important intellectual content. All authors read and approved the final manuscript.

Author details
[1]Department of Anesthesiology and Pain medicine, Seoul St. Mary's Hospital, College of Medicine, The Catholic University of Korea, 222, Banpo-daero, Seocho-gu, Seoul 06591, Republic of Korea. [2]Department of Radiology, Seoul St. Mary's Hospital, College of Medicine, The Catholic University of Korea, Seoul, Republic of Korea. [3]Department of Surgery, Seoul St. Mary's Hospital, College of Medicine, The Catholic University of Korea, Seoul, Republic of Korea.

References
1. Kaido T, Ogawa K, Fujimoto Y, Ogura Y, Hata K, Ito T, et al. Impact of sarcopenia on survival in patients undergoing living donor liver transplantation. Am J Transplant. 2013;13:1549–56.
2. Englesbe MJ, Patel SP, He K, Lynch RJ, Schaubel DE, Harbaugh C, et al. Sarcopenia and mortality after liver transplantation. J Am Coll Surg. 2010;211:271–8.
3. Chae MS, Moon KU, Jung JY, Choi HJ, Chung HS, Park CS, et al. Perioperative loss of psoas muscle is associated with patient survival in living donor liver transplantation. Liver Transpl. 2018;24:623–33.
4. Durand F, Buyse S, Francoz C, Laouenan C, Bruno O, Belghiti J, et al. Prognostic value of muscle atrophy in cirrhosis using psoas muscle thickness on computed tomography. J Hepatol. 2014;60:1151–7.

5. Kahn J, Wagner D, Homfeld N, Muller H, Kniepeiss D, Schemmer P. Both sarcopenia and frailty determine suitability of patients for liver transplantation-a systematic review and meta-analysis of the literature. Clin Transpl. 2018;32:e13226.

6. Biancofiore G, Tomescu DR, Mandell MS. Rapid recovery of liver transplantation recipients by implementation of fast-track care steps: what is holding us Back? Semin Cardiothorac Vasc Anesth. 2018;22:191–6.

7. Lai JC. Defining the threshold for too sick for transplant. Curr Opin Organ Transplant. 2016;21:127–32.

8. van Vugt JLA, Alferink LJM, Buettner S, Gaspersz MP, Bot D, Darwish Murad S, et al. A model including sarcopenia surpasses the MELD score in predicting waiting list mortality in cirrhotic liver transplant candidates: a competing risk analysis in a national corhot. J Hepatol. 2017;68:707–14.

9. Stock PG, Payne WD. Liver transplantation. Crit Care Clin. 1990;6:911–26.

10. Cohen J, Loewinger J, Hutin K, Sulkes J, Zelikovski A, Singer P. The safety of immediate extubation after abdominal aortic surgery: a prospective, randomized trial. Anesth Analg. 2001;93:1546–9 table of contents.

11. Lanuti M, de Delva PE, Maher A, Wright CD, Gaissert HA, Wain JC, et al. Feasibility and outcomes of an early extubation policy after esophagectomy. Ann Thorac Surg. 2006;82:2037–41.

12. Mandell MS, Lezotte D, Kam I, Zamudio S. Reduced use of intensive care after liver transplantation: influence of early extubation. Liver Transpl. 2002;8:676–81.

13. Aniskevich S, Pai SL. Fast track anesthesia for liver transplantation: review of the current practice. World J Hepatol. 2015;7:2303–8.

14. Biancofiore G, Bindi ML, Romanelli AM, Boldrini A, Bisa M, Esposito M, et al. Fast track in liver transplantation: 5 years' experience. Eur J Anaesthesiol. 2005;22:584–90.

15. Biancofiore G, Romanelli AM, Bindi ML, Consani G, Boldrini A, Battistini M, et al. Very early tracheal extubation without predetermined criteria in a liver transplant recipient population. Liver Transpl. 2001;7:777–82.

16. Glanemann M, Langrehr J, Kaisers U, Schenk R, Muller A, Stange B, et al. Postoperative tracheal extubation after orthotopic liver transplantation. Acta Anaesthesiol Scand. 2001;45:333–9.

17. Mandell MS, Stoner TJ, Barnett R, Shaked A, Bellamy M, Biancofiore G, et al. A multicenter evaluation of safety of early extubation in liver transplant recipients. Liver Transpl. 2007;13:1557–63.

18. Skurzak S, Stratta C, Schellino MM, Fop F, Andruetto P, Gallo M, et al. Extubation score in the operating room after liver transplantation. Acta Anaesthesiol Scand. 2010;54:970–8.

19. Feltracco P, Carollo C, Barbieri S, Pettenuzzo T, Ori C. Early respiratory complications after liver transplantation. World J Gastroenterol. 2013; 19:9271–81.

20. Cash WJ, McConville P, McDermott E, McCormick PA, Callender ME, McDougall NI. Current concepts in the assessment and treatment of hepatic encephalopathy. Qjm. 2010;103:9–16.

21. Chae MS, Jeon YK, Kim DG, Na GH, Yi YS, Park CS. Cardiac tamponade due to Suprahepatic surgical exploration in liver Retransplantation: a case report. Transplant Proc. 2016;48:3181–5.

22. Chae MS, Koo JM, Park CS. Predictive role of intraoperative serum brain natriuretic peptide for early allograft dysfunction in living donor liver transplantation. Ann Transplant. 2016;21:538–49.

23. Practice guidelines for perioperative blood management: an updated report by the American Society of Anesthesiologists Task Force on perioperative blood management*. Anesthesiology. 2015;122:241–75. https://doi.org/10.1097/ALN.0000000000000463.

24. Hong SH, Park CS, Jung HS, Choi H, Lee SR, Lee J, et al. A comparison of intra-operative blood loss and acid-base balance between vasopressor and inotrope strategy during living donor liver transplantation: a randomised, controlled study. Anaesthesia. 2012;67:1091–100.

25. Baek SD, Jang M, Kim W, Yu H, Hwang S, Lee SG, et al. Benefits of intraoperative continuous renal replacement therapy during liver transplantation in patients with renal dysfunction. Transplant Proc. 2017;49:1344–50.

26. Douthitt L, Bezinover D, Uemura T, Kadry Z, Shah RA, Ghahramani N, et al. Perioperative use of continuous renal replacement therapy for orthotopic liver transplantation. Transplant Proc. 2012;44:1314–7.

27. Lentine KL, Kasiske BL, Levey AS, Adams PL, Alberu J, Bakr MA, et al. KDIGO clinical practice guideline on the evaluation and Care of Living Kidney Donors. Transplantation. 2017;101:S1–s109.

28. Hilmi I, Horton CN, Planinsic RM, Sakai T, Nicolau-Raducu R, Damian D, et al. The impact of postreperfusion syndrome on short-term patient and liver allograft outcome in patients undergoing orthotopic liver transplantation. Liver Transpl. 2008;14:504–8.

29. Shirai H, Kaido T, Hamaguchi Y, Yao S, Kobayashi A, Okumura S, et al. Preoperative low muscle mass has a strong negative effect on pulmonary function in patients undergoing living donor liver transplantation. Nutrition. 2018;45:1–10.

30. Izumi T, Watanabe J, Tohyama T, Takada Y. Impact of psoas muscle index on short-term outcome after living donor liver transplantation. Turk J Gastroenterol. 2016;27:382–8.

31. Olthoff KM, Kulik L, Samstein B, Kaminski M, Abecassis M, Emond J, et al. Validation of a current definition of early allograft dysfunction in liver transplant recipients and analysis of risk factors. Liver Transpl. 2010;16:943–9.

32. Collins GS, Reitsma JB, Altman DG, Moons KG. Transparent reporting of a multivariable prediction model for individual prognosis or diagnosis (TRIPOD): the TRIPOD statement. Br J Surg. 2015;102:148–58.

33. Martin DS, Grocott MP. Oxygen therapy in critical illness: precise control of arterial oxygenation and permissive hypoxemia. Crit Care Med. 2013;41:423–32.

34. Miller CM, Quintini C, Dhawan A, Durand F, Heimbach JK, Kim-Schluger HL, et al. The international liver transplantation society living donor liver transplant recipient guideline. Transplantation. 2017;101:938–44.

35. Shirai H, Kaido T, Hamaguchi Y, Kobayashi A, Okumura S, Yao S, et al. Preoperative low muscle mass and low muscle quality negatively impact on pulmonary function in patients undergoing hepatectomy for hepatocellular carcinoma. Liver Cancer. 2018;7:76–89.

36. Yamashita M, Kamiya K, Matsunaga A, Kitamura T, Hamazaki N, Matsuzawa R, et al. Prognostic value of psoas muscle area and density in patients who undergo cardiovascular surgery. Can J Cardiol. 2017;33:1652–9.

37. Wagner D, DeMarco MM, Amini N, Buttner S, Segev D, Gani F, et al. Role of frailty and sarcopenia in predicting outcomes among patients undergoing gastrointestinal surgery. World J Gastrointest Surg. 2016;8:27–40.

38. Piriyapatsom A, Williams EC, Waak K, Ladha KS, Eikermann M, Schmidt UH. Prospective observational study of predictors of re-intubation following Extubation in the surgical ICU. Respir Care. 2016;61:306–15.

39. Montano-Loza AJ. Clinical relevance of sarcopenia in patients with cirrhosis. World J Gastroenterol. 2014;20:8061–71.

40. Miller AE, MacDougall JD, Tarnopolsky MA, Sale DG. Gender differences in strength and muscle fiber characteristics. Eur J Appl Physiol Occup Physiol. 1993;66:254–62.

10

Effect of ketofol versus propofol as an induction agent on ease of laryngeal mask airway insertion conditions and hemodynamic stability in pediatrics

Bacha Aberra[1]* ⓘ, Adugna Aregawi[2], Girmay Teklay[1] and Hagos Tasew[1]

Abstract

Background: Laryngeal mask airway is a supraglottic airway device which has led to a fundamental change in the management of modern general anesthesia. In the present study; we evaluated the laryngeal mask airway insertion conditions and hemodynamic changes comparing ketamine-propofol mixture (ketofol) with propofol. The study was to compare the ketamine–propofol mixture (ketofol) with propofolon the ease of laryngeal mask airway insertion conditions and hemodynamic effects for induction of general anesthesia.

Methods: One hundred twenty pediatric patients were recruited and assigned to two groups (60 each). Group KP = ketofol, group P = propofol. Insertion conditions were compared using a Chi-square test while hemodynamic variables were compared using the independentt-test. Statistical significance was stated at p-value< 0.05.

Results: Laryngeal mask airway insertion summed score was nearly similar between the two groups. Mean blood pressure and heart rate were maintained higher in ketofol group while a significant drop was observed in the propofol group. The time from the Laryngeal mask airway placement to the return of spontaneous ventilation was significantly longer in propofol group (240 s [range = 60–360 s]) compared with ketofol group (180 s [range = 30–320 s]) ($p = 0.005$).

Conclusions: Laryngeal mask airway insertion condition summed score was comparable in both ketofol and propofol group. Ketofol provided equivalent laryngeal mask airway insertion conditions while maximizing hemodynamics and minimizing apnea time. Ketofol can be used as an alternative to propofol for laryngeal mask airway insertion in pediatrics.

Keywords: Hemodynamics, Ketofol, Laryngeal mask airway insertion, Propofol

Background

The most important duty of an anesthetist is the management of airway to deliver sufficient ventilation to the patient by securing airway while general anesthesia is administered. As such, no anesthesia is safe unless meticulous efforts are devoted to maintain an intact and functional airway [1, 2]. Effective insertion of the LMA entails optimum anesthetic depth to elude undesirable airway reflexes such as swallowing, gagging, coughing or involuntary movements to severe problems such as laryngospasm [3, 4].

Adequate anesthetic induction situations are paramount delivered by propofol compared to other intravenous induction agents [4]. Nevertheless, when propofol is used as a single induction agent without premedication, doses greater than 3 mg/kg is necessary for smooth LMA insertion [5, 6]. On the other hand, increased propofol doses are not required as undesirable cardio-respiratory depression is dose-dependent [7, 8]. Several combinations of pharmacological agents have

* Correspondence: bcabera11@gmail.com
[1]Aksum University, PO box 298, Aksum City, Tigray, Ethiopia

been introduced to decrease the hemodynamic instability in anesthesia [9, 10]. Ketamine is well known for its airway reflexes maintaining activity and sympathetic cardiorespiratory stimulant so as to causes little or no cardiorespiratory depression and unlike propofol has pain relieving properties [11, 12].

Hemodynamic stability can be maintained using a combination of ketamine and propofol (ketofol), as there is additive effect of Gamma-aminobutyric acid (GABA) agonism by propofol and N-Methyl-D-Aspartate (NMDA) antagonism by ketamine leading to lesser doses of propofol required along with ketamine [13]. The effectiveness of the two agents, propofol and ketamine, may provide the best induction agent with favorable hemodynamics and decreased side effects attributed to either drug as clinical effects of propofol and ketamine seem to be complementary [14].

Therefore the finding of this research will help anesthesia professionals to provide safe and effective alternative induction agent for better LMA insertion conditions and improved hemodynamic stability. It also helps health administrators to work on quality improvement, enhancing good patient outcome, supplying cost-effective anesthetic drugs with the better patient outcome and enhancing income generation and cost reduction.

Methods
Study objective
The aim of this study was to compare the effect of the ketamine-propofol mixture (ketofol) and propofol on the insertion conditions of laryngeal mask airway and hemodynamic stability in pediatrics.

Study design
An observational prospective cohort study was employed from Jan 25-March, 25, 2017 after ethical approval (No-11/2009, Dec 1, 2016) was obtained from the Addis Ababa University Ethical committee.

Study setting
This study was conducted at Menelik-II Hospital. Menelik II hospital is one of the largest hospitals in the country. Menelik-II Hospital is now the main health provider center that offers high-quality comprehensive health services to the patient from all over the region of Ethiopia and there are two main operation departments, from which ophthalmic operation room has six operation tables. One of these is pediatric operation room table, which on average, 1920 pediatric patients operated under general anesthesia per year. The study was conducted from January 25–March 25, 2017.

Study participants
Patients of ASA class I and II, age ranging from 2 to 15 years and undergoing elective surgical procedures under GA using LMA were included in the study. Patients with hyper-reactive airway disease anticipated difficult airway, on regular sedatives and on β-blockers were excluded from the study.

Study variables
In this study, the dependent variables were ease of LMA insertion and hemodynamic changes. The independent variables were socio-demographic and operative data (Age, Sex Weight, ASA, and Mallampati class) and another exposure variable (a type of anesthesia drugs used (ketofol vs. propofol)) Table 1.

Sample size and sampling techniques determination
StatCalc EPI info 7.1.1 (Fleiss) was used based on ease of LMA insertion conditions among two groups to calculate the sample size for each group. The following assumptions were considered to estimate the sample size required for the study. A 95% confidence level and 80% power, equal sample size for two groups, a proportion of

Table 1 operational definitions

Operational Definitions		
Apnea		The absence of spontaneous respiration for < 20 s after induction
Ease of insertion	Easy	No adverse response, i.e., gagging or coughing, movement or laryngospasm
	Difficult	Moderate to severe adverse responses requiring additional boluses of drugs or more than two attempts are required for LMA insertion
Laryngospasm	Complete	when there are laryngeal spasm and no air entry on ventilation
	Incomplete	when there is laryngeal spasm but there is air entry
Coughing	Slight	coughing which can occur immediately after LMA and subside by itself
	Gross	coughing which needs deepening of anesthesia to be relieved
Gagging [23]	Slight	Gagging which stays for short seconds can relieve on its own
	Gross	Gagging which needs deepening of anesthesia to be relieved
Patient movement	Slight	Movement from small muscles which can allow insertion of LMA without an additional dose of the drugs
	Gross	The movement which cannot be relieved without an additional dose of the drugs
Insertion condition summed score		Summing the insertion score for each patient then totaling the score for all patients in the groups and taking the mean

subjects with poor insertion conditions were 41.66 and 18.33% in propofol (unexposed) and ketofol (exposed) group respectively in a recent study [15, 16]. A total of 60 ASA I and II pediatric patients age 2–15 were assigned to each group.

Sampling technique

From situational analysis mean of midyear population was used to get a total number of ophthalmic pediatric patients who underwent operation under general anesthesia using LMA in 2 months duration. The mid-year population from the situational analysis was 960. So, the size of the population in 2 months was 960 divided by three gives us 320. The study participants were selected using a systematic sampling technique every two participants from daily operation schedule list until the required sample size was obtained. The first study participants were selected by lottery method. We spent two extra weeks to reach the number of propofol group is equal to ketofol group to get an equal sample size in both groups.

Intraoperative procedure

After preoperative preparation, patients were shifted to the operation room, standard monitoring applied as routine. Baseline vitals were recorded and I.V. fluids were administered. Patients were preoxygenated with 6 L/min of Oxygen via a face mask, for 3 min and given injection atropine 0.02 mg/kg I.V. and fentanyl 1 μg/kg I. V prior to induction as the standard of care.

LMA insertion was performed 60 s after induction of anesthesia [1]. Following insertion, the position of LMA was assessed by observing movement of chest and reservoir bag through use of both spontaneous and assisted ventilation. After successful insertion of LMA, patients were allowed to breathe spontaneously. Assisted manual ventilation provided when the apnoea period is longer than 20 s from the time of LMA insertion to ensure that SpO2 remained above 95%. Manual ventilation was stopped when sufficient spontaneous respiration returned. Thereafter, anesthesia was maintained with isoflurane 2% and oxygen 100% with a flow rate of 3 L/min.

The patients were either induced with ketofol (0.5mg/kg of ketamine plus 3.0mg/kg of propofol) or 3.5mg/kg or propofol alone. If the patients respond to stimulus after induction, further increments of propofol 0.5–1 mg/kg were given until loss of consciousness and loss of eyelash reflex in either technique. All patients who were exposed to either ketofol or propofol were compared to see different outcomes of both agents as an induction agent on ease of laryngeal mask airway insertion and hemodynamic stability. Insertion condition was graded by the same anesthetist who performs the procedure as [9].

a) Mouth opening: 1 – Full, 2 – Partial, 3 – Nil
b) Coughing: 1 – Nil, 2 – slight, 3 – gross
c) Swallowing: 1 – Nil, 2 – slight, 3 – gross
d) Movement: 1 – Nil, 2 – slight, 3 – gross
e) Laryngospasm: 1 – Nil, 2 – Mild, 3– Severe
f) Ease of LMA insertion: 1-Easy, 2-Difficult, 3-Impossible

Mean blood pressure and heart rate were recorded one minute before induction (baseline), immediately after induction, immediately after LMA insertion, then at every minute for up to 3 min. The duration of apnoea was recorded via a digital timer as the time from the end of induction of anesthesia until the return of adequate spontaneous ventilation. Afterward, all patients who were scheduled for ophthalmic surgical operation under general anesthesia with LMA were enrolled in the study and assigned to either ketofol or propofol group randomly. Our study used those patients induced with propofol as a cohort group, where the same checklist was used to observe the case.

Data collection technique and instrument

Data were collected using a pretested observational checklist. Data collectors were three bachelor degree holder anesthetist and they supervised by one master degree holder anesthetist. All anesthetists participating in the study including anesthetists who inserts the LMAs and administers the medications had at least 2 years of experience in conducting anesthesia.

Data quality assurance

Before recruiting patients into the study, training and orientation about the objective and process of data collection were provided by the principal investigator. To ensure the quality of data, a pre-test of the checklist was performed in Cure International Hospital before the actual data collection time. The completed checklist was submitted and reviewed on daily basis. Close supervision and daily information exchange were used as a means to correct problems during the course of data collection.

Consent for the survey was obtained from Addis Ababa University College of health sciences and confidentiality assured to improve the quality of data. Variables were checked by the expert before the actual data collection period for the purpose of consistency.

Statistical methods

All data were analyzed by SPSS statistical package program (Version 20). Within the groups, the normality of variables was measured using the Shapiro-Wilk test. Differences of numerical data between groups were evaluated using student's t-test and Mann–Whitney

U-test when appropriate. Categorical data were analyzed with the Chi-Square test. A p value of < 0.05 with the power of 80% was regarded as statistically significant.

Results

Socio-demographic features and operative conditions

A total of 120 patients were enrolled and none were excluded from the study as there was no incidence of failed LMA insertion. There were no statistically significant differences in age, sex, weight, and ASA or mallampati class between groups [Table 2].

Comparison of ease of insertions conditions

In 12 (20%) of the propofol group patients, additional 0.5–1 mg/kg) propofol was required as compared to nine (15%) of those in the ketofol group. However, no significant difference was noted between the two groups ($p = 0.631$). The time from the LMA placement to the return of spontaneous ventilation was significantly longer in propofol group (240 s [range = 60–390 s]) compared with a ketofol group (180 s [range = 30–380 s]) ($p = 0.005$), expressed in median and range respectively. The LMA was inserted successfully and positioned correctly on the first attempt in 95% of patients receiving ketofol compared with 96.67% in patients receiving propofol [Table 3].

LMA insertion summed score was nearly similar between the two group, which were statistically insignificant ($p = 0.511$). No patient developed laryngospasm in the ketofol group while 2 patients (3.33%) developed partial laryngospasm in propofol group but not statistically significant ($p = 0.154$) [Table 4].

Table 2 Socio-demographic features of the patients

Patient characteristics	Group KP (n = 60)	Group P (n = 60)	P-value
Age in years (median, IQR[a])	5.5 (3–9)	7 (4–11)	0.18
Gender (n, %)			1.00
Male	34 (56.7)	35 (58.3)	
Female	26 (43.3)	25 (41.7)	
Weight (median, IQR*) (in Kgs[b])	19.5 (14–25)	26 (15–30)	0.14
ASA (n, %)			0.611
I	57 (95.0)	59 (98.3)	
II	3 (5.0)	1 (1.7)	
Mallampati class (n, %)			0.756
Can't be assessed[c]	18 (30)	16 (26.7)	
I	40 (66.7)	43 (71.7)	
II	2 (3.3)	1 (1.7)	

[a] = Interquartile range, [b] = kilograms, [c] = (< 4 years of age, uncooperative)

Table 3 Requirement of Additional propofol, duration of apnea and attempts of LMA

	Group KP	Group P	p-value
The requiredtop-up dose of propofol (n, %)	9 (15)	12 (20)	0.631
Duration of apnea (seconds)	180[a](30–380[b])	240[a](60–390[b])	0.005
Attempts of LMA insertion(1/2/3)	57/3/0	58/2/0	0.648

[a] =Median, [b] = range

Comparison of hemodynamic characteristics

Patients in both groups were comparable with respect to preoperative baseline hemodynamic conditions. The mean arterial pressure difference between the group is not significantly different before induction (p-value = 0.263; is insignificant). With the induction of anesthesia, a significant drop in mean arterial blood pressure was observed in propofol group from baseline while in the ketofol group, there was a rise in mean arterial pressure at all measurement times ($P < 0.001$) [Fig. 1]. Maximum mean blood pressure was 81.5 ± 11.02 mmHg with a ketofol group seen immediately after induction [Table 5].

Preoperatively there was no statistically significant difference (p-value> 0.05) between the heart rate of both groups. P values at all levels after induction were < 0.05 and statistically significant. With the induction of anesthesia, a significant rise in heart rate was observed in the ketofol group from baseline while in propofol group, there was a drop in heart rate at all measurement times ($P < 0.05$) [Fig. 2]. The increment in heart rate was seen immediately after induction compared with baseline. Maximum heart rate was 118.55 ± 24.86 beat/min with a ketofol group seen immediately after LMA insertion. Minimum heart rate (99.62 ± 25.071) was seen in propofol group 3 min after LMA insertion [Table 6].

Table 4 Comparison of insertion conditions of LMA between the ketofol and propofol groups

Assessment grades	Group KP	Group P	p value
Mouth opening (Full / Partial/None)	54/6/0	53/7/0	0.769
Coughing or gagging (Nil / Slight/Gross)	54/6/0	52/7/1	0.573
Swallowing (Nil / Slight/Gross)	55/5/0	54/5/1	0.604
Laryngospasm (Nil / Partial/Complete)	60/0/0	58/2/0	0.496
Ease of LMA insertion (easy/difficult/impossible)	59/1/0	58/2/0	0.956
Head or limbs movement (Nil / Slight/Gross)	57/3/0	58/2/0	0.648
Insertion condition summed score	6.35 (6–10)	6.48 (6–13)	0.607

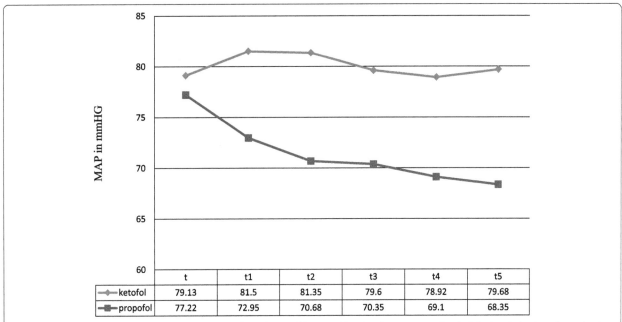

Fig. 1 Changes in mean arterial pressure between ketofol and propofol group. NB: t, baseline, t1, immediately following induction of anesthesia, t2, immediately after LMA placement, t3, t4, and t5,1,2 and 3 min after LMA placement

Discussion

In our study, LMA insertion summed score for ketofol and propofol group were nearly similar. This result coincides with the studies done by Goh et al. in their study of randomized double-blind comparison of ketamine-propofol, fentanyl-propofol and propofol-saline on hemodynamics and laryngeal mask airway insertion conditions [17].

In our study, in ketofol group, we observed a decrease in the requirement of an additional dosage of propofol for induction, although it was not statistically significant ($p > 0.05$). Consistent with our results, many researchers observed that there was a significant decrease in additional requirement of propofol for induction, loss of consciousness and LMA insertion in ketofol group than propofol group. This less requirement of additional propofol dose is due to the combined effect of ketamine and propofol at both hypnotic and anesthetic endpoints [2, 12, 18]. However, the reason for the insignificant result in our study might have been due to the use of 3.5 mg/kg (high dose) of propofol for induction unlike Yousef et al. [12]. They administered initial 2 mg/kg propofol and incremental doses of propofol until the target level of the Bispectral index of 40 was obtained.

This study also spectacles that, apnea time was significantly longer in propofol group (median = 240 s [range = 60–390 s]) compared with ketofol group (median = 180 s [range = 30–380 s]) ($p = 0.005$). Consistent with our study [19] in their study of comparison of propofol and ketofol on laryngeal tube-suction II circumstances and hemodynamics showed that apnea duration was longer in group P (median = 385 s [range = 195–840 s]) compared with group KP (median = 325.5 s [range = 60–840 s]) but was not statistically significant [19]. In their study, the overall apnea time was higher than ours. This difference might have been due to the use of remifentanil (1 µg/kg) 60 s after pre-oxygenation because remifentanil is known to have prolonged apnea time than fentanyl [13].

Table 5 Comparing the Mean of data on mean arterial blood pressure between ketofol and propofol groups

	Mean arterial pressure (in mmHg)		P value
	Group KP (Mean ± SD)	Group P (Mean ± SD)	
Baseline MAP	79.13 ± 8.96	77.22 ± 9.69	0.263
Immediately after induction	81.50 ± 11.02	72.95 ± 12.349	< 0.001
Immediately after LMA insertion	81.35 ± 11.339	70.68 ± 11.620	< 0.001
One minute after LMA insertion	79.60 ± 11.036	70.35 ± 10.844	< 0.001
Two minute after LMA insertion	78.92 ± 11.794	69.10 ± 10.188	< 0.001
Three minute after LMA insertion	79.68 ± 11.978	68.35 ± 9.295	< 0.001

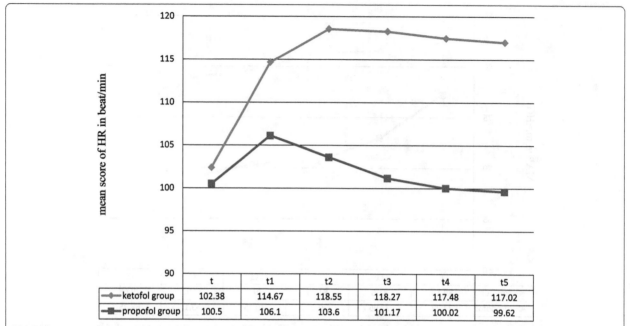

Fig. 2 Changes in heart rate between ketofol and propofol group. NB: t, baseline, t1, immediately following induction of anesthesia, t2, immediately after LMA placement, t3, t4, and t5,1,2 and 3 min after LMA placement

A comparative study done in Malaysia to compare the effects of ketamine and midazolam as co-induction agents with propofol for proseal™ laryngeal mask airway insertion showed that the ketamine-propofol combination had a shorter duration of apnoea, better mouth opening, and hemodynamic profile as compared to the combination midazolam-propofol [1].

Another Randomized double-blind comparative study of ketamine-propofol and fentanyl-propofol for LMA insertion in children showed that the conditions of LMA insertion were superior in the combination of ketamine (0.5 mg/kg and propofol than propofol and fentanyl [20].

Hemodynamic parameters can increase 20% after LMA insertion, with an additional 30% after orotracheal intubation [1]. In our study, we observed that ketofol preserved mean arterial pressure at all measurement times while a significant drop in mean arterial blood pressure was seen in the propofol group. Similarly,

several studies concluded that ketofol is superior to propofol and propofol–thiopentone mixture because of its better hemodynamic stability [11, 17, 21, 22]. With the induction of anesthesia, a significant rise in heart rate was observed in ketofol group from baseline while in propofol group, there was a drop in heart rate at all measurement times ($P < 0.05$). The cardiovascular stimulant effect of ketofol is desirable especially in pediatric anesthesia while the unduly depressant effect of propofol is unwanted [11, 12].

Limitations

This study was unable to measure anesthetic depth. Therefore the LMA insertion conditions may have been adversely affected and hemodynamic parameters change might be observed. Use of fentanyl in both groups before induction may have affected the hemodynamic effects of the agents.

Table 6 Comparing the Mean of data on heart rate between ketofol and propofol group

	Heart rate (beat per minute)		P value
	Group KP (Mean ± SD)	Group P (mean ± SD)	
Baseline heart rate	102.38 ± 16.368	100.50 ± 17.070	0.539
Immediately after induction	114.67 ± 21.972	106.10 ± 21.802	0.034
Immediately after LMA insertion	118.55 ± 24.863	103.60 ± 23.449	< 0.001
One minute after LMA insertion	118.27 ± 22.823	101.17 ± 24.668	< 0.001
Two minute after LMA insertion	117.48 ± 20.994	100.02 ± 25.780	< 0.001
Three minute after LMA insertion	117.02 ± 21.246	99.62 ± 25.071	< 0.001

The result of this study showed that LMA insertion condition summed score was comparable in ketofol group and propofol group. There was a decrease in propofol requirement for induction in the ketofol group. There was a more stable MAP picture in the ketofol group when compared to that of propofol group.

Abbreviations

ASA: American Society of Anesthesiologists; GABA: Gamma-aminobutyric acid; HR: Heart rate; KP: Ketofol; LMA: Laryngeal Mask Airway; MAP: Mean Arterial Pressure; NMDA: N-Methyl-D-Aspartate; P: Propofol

Acknowledgments

The authors acknowledge Addis Ababa University, the supervisors, data collectors, and study participants for their invaluable support.

Author's contributions

BA: Conceive of data and designed the study, supervised the data collection, performed the analysis, interpretation of data, drafted the manuscript and final approval of the revision for publication. AA: Assisted in designing the study, data interpretation and critically reviewed the manuscript. HT: Assisted in designing the study, data analysis, data interpretation and reviewed the manuscript critically. GT: Assisted in analysis, methodology, and interpretation of the data with the statistics and reviewed the manuscript critically. Agreement to be accountable for all aspects of the work in ensuring that questions related to the accuracy or integrity of the work are appropriately investigated and resolved. All authors also read and approved the final manuscript.

Author details

[1]Aksum University, PO box 298, Aksum City, Tigray, Ethiopia. [2]Addis Ababa University, PO box 811/1000, Addis Ababa, Ethiopia.

References

1. Mohamad RL, Tang S, Yahya N, Izaham A, Yusof AM, Manap NA. Comparison between effects of ketamine and midazolam as co-induction agents with propofol for prosealTM laryngeal mask insertion. Sri Lankan J Anaesthesiol. 2016;24(1).
2. Pavani Kalyanam HLBR, Praveen Kumar M, Rangarao D. Comparison of Propofol versus Propofol + ketamine for LMA insertion in children undergoing elective eye surgery. Int J Adv Health. 2015;2(5):592–601.
3. Benumof JL. Laryngeal mask airway and the ASA difficult airway algorithm. Int Anesthesiol Clin. 1998;36(2):61–90.
4. Brain A, McGhee T, McAteer E, Thomas A, Abu-Saad M, Bushman J. The laryngeal mask airway. Development and preliminary trials of a new type of airway. Anaesthesia. 1985;40(4):356–61.
5. Scanlon P, Carey M, Power M, Kirby F, Brown BR Jr. Patient response to laryngeal mask insertion after induction of Anaesthesia with Propofol or Thiopentone. Surv Anesthesiol. 1994;38(4):194.
6. Eftekhari J, Haki BK, Tizro P, Alizadeh V. A comparison to facilitate insertion of the laryngeal mask: term of recovery and postoperative nausea and vomiting after anesthesia with propofol-atracurium and thiopental-atracurium. Acta Medica Iranica. 2015;53(2):117–21.
7. Seyedhejazi M, Eydi M, Ghojazadeh M, Nejati A, Ghabili K, Golzari SE, et al. Propofol for laryngeal mask airway insertion in children: effect of two different doses. Saudi J Anaesth. 2013;7(3):266.
8. Gupta A, Kaur S, Attri JP, Saini N. Comparative evaluation of ketamine-propofol, fentanyl-propofol and butorphanol-propofol on haemodynamics and laryngeal mask airway insertion conditions. J Anaesthesiol Clin Pharmacol. 2011;27(1):74.
9. Hosseinzadeh H, Eidi M, Ghaffarlou M, Torabi E, Ghabili K, Golzari S. Comparison of remifentanil with esmolol to blunt the cardiovascular response to tracheal extubation in patients undergoing neurosurgical procedures for intracranial masses. J Pak Med Assoc. 2013;63(8): 950–4.
10. Hosseinzadeh H, Eidy M, Ghaffarlou M, Ghabili K, Golzari SE. Esmolol: a unique beta-blocker in maintaining cardiovascular stability following neurosurgical procedures. Adv Pharm Bull. 2012;2(2):249.
11. Furuya A, Matsukawa T, Ozaki M, Nishiyama T, Kume M, Kumazawa T. Intravenous ketamine attenuates arterial pressure changes during the induction of anaesthesia with propofol. Eur J Anaesthesiol. 2001;18(2): 88–92.
12. Yousef GT, Elsayed KM. A clinical comparison of ketofol (ketamine and propofol admixture) versus propofol as an induction agent on quality of laryngeal mask airway insertion and hemodynamic stability in children. Anesth Essays Res. 2013;7(2):194.
13. Gül R, Hizli Ş, Kocamer B, Koruk S, Şahin L, Kilinçaslan H, et al. The safety and efficacy of remifentanil compared to fentanyl in pediatric endoscopy. Turkish J Med Sci. 2013;43(4):611–6.
14. Smischney NJ, Beach ML, Dodds TM, Koff MD. Ketofol as a sole induction agent is associated with increased hemodynamic indices in low-risk patients. Anesthesiology. 2011;16:A485.
15. Ghatak T, Singh D, Kapoor R, Bogra J. Effects of addition of ketamine, fentanyl and saline with Propofol induction on hemodynamics and laryngeal mask airway insertion conditions in oral clonidine premedicated children. Saudi J Anaesth. 2012;6(2):140.
16. Khutia SK, Mandal MC, Das S, Basu S. Intravenous infusion of ketamine-propofol can be an alternative to intravenous infusion of fentanyl-propofol for deep sedation and analgesia in paediatric patients undergoing emergency short surgical procedures. Indian J Anaesth. 2012;56(2):145.
17. Goh P, Chiu C, Wang C, Chan Y, Loo P. Randomized double-blind comparison of ketamine-propofol, fentanyl-propofol and propofol-saline on haemodynamics and laryngeal mask airway insertion conditions. Anaesth Intensive Care. 2005;33(2):223.
18. Hui T, Short T, Hong W, Suen T, Gin T, Plummer J. Additive interactions between Propofol and ketamine when used for anesthesia induction in female patients. Surv Anesthesiol. 1996;40(2):81.
19. Ozgul U, Begec Z, Karahan K, Erdogan MA, Aydogan MS, Colak C, et al. Comparison of propofol and ketamine-propofol mixture (Ketofol) on laryngeal tube-suction II conditions and hemodynamics: a randomized, prospective, double-blind trial. Curr Ther Res. 2013;75:39–43.
20. Singh R, Arora M, Vajifdar H. Randomized double-blind comparison of ketamine-propofol and fentanyl-propofol for the insertion of laryngeal mask airway in children. J Anaesthesiol Clin Pharmacol. 2011;27(1):91.
21. Goel S, Bhardwaj N, Jain K. Efficacy of ketamine and midazolam as co-induction agents with propofol for laryngeal mask insertion in children. Pediatr Anesth. 2008;18(7):628–34.
22. Begec Z, Demirbilek S, Onal D, Erdil F, Ilksen Toprak H, Ozcan Ersoy M. Ketamine or alfentanil administration prior to propofol anaesthesia: the effects on ProSeal™ laryngeal mask airway insertion conditions and haemodynamic changes in children. Anaesthesia. 2009;64(3):282–6.
23. Ghafoor HB, Afshan G, Kamal R. General anesthesia with laryngeal mask airway: etomidate vs propofol for hemodynamic stability. Open J Anesthesiol. 2012;2(4):161–5.

11

High-flow nasal cannula improves clinical efficacy of airway management in patients undergoing awake craniotomy

Ping Yi[1†], Qiong Li[2†], Zhoujing Yang[1], Li Cao[1], Xiaobing Hu[1] and Huahua Gu[1*]

Abstract

Background: Awake craniotomy requires specific sedation procedure in an awake patient who should be able to cooperate during the intraoperative neurological assessment. Currently, limited number of literatures on the application of high-flow nasal cannula (HFNC) in the anesthetic management for awake craniotomy has been reported. Hence, we carried out a prospective study to assess the safety and efficacy of humidified high-flow nasal cannula (HFNC) airway management in the patients undergoing awake craniotomy.

Methods: Sixty-five patients who underwent awake craniotomy were randomly assigned to use HFNC with oxygen flow rate at 40 L/min or 60 L/min, or nasopharynx airway (NPA) device in the anesthetic management. Data regarding airway management, intraoperative blood gas analysis, intracranial pressure, gastric antral volume, and adverse events were collected and analyzed.

Results: Patients using HFNC with oxygen flow rate at 40 or 60 L/min presented less airway obstruction and injuries. Patients with HFNC 60 L/min maintained longer awake time than the patients with NPA. While the intraoperative PaO_2 and SPO_2 were not significantly different between the HFNC and NPA groups, HFNC patients achieved higher PaO_2/FiO_2 than patients with NPA. There were no differences in Brain Relaxation Score and gastric antral volume among the three groups as well as before and after operation in any of the three groups.

Conclusion: HFNC was safe and effective for the patients during awake craniotomy.

Keywords: Awake craniotomy, High-flow nasal cannula (HFNC); nasopharyngeal airway (NPA), Gastric antral volume, Adverse events, Intracranial pressure

Background

Awake craniotomy is commonly performed for resection of epileptic lesions or tumors located close to or into the functionally essential motor, cognitive, or sensory cortical areas [1]. It allows continuous monitoring of patients' neurological functions throughout the surgery to minimize iatrogenic language or motor deficits. However, this technique brings challenges both to the neurosurgeon and anesthesiologist. The anesthetic management for this type of surgery must include sedation, analgesia, respiratory and hemodynamic control, and a responsive, co-operative patient for neurologic testing intra-operatively. There is a growing trend of preference for awake craniotomy as the approach for the removal of tumors in the sensitive cortical area has been established over the last few decades.

* Correspondence: ghhmzk@sina.com
†Ping Yi and Qiong Li contributed equally to this work.
[1]Department of Anesthesiology, Huashan Hospital, Fudan University, No.12 Wulumuqi Zhong Road, Shanghai 200040, China

Airway management in the anesthesia for awake craniotomy is always concerned by anesthesiologists. Up to date, a series of venting devices including nasal cannula [2], simple facemask [3], bilateral nasopharyngeal [4], laryngeal mask [5], and endotracheal tube [6] have been used in the awake craniotomy. When these methods were applied, the patient's head is fixed during the surgical procedure, and potential laryngospasm or cough occur when the patient is awake, which may result in surgical bleeding, increased intracranial pressure or neurological injury. Thus, endotracheal intubation or laryngeal mask, and a deeper grade of sedation/anesthesia (BIS value at 40–60) are required for the patients to prevent coughing and laryngospasm. Consequently, it takes a longer time for the patient to recover from anesthesia. Furthermore, it is difficult to re-establish the airway when the patient is inducted into the state of being asleep again [6–8]. The spontaneous breathing can be maintained under mild to moderate sedation (BIS value 60–80) through nasopharynx or oropharyngeal airways. However, nasopharyngeal or oropharyngeal airways could not completely relieve upper airway obstruction, and concentration of inhaled oxygen cannot be adjusted. In addition, nasopharyngeal airway may cause injury to nasopharynx, and the airway may be obstructed by secretions or blood clot. Furthermore, some patients may have difficulty in tolerating the nasopharyngeal or oropharyngeal airways or feel uncomfortable due to the dry airway.

Currently, while there is still no consensus or any established protocol for the best airway management for awake craniotomy, in recent years, a novel oxygen supply device, a high-flow nasal cannula (HFNC), has been introduced into medical practice [9–11]. HFNC is capable of delivering humidified (100% humidity) and heated (37 °C) oxygen at a maximum flow rate of 60 L/min [11, 12]. HFNC has presented many potential advantages over traditional oxygen supply devices, including decreased nasopharyngeal resistance, washing out of the nasopharyngeal dead space, generation of positive pressure in the pharynx, increasing alveolar recruitment in the lungs, humidification of the airways, increased fraction of inspired oxygen and improved mucociliary clearance [13–18]. Emerging evidence indicates that HFNC is effective in various clinical settings, such as acute respiratory failure [11, 19, 20], acute heart failure [21, 22], postoperative hypoxemia after cardiac surgery [23, 24], during sedation and analgesia [25]. However, there is no published study on the investigation of clinical efficacy and safety of HFNC in patients undergoing awake craniotomy. Therefore, we designed this study to evaluate the clinical outcomes of HFNC by comparing HFNC with NPA in the anesthesia management for awake craniotomy. The primary endpoint of this study was to determine if HFNC could be safely used during awake craniotomy, and secondary endpoint was to determine if HFNC is superior to the traditional NPA in terms of outcomes and safety in the awake craniotomy.

Methods

Study population

We collected medical data of patients who underwent awake craniotomy at our hospital from June 2018 to July 2019. This manuscript adheres to the applicable CONSORT guidelines. This clinical trial was approved by the Institutional Ethics Committee (approval number: KY2018–232) and registered at http://www.chictr.org.cn/index.aspx (registration number: CHiCTR1800016621).

The inclusion criteria: 1). Patients were 14–70 years of age. No gender preference; 2). Intracranial tumors or epileptic lesions located in the eloquent brain areas and its peripheral areas, wake-up anesthesia was required in craniotomy; 3). American Society of Anesthesiologists (ASA) physical status: Grade I or II; 4). Patients had no aphasia or changes in muscle strength before surgery.

The exclusion criteria: 1). Patients had severe organ diseases and were in decompensation (such as medical severe complications: a. Cardiac functional capacity ≥ class III; b. Respiratory failure; c. Hepatic and renal dysfunction; d. Hematological diseases; e. Uncontrolled hypertension; f. Patients with a history of COPD, pulmonary fibrosis, or long-term heavy smoking before surgery; g. Patients with severe intracranial hypertension, or even had cerebral herniation before surgery); 2). Patients who were extremely fear of surgery and were expected to have difficulty in cooperating during the operation; 3). Patients with conscious or cognitive dysfunction before surgery; 4). Patients who were unable to communicate well before surgery; 5). Patients with morbid obesity (BMI ≥ 40) accompanied by obstructive sleep apnea syndrome; 6). Patients had difficult airways; 7). Patients suffered from glioma along with other tumors outside the nervous system; 8). Pregnant women; 9). Patients involved in other clinical trials in the past three months.

Sixty-five patients were eventually enrolled in this study. They were randomly assigned into the following three groups according to the airway management during anesthesia: Group 1 ($n = 22$), patients used HFNC device with an oxygen flow rate of 40 L/min (HFNC 40); Group 2 ($n = 20$), patients used HFNC device with an oxygen flow rate of 60 L/min (HFNC 60); Group 3 ($n = 23$), patients used nasopharyngeal airway (NPA). Patients were evaluated during the pre-operative visit by the anesthesiologist and the procedure was explained in detail.

Anesthesia management

In the operating room, the peripheral intravenous catheters were set up, and standard monitors such as electrocardiograph, pulse oximeter, and non-invasive blood pressure measurement devices were connected. Invasive blood pressure was monitored after arterial cannulation with local antiesthetic (LA) infiltration in radial or dorsalis pedis artery. Bispectral index (BIS®) monitoring (A-2000; Aspect

Medical Systems, Newton, MA, USA) was connected to ti-trate the amount of sedatives and hypnotics. Sedative drugs were injected by a pump in the following sequence: 1). A loading dose of 0.6 µg/kg dexmedetomidine was infused within 15 min. Then, dexmedetomidine was maintained at 0.1 µg/kg/h. 2). Remifentanil Target controlled Infusion model (TCI) (Ce) was maintained at 0.5–2.0 ng/ml, which started from 0.5 µg and increased by 0.5 µg every 5–10 min till respiration frequence was at least 12 times/min. When respiration was nearly 12 times/min, TCI increased by 0.25 µg till stabilized. After the scalp nerve was blocked with 20 mL of 0.75% ropivacaine + 10 mL of 2% lidocaine + 1: 200,000 of epinephrine, propofol was infused under TCI (Ce) model at the dose of 1.0–2.0 µg/ml. Specifically, titration target of propofol was to reach BIS: 60–70, and respiration frequency: 10–20 times/min. Propofol TCI was set to 1.0–2.0 µg/mL, which started from 1.0 µg and in-creased by 0.5 µg every 10–15 min till BIS reached 70. If BIS decreased to 60, TCI concentration increased by 0.25 µg till stabilized. Three ways of oxygen delivery were established. 1). Group I- HFNC 40, high-flow nasal cannula (HFNC) device was used, and oxygen flow rate was set at 40 L/ min, FiO_2 60%, airway humidified temperature was set at 34°C; 2); Group II- HFNC 60, high-flow nasal cannula (HFNC) device was used, and oxygen flow rate was set at 60 L/ min, FiO_2 60%, airway humidified temperature was set at 34°C; 3). Group III-nasopharyngeal airway (NPA): nasopharynx airway device was used. The end of the naso-pharyngeal airway was connected to the threaded tube of anesthesia machine. The oxygen flow rate was set at 6 L/min, FiO_2 60% with no humidification.

When BIS value was maintained at 60–70 and the respiratory rate was maintained at 12–20 times/min by titration of propofol and remifentanil, induction of anesthesia was considered as completed. A urinary cath-eter was inserted. The head of the patient was fixed with a Mayfield head clamp. The body was adjusted to a com-fortable position; with the head slightly elevated in order to avoid jugular venous flow compression. Such position prevents airway occlusion when the patient was asleep. The patient was asleep during the processes of scalp in-cision, bone flap removal, and dura suspending. Before bone flap removal, mannitol was administrated at the dose of 1.0 g/kg for 20 min. The intracranial pressure was assessed by the surgeons five seconds after removing the bone flap using Brain Relaxation Score (BRS). Specif-ically, by palpating and feeling the tension of the dura mater, BRS was subjectively scored by the surgeons from 1 to 10, with 10 was the most satisfied intracranial pres-sure control. After the dura suspending was done, pro-pofol infusion was stopped, and the patient was allowed to wake up spontaneously. If the patient could not be awoken in 10 min after stopping propofol infusion, dex-medetomidine infusion would be decreased or stopped.

After the BIS value was maintained above 90, cortical functional mapping was achieved using NIM-ECLIPSE® System (Medtronic Xomed Inc., Jacksonville, FL, USA) with a monopolar probe, delivering stimuli with a single 1 ms pulse with a 60 Hz frequency during surgical tumor re-section. Upon the requirement of surgeons, the deep sed-ation was induced again by the titration of propofol, dexmedetomidine, and remifentanil. BIS value at 60–70 and the respiratory rate at 12–20 times/min could be con-sidered as the completion of re-induction of anesthesia.

Study variables

The baseline characteristics including age, gender, body mass index (BMI) and ASA physical status was collected. The following intraoperative data were collected: 1). Blood gas analysis at 6 different time points (before induction of anesthesia; 15 min after induction of anesthesia, 15 min after the adjustment of comfortable body position, dura suspen-sion was completed, functional mapping was being per-formed, 15 min after re-induction of anesthesia). 2). Vital signs (heart rate, blood pressure, SpO_2, and respiratory rate were measured every 5 min). 3). Depth of sedation/ anesthesia (BIS value and OAA/S score). 4). Brain Relaxation Score, which was assessed every 15 min. 5). The time that patients took to wake up spontaneously. 6). The total time that patients were awake. 7). Total dose of each sedative drug. 8). Total anesthesia time. 9). Gastric antral volume be-fore and after surgery. 10). Incidence of adverse events. The gastric antral volume was evaluated by measuring the cross-sectional area (CSA) of the antrum using the ultrasound [26]. The head to sacral (CC) and anteroposterior (AP) diam-eter of the antrum was measured. The CSA was calculated by the formula CSA = AP x CC x π/4.

Adverse events

Information of the following adverse events was col-lected. 1). The incidence of respiratory tract obstruction, which was defined as no airflow, apnea, or snoring due to partial airway obstrction. 2). Airway injury, which was defined as blood or bloody secretion found on the tube of NPA or in the patients' mouth. 3). Increased intracra-nial pressure that required instant treatment.

Statistical analysis

The sample size was calculated using PASS11 software. By ANOVA, took SPO_2 as major parameter, that is, gave SPO_2 as 100, 95, and 97 for HFNC 40, HFNC 60 and NPA, respectively, and a was 0.05. Sample number was from 5 to 40 with 5 as interval, and standard deviations were 2, 4, and 5. Statistical power and sample size were then calculated. When sample number was 20 and SD was 5, 0.8 of the statistical power was obtained; if SD was 2, 1 statistical power was obtained. Therefore, 20 was chosen as the sample size of each group.

Table 1 Baseline characteristics of the participants

Variables	Index of variables	HFNC 40 (n = 22)	HFNC 60 (n = 20)	NPA (n = 23)
Age (years)	Mean ± SD	37.32 ± 15.28	41.25 ± 13.89	40.43 ± 10.16
Body Mass Index (kg/m^2)	Mean ± SD	23.71 ± 3.68	23.45 ± 4.16	21.81 ± 2.29
Gender	Male	11 (50.00)	13 (65.00)	11 (47.83)
	Female	11 (50.00)	7 (35.00)	12 (52.17)
ASA physical status	I	10 (45.45)	11 (55.00)	16 (69.57)
	II	12 (54.55)	9 (45.00)	7 (30.43)
Epilepsy	No	18 (81.82)	18 (90.00)	18 (78.26)
	Yes	4 (18.18)	2 (10.00)	5 (21.74)
Hypertension	No	20 (90.91)	19 (95.00)	23 (100.0)
	Yes	2 (9.09)	1 (5.00)	0 (0.00)
Surgery type	Other surgery	4 (18.18)	1 (5.00)	2 (8.70)
	Right-sided glioma resection	7 (31.82)	2 (10.00)	7 (30.43)
	Left-sided glioma resection	11 (50.00)	17 (85.00)	14 (60.87)

HFNC high-flow nasal cannula, *NPA* nasopharyngeal airway, *ASA* American Society of Anesthesiologists

The categorical variables were expressed as the frequency (%), and the Chi-square test was used for comparison. The measurable variables were expressed as mean ± SD, representation or median (interquartile range). Differences between groups were compared using One-way ANOVA when normal distribution was achieved, followed by Student-Newman-Keuls (SNK) test. If the normal distribution was not achieved, the Kruskal-Wallis test was used. Comparison within group, that is, before and after operation, was performed by Paired Student t test. All tests were two-tailed and statistical significance was accepted at $P < 0.05$. All statistical analysis was performed with SAS 9.2.

Table 2 Intraoperative blood gas analysis among three groups

Variables	Sample collection time point	HFNC 40 (n = 22)	HFNC 60 (n = 20)	NPA (n = 23)
SpO$_2$	Before induction of anesthesia	98.2 ± 1.4	97.4 ± 2.0	97.5 ± 1.2
	15 min after induction of anesthesia	99.4 ± 1.0	99.6 ± 0.5	99.8 ± 0.4
	15 min after achieving position	99.6 ± 0.7	99.5 ± 0.6	99.7 ± 0.6
	End of dura suspension	99.6 ± 0.7	99.6 ± 0.5	99.8 ± 0.4
	Cortical functional mapping	99.5 ± 0.8	99.8 ± 0.3	99.9 ± 0.2
	15 min after re-induction	99.7 ± 0.7	99.6 ± 0.6	99.7 ± 0.5
PaCO$_2$	Before induction of anesthesia	39.4 ± 3.7	38.6 ± 4.7	39.5 ± 4.9
	15 min after induction of anesthesia	46.2 ± 4.6	45.8 ± 7.3	49.6 ± 6.6
	15 min after achieving position	48.0 ± 4.3	47.9 ± 6.3	50.7 ± 6.2
	End of dura suspension	50.2 ± 4.1	49.2 ± 6.1	51.7 ± 6.2
	Cortical functional mapping	44.1 ± 2.8	42.3 ± 4.9	43.6 ± 5.9
	15 min after re-induction	47.0 ± 4.3	46.0 ± 5.0	48.3 ± 5.4
PaO$_2$/FiO$_2$	Before induction of anesthesia	451.8 ± 69.4	421.9 ± 112.7	447.8 ± 64.9
	15 min after induction of anesthesia	475.5 ± 81.7	496.00 ± 80.54	332.1 ± 115.0[*#]
	15 min after achieving position	500.5 ± 93.6	499.45 ± 73.21	376.9 ± 92.1[*#]
	End of dura suspension	477.6 ± 103.8	464.2 ± 90.8	384.3 ± 98.6[*#]
	Cortical functional mapping	475.0 ± 106.1	465.4 ± 78.0	275.1 ± 92.8[*#]
	15 min after re-induction	488.1 ± 100.4	494.7 ± 81.0	315.6 ± 93.9[*#]

Data were expressed as mean ± SD. *$P < 0.05$ compared with HFNC 40 group; #$P < 0.05$ compared with HFNC 60 group. HFNC: high-flow nasal cannula; NPA: nasopharyngeal airway

Table 3 $PaCO_2$ alteration at the end of dura suspension compared to before surgery

Group	Sample Number	Difference (Mean ± SD)	Median (Interquartile range)	P value
HFNC 40	22	10.80 ± 4.40	10.75 (6.50,13.90)	< 0.001[a]
HFNC 60	20	10.60 ± 3.91	11.00 (6.95,12.85)	< 0.001[a]
NPA	23	12.25 ± 5.10	12.50 (8.10,14.90)	< 0.001[a]

[a]Compared to the value before surgery. HFNC: high-flow nasal cannula
NPA nasopharyngeal airway

Results
Baseline characteristics
This study enrolled 65 patients who underwent awake craniotomy and supplied oxygen via HFNC or NPA. Baseline characteristics of patients were presented in Table 1. There was no significant difference in age, gender ratio, BMI, presence of epilepsy or hypertension, and types of surgery among three groups (Table 1).

Intraoperative data of the patients using HFNC or NPA devices
Blood gas analysis
There were no significant differences in SpO_2 and $PaCO_2$ at various time points during surgery among HFNC 40, HFNC 60 and NPA groups (Table 2). However, patients using HFNC 40 or HFNC 60 treatment achieved higher PaO_2/FiO_2 than patients using the nasopharyngeal airway at various time points (HFNC 40 vs. NPA or HFNC 60 vs. NPA, all $P < 0.05$, Table 2). In addition, in this study, mild to moderate sedation generated high but acceptable $PaCO_2$ level in all three groups at the end of dura suspension although the differences of $PaCO_2$ before and after the anesthesia were significant in all three groups (HFNC 40: 10.80 ± 4.40; HFNC 60: 10.60 ± 3.91; NPA: 12.25 ± 5.10, $P < 0.01$, Table 3).

Brain relaxation score and gastric antral volume
There were no differences in Brain Relaxation Score at the end of the dura suspension and during the period of cortical functional mapping among the three groups (Table 4). Furthermore, no differences were noted in gastric antral volume among the three groups as well as before and after operation in any of the three groups (Table 4).

Anesthesia duration, time that patients took to wake up and the time that patients maintained awake
There were no differences in anesthesia duration and the time that patients took to wake up spontaneously among the three groups (Table 5). However, the awake time maintained in the patients receiving HFNC 60 treatment (141.5 [98.0, 198.5]) was longer than that in the patients received HFNC 40 (105.0 [75.0, 136.0], $P < 0.05$, Table 5) or NPA treatment (99.0 [85.0, 113.0], $P < 0.05$, Table 5), respectively.

Total sedative drugs used by patients
There were no differences in the total dose of dexmidiatomidine, propofol or remifentanil used throughout the whole surgery among the three groups ($P > 0.05$, Table 6).

Incidence of adverse events
The incidence of respiratory tract obstruction in NPA group was 43% (10 out of 23 patients), which was significantly higher than that in HFNC 40 (3 out of 22 patients, 13%, $P < 0.05$) or HFNC 60 group (1 out of 20 patients, 5%, $P < 0.05$, Table 7). No patient presented airway injury (blood or bloody secretion found on the tube of NPA or in the patients' mouth) in HFNC 40 or HFNC 60 group (Table 7). However, 6 patients in the NPA group suffered from airway injury, which was significantly higher than that in the patients using HFNC (all $P < 0.05$, Table 7). Three patients in HFNC 40 group, five patients in HFNC 60 group, and six patients in NPA group presented increased Brain Relaxation Score, and appropriate treatment, including mannitol infusion, body position change (head high and feet low), or decreased dose of anesthesia drugs, was required to reduce intracranial pressure. There were no differences in the incidence of intracranial pressure enhancement among the three groups ($P > 0.05$, Table 7).

Discussion
To our knowledge, this was the first study evaluating the efficacy and safety of HFNC application in the anesthesia management for awake craniotomy. As compared with NPA group, HFNC 40 or HFNC

Table 4 Brain Relaxation Score and gastric antral volume among three groups

Group	Brain Relaxation Score		Gastric antral volume (L)	
	End of dura suspension	Functional mapping	Preoperative	Postoperative
HFNC 40 (*n* = 22)	7.9 ± 1.6	8.6 ± 0.8	1.6 ± 0.9	2.0 ± 0.4
HFNC 60 (*n* = 20)	7.3 ± 1.3	8.7 ± 2.1	1.7 ± 0.4	2.1 ± 0.4
NPA (*n* = 23)	7.0 ± 1.9	8.1 ± 1.1	1.6 ± 0.3	1.9 ± 0.4

Data were expressed as mean ± SD. There was no significant difference in any pair of comparison. L: liter; HFNC: high-flow nasal cannula; NPA: nasopharyngeal airway

Table 5 Comparison of anesthesia duration, time that patients took to wake up and the time that patients maintained awake

Variables	HFNC 40 (n = 22)	HFNC 60 (n = 20)	NPA (n = 23)
Anesthesia Duration (min)	366.5 (300.0, 3933.0)	380 (321.5407.5)	385.0 (340.0,404.0)
Time patients took to wake up (min)	8.0 (6.0,12.0)	7.0 (6.0,11.0)	8.0 (7.0,13.0)
Awakening Duration (min)	105.0 (75.0,136.0)	141.5 (98.0,198.5) [*]	99.0 (85.0,113.0) [#]

Data were expressed as median (interquartile range). *$P < 0.05$ compared with HFNC 40; #$P < 0.05$ compared with HFNC 60. HFNC: high-flow nasal cannula; NPA: nasopharyngeal airway

60 treatment resulted in similar physiological response including intraoperative SpO_2 and $PaCO_2$, Brain Relaxation Score at the end of dura suspension or during the period of cortical functional mapping, and the gastric antral volume before and after anesthesia. However, both HFNC 40 and HFNC 60 treatments achieved higher PaO_2/FiO_2 ratio than NPA did. Furthermore, neither HFNC 40 nor HFNC 60 treatment caused respiratory tract injury while NPA did cause the injury. In addition, less airway obstruction occurred in the patients given HFNC 40 or 60, and longer awake time was observed in the patients with HFNC 60.

In recent years, HFNC has become a world-wide popular strategy in clinical practice for the delivery of humidified and heated oxygen in the treatment of the critically ill patient who requires high inspiratory oxygen therapy [9]. It has been reported that humidified high flow oxygen may benefit not only mucociliary clearance and mobilization of respiratory secretions [27, 28], but also increasing patient comfort and reducing mucus injury [10, 11, 18, 23, 29, 30]. Furthermore, it does not impede mobility, oral intake, or speaking [31, 32]. Consistent with these studies, in the current study, neither HFNC 40 nor HFNC 60 treatment resulted in airway injury, while 26% of patients in NPA group presented airway injury. Furthermore, patients given HFNC 40 or 60 presented lower incidence of airway obstruction as compared with patients given NPA. This advantage of HFNC may be due to the increased nasopharyngeal pressure generated by high flow oxygen. In support of this concept, a similar phenomenon was observed in McGinley's study [33]. They reported that high flow oxygen alleviated obstructive apnea-hypopnea syndrome in 11 patients [33]. This phenomenon could be associated with the enhanced nasopharyngeal pressure at the

end of exhalation, which resulted in decreased airway subsidence and subsequently relieved respiratory obstruction [15, 34, 35].

In this study, high flow oxygen generated acceptable $PaCO_2$ and desired PaO_2. Although three patients in the HFNC 40 group presented increased $PaCO_2$, it dropped to normal range when the oxygen flow was increased to 60 L/min, indicating that HFNC could generate a certain degree of continuous positive airway pressure (CPAP)-like effect, which depended on both flow rate and mouth position (open versus closed) [14]. Nevertheless, $PaCO_2$ level was significantly increased in all three treatment groups at each checking time point without significant differences among the three groups, suggesting $PaCO_2$ could be affected by multiple factors in addition to the oxygen flow amount, and thus, it should be closely monitored by the Anethesiologist during the process of awake craniotomy.

The intracranial pressure was assessed by surgeons subjectively and expressed as Brain Relaxation Score in this study. During the processes of dura suspending and tumor resection, Brain Relaxation Score in both HFNC groups was maintained at the level that surgeons desired to have, suggesting intracranial pressure was not significantly affected by high flow oxygen inhalation.

In this study, all patients maintained spontaneous breath throughout the surgical process. One of the adverse effects of high flow oxygen inhalation could be gastric discomfort. Therefore, gastric antral volumes before and after anesthesia were compared among the three groups. We found that gastric antral volume did not change after anesthesia in any of the study groups, suggesting that HFNC do not lead to gas accumulation in the stomach and cause gastric discomfort. Furthermore, none of the HFNC patient needed invasive airway device

Table 6 Total sedative medications used for the patients

Medications	HFNC 40 (n = 22)	HFNC 60 (n = 20)	NPA (n = 23)
Dexmediatomidine (μg)	76.3 (67.6,83.2)	80.5 (59.7102.4)	82.0 (63.0,115.0)
Remifentanil (mg)	0.43 (0.35,0.48)	0.39 (0.27,0.51)	0.45 (0.36,0.56)
Propofol (mg)	403.5 (318.0,575.0)	397.25 (340.0,608.0)	442.0 (273.0,500.0)

Data were expressed as median (interquartile range). HFNC: high-flow nasal cannula; NPA: nasopharyngeal airway

Table 7 Incidence of adverse events among three groups

Adverse events	Variable level	HFNC 40 (n = 22)	HFNC 60 (n = 20)	NPA (n = 23)
Obstruction of upper airway	No	19 (86.3)	19 (95.0)	13 (56.5)
	Yes	3 (13.6)*	1 (5.0)*	10 (43.5)
Airway injury	No	22 (100.0)	20 (100.0)	17 (73.9)
	Yes	0 (0.0)*	0 (0.0)*	6 (26.1)
Requiring treatment for increased Brain Relaxation Score	No	19 (86.4)	15 (75.0)	17 (73.9)
	Yes	3 (13.6)	5 (25.0)	6 (26.1)

*P < 0.05 compared with NPA. HFNC: high-flow nasal cannula; NPA: nasopharyngeal airway. "Obstruction of upper airway" was defined as no airflow, apnea or snoring due to partial airway obstruction. "Airway injury" was defined as blood or bloody secretion was found on the tube of NPA or in the patients' mouth

during the surgery. To maintain the patient's sedation depth during the surgery, doses of anesthetics were adjusted according to the BIS value and the OAA/S score, which was satisfied by the sugeons and met the requirement of anesthesia management.

We recommended that initial flow rate be set at 40 L/min, which could be increased during the operation, if the patient have upper airway obstruction or other complications. When the upper airway obstruction cannot be relieved by increasing the inspired flow or position adjustment, airway management device (such as nasopharynx or oropharyngeal airway) must be immediately applied.

Conclusion

The current study demonstrated that application of HFNC 40 or 60 during awake craniotomy resulted in higher ratio of PaO_2/FiO_2, longer awaken time (HFNC 60), but less airway injury or obstruction compared to that of NPA. These findings suggested that nasal high-flow oxygen inhalation device can be safely and effectively used in the anesthesia management for awake craniotomy. However, findings of the current study should be confirmed in the morbid obesity patients in the future.

Abbreviations
HFNC: High-flow nasal cannula; LA: Local antiesthetic; BMI: Body mass index; CSA: The cross-sectional area; CPAP: Continuous positive airway pressure

Acknowledgments
None.

Authors' contributions
HG designed the study and was involved in revising the manuscript. PY and QL were involved in writing the manuscript. PY, QL, ZY, LC, XH, HG collected the data and performed the data analysis. PY, QL, ZY contributed to the interpretation of the data and the completion of figures and tables. All authors reviewed and approved the final version of the manuscript.

Author details
[1]Department of Anesthesiology, Huashan Hospital, Fudan University, No.12 Wulumuqi Zhong Road, Shanghai 200040, China. [2]Department of Anesthesiology, Shanghai Jiahui International Hospital, Shanghai 200000, China.

References
1. Sahjpaul RL. Awake craniotomy: controversies, indications and techniques in the surgical treatment of temporal lobe epilepsy. Can J Neurol Sci. 2000;27 Suppl 1:S55–63 discussion S92–56.
2. Skucas AP, Artru AA. Anesthetic complications of awake craniotomies for epilepsy surgery. Anesth Analg. 2006;102(3):882–7.
3. Picht T, Kombos T, Gramm HJ, Brock M, Suess O. Multimodal protocol for awake craniotomy in language cortex tumour surgery. Acta Neurochir. 2006; 148(1):127–37 discussion 137-128.
4. Sivasankar C, Schlichter RA, Baranov D, Kofke WA. Awake craniotomy: a new airway approach. Anesth Analg. 2016;122(2):509–11.
5. Murata H, Nagaishi C, Tsuda A, Sumikawa K. Laryngeal mask airway supreme for asleep-awake-asleep craniotomy. Br J Anaesth. 2010;104(3):389–90.
6. Deras P, Moulinie G, Maldonado IL, Moritz-Gasser S, Duffau H, Bertram L. Intermittent general anesthesia with controlled ventilation for asleep-awake-asleep brain surgery: a prospective series of 140 gliomas in eloquent areas. Neurosurgery. 2012;71(4):764–71.
7. Cai T, Gao P, Shen Q, di Zhang Z, Yao Y, Ji Q. Oesophageal naso-pharyngeal catheter use for airway management in patients for awake craniotomy. Br J Neurosurg. 2013;27(3):396–7.
8. Audu PB, Loomba N. Use of cuffed oropharyngeal airway (COPA) for awake intracranial surgery. J Neurosurg Anesthesiol. 2004;16(2):144–6.
9. Zhang J, Lin L, Pan K, Zhou J, Huang X. High-flow nasal cannula therapy for adult patients. J Int Med Res. 2016;44(6):1200–11.
10. Spoletini G, Alotaibi M, Blasi F, Hill NS. Heated humidified high-flow nasal oxygen in adults: mechanisms of action and clinical implications. Chest. 2015;148(1):253–61.
11. Roca O, Riera J, Torres F, Masclans JR. High-flow oxygen therapy in acute respiratory failure. Respir Care. 2010;55(4):408–13.
12. Kubicka ZJ, Limauro J, Darnall RA. Heated, humidified high-flow nasal cannula therapy: yet another way to deliver continuous positive airway pressure? Pediatrics. 2008;121(1):82–8.
13. Sztrymf B, Messika J, Bertrand F, Hurel D, Leon R, Dreyfuss D, Ricard JD. Beneficial effects of humidified high flow nasal oxygen in critical care patients: a prospective pilot study. Intensive Care Med. 2011;37(11):1780–6.
14. Groves N, Tobin A. High flow nasal oxygen generates positive airway pressure in adult volunteers. Aust Crit Care. 2007;20(4):126–31.
15. Parke R, McGuinness S, Eccleston M. Nasal high-flow therapy delivers low level positive airway pressure. Br J Anaesth. 2009;103(6):886–90.
16. Moller W, Celik G, Feng S, Bartenstein P, Meyer G, Oliver E, Schmid O, Tatkov S. Nasal high flow clears anatomical dead space in upper airway models. J Appl Physiol (1985). 2015;118(12):1525–32.
17. Dewan NA, Bell CW. Effect of low flow and high flow oxygen delivery on exercise tolerance and sensation of dyspnea. A study comparing the transtracheal catheter and nasal prongs. Chest. 1994;105(4):1061–5.
18. Dysart K, Miller TL, Wolfson MR, Shaffer TH. Research in high flow therapy: mechanisms of action. Respir Med. 2009;103(10):1400–5.
19. Diaz-Lobato S, Folgado MA, Chapa A, Mayoralas Alises S. Efficacy of high-flow oxygen by nasal cannula with active humidification in a patient with acute respiratory failure of neuromuscular origin. Respir Care. 2013;58(12):e164–7.
20. Rochwerg B, Granton D, Wang DX, Helviz Y, Einav S, Frat JP, Mekontso-Dessap A, Schreiber A, Azoulay E, Mercat A, et al. High flow nasal cannula compared with conventional oxygen therapy for acute hypoxemic respiratory failure: a systematic review and meta-analysis. Intensive Care Med. 2019;45(5):563–72.

21. Kang MG, Kim K, Ju S, Park HW, Lee SJ, Koh JS, Hwang SJ, Hwang JY, Bae JS, Ahn JH, et al. Clinical efficacy of high-flow oxygen therapy through nasal cannula in patients with acute heart failure. J Thorac Dis. 2019;11(2):410–7.

22. Carratala Perales JM, Llorens P, Brouzet B, Albert Jimenez AR, Fernandez-Canadas JM, Carbajosa Dalmau J, Martinez Beloqui E, Ramos Forner S. High-flow therapy via nasal cannula in acute heart failure. Rev Esp Cardiol. 2011; 64(8):723–5.

23. Parke RL, McGuinness SP, Dixon R, Jull A. Protocol for a randomised controlled trial of nasal high flow oxygen therapy compared to standard care in patients following cardiac surgery: the HOT-AS study. Int J Nurs Stud. 2012;49(3):338–44.

24. Nicolet J, Poulard F, Baneton D, Rigal JC, Blanloeil Y. High-flow nasal oxygen for severe hypoxemia after cardiac surgery. Ann Fr Anesth Reanim. 2011; 30(4):331–4.

25. Deitch K, Chudnofsky CR, Dominici P, Latta D, Salamanca Y. The utility of high-flow oxygen during emergency department procedural sedation and analgesia with propofol: a randomized, controlled trial. Ann Emerg Med. 2011;58(4):360–4 e363.

26. Cubillos J, Tse C, Chan VW, Perlas A. Bedside ultrasound assessment of gastric content: an observational study. Can J Anaesth. 2012;59(4):416–23.

27. Chanques G, Constantin JM, Sauter M, Jung B, Sebbane M, Verzilli D, Lefrant JY, Jaber S. Discomfort associated with underhumidified high-flow oxygen therapy in critically ill patients. Intensive Care Med. 2009;35(6):996–1003.

28. Hasani A, Chapman TH, McCool D, Smith RE, Dilworth JP, Agnew JE. Domiciliary humidification improves lung mucociliary clearance in patients with bronchiectasis. Chron Respir Dis. 2008;5(2):81–6.

29. Ward JJ. High-flow oxygen administration by nasal cannula for adult and perinatal patients. Respir Care. 2013;58(1):98–122.

30. Maggiore SM, Idone FA, Vaschetto R, Festa R, Cataldo A, Antonicelli F, Montini L, De Gaetano A, Navalesi P, Antonelli M. Nasal high-flow versus Venturi mask oxygen therapy after extubation. Effects on oxygenation, comfort, and clinical outcome. Am J Respir Crit Care Med. 2014;190(3):282–8.

31. Peters SG, Holets SR, Gay PC. High-flow nasal cannula therapy in do-not-intubate patients with hypoxemic respiratory distress. Respir Care. 2013; 58(4):597–600.

32. Roca O, Hernandez G, Diaz-Lobato S, Carratala JM, Gutierrez RM, Masclans JR. Spanish multidisciplinary Group of High Flow Supportive Therapy in a: current evidence for the effectiveness of heated and humidified high flow nasal cannula supportive therapy in adult patients with respiratory failure. Crit Care. 2016;20(1):109.

33. McGinley BM, Patil SP, Kirkness JP, Smith PL, Schwartz AR, Schneider H. A nasal cannula can be used to treat obstructive sleep apnea. Am J Respir Crit Care Med. 2007;176(2):194–200.

34. Badiee Z, Eshghi A, Mohammadizadeh M. High flow nasal cannula as a method for rapid weaning from nasal continuous positive airway pressure. Int J Prev Med. 2015;6:33.

35. Jeong JH, Kim DH, Kim SC, Kang C, Lee SH, Kang TS, Lee SB, Jung SM, Kim DS. Changes in arterial blood gases after use of high-flow nasal cannula therapy in the ED. Am J Emerg Med. 2015;33(10):1344–9.

12

Impact of changes in head position during head and neck surgery on the depth of tracheal tube intubation in anesthetized children

Siyi Yan and Huan Zhang[*]

Abstract

Background: The classic formula has been used to estimate the depth of tracheal tube intubation in children for decades. However, it is unclear whether this formula is applicable when the head and neck position changes intraoperatively.

Methods: We prospectively reviewed the data of 172 well-developed children aged 2–12 years (64.0% boys) who underwent head and neck surgery under general anesthesia. The distances from the tracheal carina to the endotracheal tube tip (CT), from the superior margin of the endotracheal tube tip to the vocal cord posterior commissure (CV), and from the tracheal carina to the posterior vocal commissure (TV) were measured in the sniffing position (maximum), neutral head, and maximal head flexion positions.

Results: Average CT and CV in the neutral head position were 4.33 cm and 10.4 cm, respectively. They increased to 5.43 cm and 11.3 cm, respectively, in the sniffing position, and to 3.39 cm and 9.59 cm, respectively, in the maximal flexion position (all P-values < 0.001). TV remained unchanged and was only dependent on age. After stratifying patients by age, similar results were observed with other distances. CT and CV increased by 1.099 cm and 0.909 cm, respectively, when head position changed from neutral head to sniffing position, and decreased by 0.947 cm and 0.838 cm, respectively, when head position changed from neutral head to maximal flexion.

Conclusion: Change in head position can influence the depth of tracheal tube intubation. Therefore, the estimated depth should be corrected according to the surgical head position.

Keywords: Head and neck surgery, Depth of Oral trachea cannula, Position changes, Tracheal tube intubation, Children

Background

Inappropriate placement of tracheal tube can lead to incidences of perioperative respiratory complications in pediatric patients [1, 2]. If the tracheal tube is placed too shallow, the catheter cuff is directly clamped onto the vocal cords, causing air leakage during mechanical ventilation, leakage of oropharynx secretions, and entry of blood from the surgical field into the airway, which results in

aspiration pneumonia or vocal cord damage, and even hoarseness. In contrast, if the tracheal tube is placed too deep, it might damage the tracheal carina or cause endobronchial intubation, possibly resulting in single lung ventilation, hypoxemia, and finally, lung damage.

There are several simple formulas to calculate the depth of orotracheal intubation in children over 1 year of age, which are mainly based on body weight, body length, and age. All these formulas have been widely used in clinical practice for many decades. However, a recent meta-analysis of 16 published studies found that

* Correspondence: btchmz@163.com
Department of Anesthesiology, Beijing Tsinghua Changgung Hospital, No.168, LiTang Road, ChangPing District, Beijing, China

only 81% of catheter placements after orotracheal cannulation were appropriate when using the advanced pediatric life support (APLS) [3], and that the rate of catheter tip malposition was up to 74% [4]. It has been reported that intraoperative changes in head position might be one of the causes for tracheal tube shifts [5–7]. In general, in the head flexion position, if the tip of the tracheal tube moves toward the tracheal carina, it may cause endobronchial intubation and single lung ventilation. In contrast, in the maximal head flexion position, if the tracheal tube shifts toward the glottis, tracheal tube prolapse may occur. Moreover, the available formulas are only appropriate for intubation under relatively fixed head-neck positions, mostly the neutral head position. Moreover, to date, there is no specific formula to estimate the intubation depth for pediatric patients when the head-neck position changes during surgery. Therefore, we conducted a prospective study on 172 Chinese children to quantify the impacts of intraoperative head-neck position changes on the depth of oral tracheal tube intubation and attempted to create an appropriate formula for those surgical situations. All included children were in the top 3 percentile of growth.

Methods

Participants

This was a prospective study, which included 172 children aged 2–12 years (110 boys and 62 girls) who underwent head and neck surgery with elective general anesthesia in Beijing Tsinghua Chang Gung Hospital from December 2015 to December 2017. For each age group, 13–19 children were included. All children were well-developed, and their height and weight were above the 3rd percentile of the growth curve according to the growth and development study of children in China [8]. Among them, 160 underwent ear, nose, and throat surgery, 7 children underwent orthopedic surgery (facial excision, skin dilator implantation), and 5 children underwent external surgery (intracranial tumor resection). Children who had at least one of the following conditions were excluded: 1) limited head movement, 2) had airway dysplasia (such as airway stenosis, tracheoesophageal fistula), 3) American Society of Anesthesiologists score of III or more.

The study protocol complied with the Helsinki Declaration and was discussed and approved by the ethics committee of Beijing Tsinghua Chang Gung Hospital. The guardian of each child provided signed informed consent.

Data collection and measurements

We extracted and collected the following general information from the electronic medical records of the patients during the perioperative period: sex, age, height, body weight, surgical type, and adverse effects. Routine records and measurements taken before and during the operation, including vital signs, electrocardiography information, percutaneous oxygen saturation, and noninvasive blood pressure, were also recorded.

Routine general anesthesia was induced in for each patient by slow intravenous injection of sufentanil (0.2–0.3 µg/kg), propofol (2 mg/kg), and rocuronium (0.6 mg/kg). The tracheal tube was inserted according to the depth calculated using the APLS formula—(age/2 + 12) cm—and fixed using tape. Anesthesia was maintained with 1.5–3.0% sevoflurane inhalation (minimum alveolar concentration was maintained between 1.5–2.0), as well as continuous infusion of 2–4 mg/kg/h propofol and 0.1 µg/kg/min of remifentanil using a microinjection pump; sufentanil was injected intermittently. The following breathing parameters were set: tidal volume, 8–10 mL/kg; respiratory rate, 16–26 times/min; end-tidal carbon dioxide, 35–45 mmHg, and intraoperative oxygen concentration, 60%.

The children were in the supine position and underwent a fiberoptic bronchoscopy. The distances from the tracheal carina to the endotracheal tube tip (CT), from the superior margin of the endotracheal tube tip cuff to the vocal cord posterior commissure (CV), and between the trachea carina and the posterior vocal commissure (TV or airway length), were measured in the sniffing, median head-neck, and maximum flexion head-neck positions. The surgical head positions are shown in Fig. 1, while the measured distances are shown in Fig. 2.

Statistical analyses

We calculated the mean ± standard deviation or median (interquartile range) for continuous variables (age, weight, height, BMI, depth of intubation, CT, and TV/airway length) and frequency (percentage) for categorical variables (sex, type of surgery, tracheal prolapse, postoperative hoarseness, and bronchial intubation/single lung ventilation). We compared the differences between the distance (CT, CV, and TV) in the sniffing and maximal head flexion positions with those in the neutral head position using paired t-test. Considering the multiple comparisons, significance was set at P-value < 0.025 (Bonferroni correction). Linear regression models were used to fit the estimated models of distance on age. R-square values were calculated to evaluate the goodness of fit.

All analyses were conducted using SPSS 18.0 software (IBM, Chicago). Two-tailed P-value < 0.05 was considered statistically significant.

Results

A total of 172 children were enrolled in the study, including 110 boys and 62 girls (age, 7 years [range, 2–12

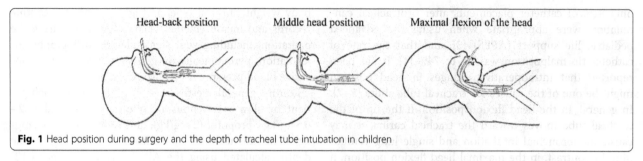

Fig. 1 Head position during surgery and the depth of tracheal tube intubation in children

years]) (Table 1). Among them, 160 children (93.0%) underwent ENT surgeries (adenotonsillectomy, myringotomy), 7 (4.07%) children underwent orthopedic surgeries (facial nevi excision, skin expander implantation), and 5 (2.91%) children underwent extracranial surgery (craniocerebral tumorectomy). All participants were well-developed children, with a median weight of 24.8 kg (11–84 kg), a median height of 128 cm (87–176 cm), and a mean BMI of 17.17 kg/m² (±3.81 kg/m²).

Distances with different intraoperative head and neck positions
In the neutral head position, the mean values of CT, CV, and TV were 4.33 cm ± 1.37 cm, 10.4 cm ± 1.47 cm, and 6.11 cm ± 1.25 cm, respectively. In the sniffing position, CT and CV values increased significantly to 5.43 cm ± 1.46 cm and 11.3 cm ± 1.49 cm, respectively, and TV shortened to 5.90 cm ± 1.20 cm (all P-values < 0.025). In contrast, under maximal head flexion position, CT and CV significantly shortened to 3.39 cm ± 1.35 cm and 9.59 cm ± 1.47 cm (all P-values < 0.025), respectively, whereas TV increased slightly to 6.20 cm ± 1.26 cm (P = 0.048) (Table 2).

On stratification by age (Fig. 3), both CT and CV increased with age. The CT and CV values increased significantly when the head position changed from neutral

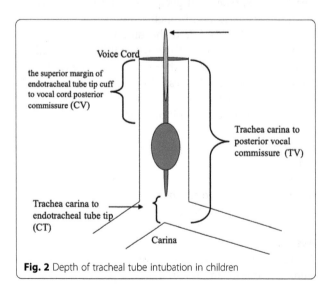

Fig. 2 Depth of tracheal tube intubation in children

head to sniffing position, while CT and CV decreased significantly when the head position changed from neutral head to maximal flexion position. The increments and reductions in CT and CV in different age groups were similar.

Effect of changes in head and neck position on airway length
Results from our linear regression models suggested that TV did not change with change in head position, but was only dependent on age—TV (cm) = 5 + 0.1 × age. P-values for all position changes in the regression models were larger than 0.05, which suggested that the position change might have no effect on TV distance (Table 3; Fig. 4). In contrast, CT and CV changed not only with age but also with the different head positions. When head position was changed from neutral head to sniffing position, both CT and CV increased by 1.099 cm (standard error, 0.122 cm) and 0.909 cm (standard error, 0.094 cm) (all P-values < 0.05), respectively. An increment in each year of age was related with an increase of 0.277 cm (standard error, 0.020 cm) of CT and 0.390 cm (standard error, 0.015 cm) of CV. When the head position was changed from middle to maximal head flexion, the reductions in CT and CV were 0.947 cm (standard error, 0.122 cm) and 0.838 cm (standard error, 0.098 cm), respectively (all P-values < 0.05). Moreover, each 1-year increase in age was related with a 0.246-cm (standard error, 0.020 cm) and 0.370-cm (standard error, 0.016 cm) increase in CT and CV values, respectively.

Adverse effects
Tracheal prolapse occurred in 9 children (5.2%), all of whom underwent ENT surgery for adenotonsillectomy and sniffing position. After increasing the intubation depth by 1–2 cm, no tracheal prolapse occurred, and all 9 patients showed good postoperative recovery; no aspiration pneumonia or hoarseness occurred postoperatively. Single lung ventilation due to excessively deep tracheal tube tip position was not observed in any of the 172 children examined.

Discussion
In this study, we compared the CT, CV, and TV values in 3 common head positions during head and neck

Table 1 Characteristics of 172 children included in this study

Characteristics	Total
n	172
Age, year	7 (2–12)
Boys, n (%)	110 (63.95)
Weight, kg	24.8 (11–84)
Height, cm	128 (87–176)
BMI, kg/m^2	17.17 ± 3.81
Types of surgery, n (%)	
ENT surgery	160 (93.0)
Orthopedic surgery	7 (4.07)
Extracranial surgery	5 (2.91)
Insertion depth (Age/2 + 12 cm), cm	15.5 (14.4, 16.9)
Distance of trachea carina to endotracheal tube tip, cm	4.1 (1.7–9.2)
Distance between trachea carina to posterior vocal commissure, cm	10.5 (7.6–13.5)
Tracheal prolapsing, n (%)	9 (5.23)
Hoarseness after surgery, n (%)	0
Bronchial intubation/single lung ventilation, n (%)	0

surgery in children. We found that CT and CV values changed significantly when the head position shifted from neutral head to sniffing position or maximal flexion. However, TV remained unchanged and was only dependent on age.

Currently, the commonly used formulas for calculating the depth of oro-tracheal intubation in children include the APLS formula, tube diameter formula, tube withdrawal method, and marker method [9, 10]. According to previous reports, the positional suitability rate of the APLS method ranges from 67.9–81% [3, 10, 11], while that reported by another study was only 26% [4]. For the tube diameter formula method, suitability rate ranged between 42 and 76.5%, while it was 73% for the tube withdrawal method [10, 11] and 53% for the catheter marker method [8, 11]. Mariano et al. [10] considered that the tube withdrawal method was more suitable than the formula and marker methods; however, the major complication is the cumbersome operation of the tube withdrawal method. Briefly, the tracheal tube is first inserted into one side of the bronchus; if the breath sound on auscultation is judged to be single lung

ventilation, then the tracheal tube is slowly withdrawn. When breath sounds of both lungs are heard on auscultation, the tracheal tube tip is placed on the carina, and the tube is further withdrawn for 2 cm to achieve a suitable depth. Another complication of this method is airway stimulation by the tracheal tube, induction of airway spasm, and airway damage; therefore, it is not a preferred procedure. The easiest intubation method is to place the black marker line of the tracheal tube on the glottis under direct vision. Since the parameter of the catheter from different manufacturers were designed according to the parameters of growth and development of the child. Therefore, whether the depth of the catheter is appropriate dependent on the parameters used, which affects the safety of intubation [12].. However, the data used by tracheal tube manufacturers are mostly derived from European and American children. Because of the ethnic differences on growth and development in children, whether these data are suitable for Chinese children remain unclear.

Our study found that the CT and CV values were dependent on the children's age and the head-neck position, and that TV remained stable and did not change with changing head positions. Generally, each 1-year increase in age was related with a 0.2-cm, 0.4-cm, and 0.1-cm increase in CT, CV, and TV values, irrespective of the head position. When the head position changed from neutral head to sniffing position, CT and CV values increased by 1 cm; in contrast, the distances decreased by 1 cm when the head position shifted from neutral head to maximal flexion. Our result was similar to that of a previous study [13],which reported that the main airway length increased by 0.95 ± 0.43 cm when the head was at the maximum hypokinesis, and the distance between the endotracheal tube tip and glottis reduced by 1.08 ± 0.47 cm, while the CT increased by 2.02 ± 0.58 cm. All these data indicate that when the head was at a sniffing position, the increased distances for the carina at the tip of the catheter was greater than the increased distance of the airway length. The length of the airway increased, but not proportionate to the movement of the tracheal tube, which caused tracheal tube prolapse after the head position changed.

In this study, 9 children (5.2%) experienced tracheal tube prolapses, all of which were during otolaryngeal surgeries. This surgery required head-neck hypokinesis

Table 2 Measured and calculated distances at 3 surgery positions in 172 children

Distances, cm (mean ± SD)	Head-back position (calculated by APLS formula)	Middle head position	Maximal flexion of the head	P-value for HB vs. MH	P-value for MF vs. MH
CT, cm	5.43 ± 1.46	4.33 ± 1.37	3.39 ± 1.35	< 0.0001	< 0.0001
CV, cm	11.3 ± 1.49	10.4 ± 1.47	9.59 ± 1.47	< 0.0001	< 0.0001
TV, cm	5.90 ± 1.20	6.11 ± 1.25	6.20 ± 1.26	< 0.0001	0.048

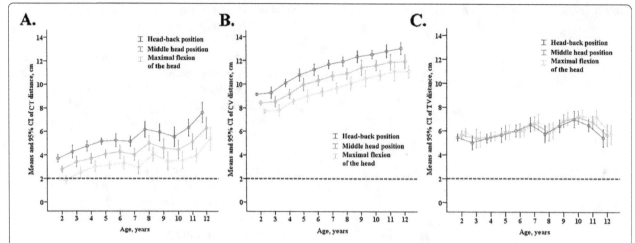

Fig. 3 Average distance from the tracheal carina to the endotracheal tube tip (**a**), distance between the tracheal carina to the posterior vocal commissure (**b**), and the distance from the superior margin of the endotracheal tube tip cuff to the vocal cord posterior commissure (**c**) in children with different ages under 3 surgical head positions. The red dotted line indicates that the distance from tip of the tube to bulge is 2 cm, which is the ideal position for the endotracheal tube tip. The error bars represent 95% CIs

for a good surgical view. J Lu et al. [14] reported that the incidence of prolapse in children undergoing adenoidectomy was 1.45% (4/276), while Wagner et al. [15] found that prolapse rate was 0.03% during extracranial surgery. During extracranial surgery, the head and neck are fixed, whereas during otolaryngeal surgeries, the surgeon often needs to change the patients' head position, which was the reason for the high rate of tracheal tube prolapse during this type of surgery. To date, much research has focused on prolapse in children with long-term intubation with a tracheal tube at NICU. Several studies have reported that 3.39–5.3% of children had unplanned extubation [16, 17], and 0.59–0.61% unplanned extubating events/100 intubation days. This evidence suggested that the high-risk factors for unplanned extubation were similar to those of intraoperative prolapse, when tracheal tube was improperly fixed with incomplete patient sedation or lack of operational expertise. This also suggested that for surgeries involving head-

neck hypokinesis changes, intubation depth calculated by the APLS formula was shallow, and that the risk of tracheal tube prolapse was higher. The required depth of tracheal tube can be deeper than the original APLS formula.

In medical practice, physicians tend to insert the tracheal tube more deeply than that recommended by the APLS formula [18]. Nicky Lau et al. [5] compared the intubation depth calculated by the classic formula by recording the actual clinical intubation depth in the neutral head position for 137 children aged 1–16 years who underwent oro-tracheal intubation, and considered the following new formula: intubation depth (cm) = age / 2 + 13, which conferred better clinical safety and practicality. However, they did not address the effect of head and neck activity on tracheal tube position. In this study, when a patient's head was flexed, the tracheal tube could be displaced to the tracheal carina, which may cause endobronchial intubation and single lung ventilation. In

Table 3 Linear regression models for 3 distances with age under 3 different surgical positions

Distances, cm	Positions		
	Head-back position	Middle head position	Maximal flexion of the head
CT, cm	CT = 3.236 + 0.298 × age	CT = 2.443 + 0.256 × age	CT = 1.650 + 0.236 × age
CV, cm	CV = 8.362 + 0.403 × age	CV = 7.647 + 0.377 × age	CV = 6.902 + 0.364 × age
TV, cm	TV = 5.125 + 0.105 × age	TV = 5.291 + 0.111 × age	TV = 5.252 + 0.129 × age
		Position changes	
	Middle head position to be Head-back position		Middle head position to be Maximal flexion of the head
CT, cm	CT = 2.290 + 0.277 × age* + 1.099 × Position change*		CT = 2.520 + 0.246 × age*-0.947 × Position change *
CV, cm	CV = 7.550 + 0.390 × age* + 0.909 × Position change *		CV = 7.693 + 0.370 × age*-0.838 × Position change *
TV, cm	TV = 5.312 + 0.108 × age*-0.208 × Position change		TV = 5.226 + 0.120 × age* + 0.90 × Position change

*P-value for regression coefficients < 0.05

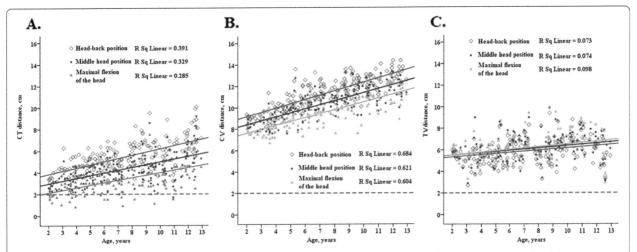

Fig. 4 Scatter plot of distance between the tracheal carina to the endotracheal tube tip (**a**), distance from the superior margin of the endotracheal tube tip cuff to the vocal cord posterior commissure (**b**), and the distance between the tracheal carina to the posterior vocal commissure (**c**) with age in children with 3 different intraoperative head positions. The red dotted line indicates that the distance from tip of the tube to the bulge is 2 cm, which is the ideal position for the endotracheal tube tip

fact, we demonstrated that during head flexion, CT shortened by 0.947 (± 0.122) cm. If an extra 1 cm depth was added to the APLS formula, the safety of the airway cannot be guaranteed.

Conclusions

Our study found that the length of the airway was dependent on children's age and position of the head and neck. Especially in children undergoing common surgery of the ear, nose, and throat, involving the head and neck hypokinesis, the incidence of tracheal tube prolapse was high. When the head position was changed from neutral head to sniffing position, a 1-cm increase was needed for CT and CV; in contrast, a 1-cm decrease was needed if head position was changed from neutral head to maximal head flexion. Additional well-designed large-scale clinical trials are warrant to confirm our conclusions.

Abbreviations
CT: the distance from the trachea carina to the endotracheal tube tip; CV: the superior margin of the endotracheal tube tip cuff to the vocal cord posterior commissure; TV: the distance from the trachea carina to the posterior vocal commissure; ASA: American Society of Anesthesiologists; SD: standard deviation

Acknowledgements
Not applicable.

Authors' contributions
YSY designed the plan, analyzed and interpreted the patient data, and collect the patients. ZH arranged the trial and manage the patients' data. They were major contributor in writing the manuscript. All authors read and approved the final manuscript.

References
1. Dronen S, Chadwick O, Nowak R. Endotracheal tip position in the arrested patient. Ann Emerg Med. 1982;11(2):116–7.
2. McCoy EP, Russell WJ, Webb RK. Accidental bronchial intubation. An analysis of AIMS incident reports from 1988 To 1994 inclusive. Anaesthesia. 1997; 52(1):24–31.
3. Boensch M, Schick V, Spelten O, Hinkelbein J. Estimation of the optimal tube length: systematic review article on published formulae for infants and children. Anaesthesist. 2016;65(2):115–21.
4. Volsko TA, McNinch NL, Prough DS, Bigham MT. Adherence to endotracheal tube depth guidelines and incidence of malposition in infants and children. Respir Care. 2018;63(9):1111–7.
5. Bloch EC, Ossey K, Ginsberg B. Tracheal intubation in children: a new method for assuring correct depth of tube placement. Anesth Analg. 1988; 67(6):590–2.
6. Weiss M, Knirsch W, Kretschmar O, Dullenkopf A, Tomaske M, Balmer C, Stutz K, Gerber AC, Berger F. Tracheal tube-tip displacement in children during head-neck movement--a radiological assessment. Br J Anaesth. 2006; 96(4):486–91.
7. Wang QS. Determination of the position of the tracheal catheter displacement caused by changes by Fiberoptic bronchoscopy in head position during pediatric anesthesia. J Clin Anesthesiol. 2001;17.
8. Li H, Ji CY, Zong XN, Zhang YQ. Height and weight standardized growth charts for Chinese children and adolescents aged 0 to 18 years. Zhonghua er ke za zhi = Chinese Journal of Pediatrics. 2009;47(7):487–92.
9. Advanced Life Support Group, Advanced Paediatric Life Support: The practical approach, 3rd edn. London; 2001.
10. Mariano ER, Ramamoorthy C, Chu LF, Chen M, Hammer GB. A comparison of three methods for estimating appropriate tracheal tube depth in children. Paediatr Anaesth. 2005;15(10):846–51.
11. Lee SU, Jung JY, Kim DK, Kwak YH, Kwon H, Cho JH, Park JW, Choi YJ. New decision formulas for predicting endotracheal tube depth in children: analysis of neck CT images. Emerg Med J. 2018;35(5):303–8.
12. Weiss M, Gerber AC, Dullenkopf A. Appropriate placement of intubation depth marks in a new cuffed paediatric tracheal tube. Br J Anaesth. 2005; 94(1):80–7.
13. Jin-Hee K, Ro YJ, Seong-Won M, Chong-Soo K, Seong-Deok K, Lee JH, Jae-Hyon B. Elongation of the trachea during neck extension in children: implications of the safety of endotracheal tubes. Anesthesia and analgesia. 2005;101(4):974–7 table of contents.

14. Lu J, Yu XZ, Qin W. Unplanned intraoperative Extubations in pediatric Adenotonsillectomy: analysis of 4 cases. Chin Clin Doct. 2013;41:51–3.
15. Wagner KM, Raskin JS, Carling NP, Felberg MA, Kanjia MK, Pan IW, Luerssen TG, Lam S. Unplanned intraoperative Extubations in pediatric neurosurgery: analysis of case series to increase patient safety. World Neurosurg. 2018;115: e1–6.
16. Al-Abdwani R, Williams CB, Dunn C, Macartney J, Wollny K, Frndova H, Chin N, Stephens D, Parshuram CS. Incidence, outcomes and outcome prediction of unplanned extubation in critically ill children: an 11year experience. J Crit Care. 2018;44:368–75.
17. Vats A, Hopkins C, Hatfield KM, Yan J, Palmer R, Keskinocak P. An airway risk assessment score for unplanned Extubation in intensive care pediatric patients. Pediatr Crit Care Med. 2017;18(7):661–6.
18. Schmidt AR, Ulrich L, Seifert B, Albrecht R, Spahn DR, Stein P. Ease and difficulty of pre-hospital airway management in 425 paediatric patients treated by a helicopter emergency medical service: a retrospective analysis. Scan J Trauma Resusc Emerg Med. 2016;24:22.

13

Effect of forced-air warming by an underbody blanket on end-of-surgery hypothermia: A propensity score-matched analysis of 5063 patients

Hiroshi Sumida[1,3]* ⓘ, Shigekazu Sugino[1], Norifumi Kuratani[2], Daisuke Konno[1], Jun-ichi Hasegawa[3] and Masanori Yamauchi[1]

Abstract

Background: Underbody blankets have recently been launched and are used by anesthesiologists for surgical patients. However, the forced-air warming effect of underbody blankets is still controversial. The aim of this study was to determine the effect of forced-air warming by an underbody blanket on body temperature in anesthetized patients.

Methods: We retrospectively analyzed 5063 surgical patients. We used propensity score matching to reduce the bias caused by a lack of randomization. After propensity score matching, the change in body temperature from before to after surgery was compared between patients who used underbody blankets (Under group) and those who used other types of warming blankets (Control group). The incidence of hypothermia (i.e., body temperature < 36.0 °C at the end of surgery) was compared between the two groups. A p value < 0.05 was considered to indicate statistical significance.

Results: We obtained 489 propensity score-matched pairs of patients from the two groups, of whom 33 and 63 had hypothermia in the Under and Control groups, respectively (odds ratio: 0.49, 95% confidence interval: 0.31–0.76, $p = 0.0013$).

Conclusions: The present study suggests that the underbody blanket may help reduce the incidence of intraoperative hypothermia and may be more efficient in warming anesthetized patients compared with other types of warming blankets.

Keywords: Forced-air warming, Underbody blanket, Propensity score matching, Anesthesia information management system, Body temperature, Intraoperative hypothermia

Background

Forced-air warming plays a critical role in warming patients during surgery [1–3]. This active warming prevents postoperative complications, such as cardiovascular [4] and major bleeding events [5, 6], and decreases the recovery time [7], hospital costs [8, 9], length of hospital stay [8, 9], and mortality [8]. Recent international guidelines (e.g., CG65 of the National Institute for Health and Care Excellence in the UK) strongly recommend use of a forced-air warming device from the time of anesthetic induction to maintain a patient temperature of at least 36.5° C [10, 11]. Efficient perioperative forced-air warming is achieved by convection of warmed air flow [12]. This effect depends on the difference between skin and ambient temperatures and the area of air flow at the skin surface [12, 13]. However, conventional forced-air warming using an over (full) body blanket cannot fully warm the entire body except during cranial or ear, nose, and throat surgery. Thus, upper or lower body blankets are typically used despite being approximately half as effective [14].

Underbody blankets have recently been launched in the market. As these blankets are more expensive than

* Correspondence: tthsumida@yahoo.co.jp
[1]Department of Anesthesiology and Perioperative Medicine, Tohoku University School of Medicine, 2-1, Seiryo-machi, Aoba-ku, Sendai, Miyagi 980-8575, Japan
[3]Department of Anesthesia, Katta General Hospital, 36 Shimoharaoki, Kuramoto, Fukuoka, Shiroishi, Miyagi 989-0231, Japan

conventional warming devices (e.g., overbody blankets or thermal mattresses with circulating water), the underbody blanket is still not popular. However, underbody blankets, together with surgical draping, enable efficient convection of airflow over the body. This warmed tent produces a larger body surface area that can be warmed by the blanket [15]. Although several prospective studies have recently reported that the underbody blanket is superior to the overbody blanket in preventing intraoperative hypothermia [16–18], its usefulness remains to be elucidated [19]. Those previous studies partially showed the efficacy of underbody blankets but under limited conditions: cardiac and abdominal surgeries. The ultimate aim of this study was to determine the effect of forced-air warming by underbody blankets in statistically matched patients undergoing different types of surgery.

Methods

This study was approved by the Institutional Review Board and Ethics Committee of Tohoku University School of Medicine (#2015-1-787, approved on March 17, 2016). We applied opt-out consent according to the recruitments of the human research ethics committees at the institutions and local law.

Study population

We retrospectively reviewed 8032 consecutive adult patients who underwent surgery in the operating room of Tohoku University Hospital between April 2014 and November 2015. Of these patients, 2669 whose body temperature at the bladder during surgery was not measured (e.g., for surgeries less than 1 h in duration) and 300 with inaccurate body temperature measurements during surgery (i.e., measurement of less than 30.0°C) were excluded from the study. The remaining 5063 patients were enrolled in the study (Fig. 1).

Warming of patients during surgery

After anesthetic induction, we initiated forced-air warming using two types of warming power units: the Bair Hugger Model 775 (3M Company, St. Paul, MN, USA) and Warm Touch 5300A (Medtronic, Minneapolis, MN, USA). We used the power units with one of four types of blankets: under full body (Bair Hugger Models 545, 585, and 635), over full body (Warm Touch Lower Body Blanket), over upper body (Warm Touch Upper Body Blanket), and over lower body (Warm Touch Lower Body Blanket) blankets. We defined each warming method as follows: under full cover (under full body warming by an under full body blanket), over full cover (over full body warming by an over full body blanket), over upper cover (over upper body warming by an over upper body blanket), over lower cover (over lower body warming by an over lower body blanket). In some

patients, the over full body blanket was used to cover only the right or left half of the body (over right cover and over left cover, respectively). Resistive heating blankets (SmartCare, Geratherm Medical AG, Geschwenda, Germany) were used during surgeries performed in a bioclean room (over heating cover). Thus, we used the following seven warming methods: under full cover, over full cover, over upper cover, over lower cover, over right cover, over left cover, and over heating cover. Nurses selected these seven warming methods, either alone or in combination, according to the surgical procedure performed and the appropriate patient position.

Data acquisition

Raw measurements of vital signs, including body temperature, were transferred onto a server (PRIMERGY TX200 S3, 2 Intel Xenon X5335 processors, 2 GB DIMM, 300 GB HDD) and saved in text format. An electronic anesthesia recording system (PrimeGaia, Nihon Kohden, Tokyo, Japan) was used to retrieve the data from the server at 2.5-min intervals and to display them, together with the patient's medical information obtained from the hospital information system, as an anesthesia record. Background information on age, sex, height, weight, American Society of Anesthesiology physical status, and type of surgery was obtained. All surgeries were classified into 11 categories defined by the Japanese Society of Anesthesiologists Committee on Operating Room Safety for closed claim studies [20]. The duration of anesthesia from start to end, method of warming (e.g., under full body, over lower body), and body temperature measurement at the bladder were obtained in CSV format from the data warehouse on the server. We assigned the patients warmed by the under full cover method to the Under group and those warmed by the other methods (i.e., all other patients except for those in the Under group) to the Control group (Fig. 1).

Statistical analysis

We used propensity score matching to reduce potential bias caused by the lack of randomization in this study. The probability (from 0 to 1) of allocation of use of the under full cover was estimated in each patient as a propensity score, based on a multivariate logistic regression model incorporating age, sex, height, weight, American Society of Anesthesiology physical status, type of surgery, duration of anesthesia, and use of one of the other six cover methods (excluding under full cover) as variables. Propensity score matching was performed by random selection of a patient in the Under group and identifying the patient who had the closest propensity score (within 0.03 on a scale of 0 to 1) in the Control group, as described previously [21]. Both before and after propensity score matching, numerical data such as

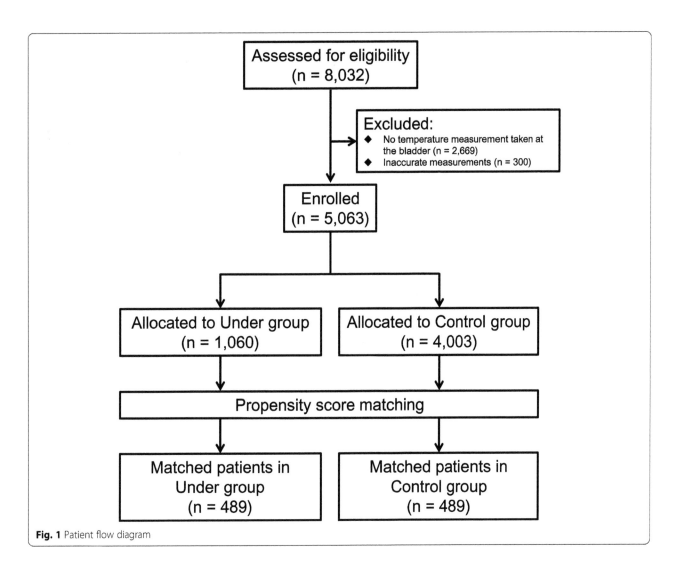

Fig. 1 Patient flow diagram

body temperature were compared between the Under and Control groups using Student's t-test or the Mann–Whitney test. Categorical data were compared between the two groups using the chi square test. The primary endpoint was the incidence of hypothermia at the end of surgery (i.e., a body temperature < 36.0°C, defined by the National Institute for Health and Care Excellence guidelines [10]), which was compared between the two groups using the chi square test. All statistical calculations were performed using SPSS software (ver. 22, IBM Corp., Chicago, IL, USA). A p value < 0.05 was considered to indicate statistical significance.

Results

Table 1 summarizes the demographic and clinical characteristics of the patients in both the Under and Control groups before propensity score matching. Figure 1 shows a flow diagram of the selection of patients into the current study. We obtained 489 propensity score-matched pairs between the Under and Control groups. Table 2 summarizes the demographic and clinical characteristics of the

patients in both groups after propensity score matching. The baseline characteristics were not significantly different between the two groups.

Of the 5063 patients in this study before matching, there were no missing data. The body temperatures [median (interquartile range)] at the start of surgery in the Under and Control groups were 36.7 (0.6)°C and 36.8 (0.6)°C, respectively (p = 0.30). In the Under group, the body temperature was 0.6°C higher at the end of surgery compared with the start of surgery. In the Control group, the temperature at the end of surgery increased 0.2°C from that at the start of surgery. There was a significant difference in body temperature at the end of surgery between the Under and Control groups (p < 0.0001, Fig. 2). After propensity score matching, 978 total matched patients were evaluated. The median (interquartile range) body temperatures of the matched patients at the start of surgery were 36.7 (0.6) and 36.8 (0.6) in the Under and Control groups, respectively (p = 0.04). At the end of

Table 1 Characteristics of the patients before propensity score matching

	Under group	Control group	Standardized difference[a]	P value
Number	1060	4003		
Age (years)	57 ± 21	54 ± 21	14%	< 0.0001
Male / female	521 / 539	2054 / 1949		0.211
Height (cm)	155 ± 21	159 ± 14	19%	< 0.0001
Weight (kg)	55 ± 17	59 ± 17	24%	< 0.0001
ASA-PS				< 0.0001
1 / 2	175 / 642	1037 / 2176		
3 / 4 / 5	231 / 12 / 0	737 / 51 / 2		
Type of surgery				< 0.0001
Craniotomy	4	330		
ENT	82	1049		
Thoracic	66	205		
Cardiovascular	81	366		
Endovascular aortic repair	72	49		
Abdominal (laparoscopic)	164	404		
Abdominal (non-laparoscopic)	447	654		
Surface of the trunk	41	387		
Orthopedic	23	380		
Spinal	71	74		
Unclassifiable	9	105		
Type of warming method				< 0.0001
Over full cover	37	1333		
Over upper cover	124	1123		
Over lower cover	237	1652		
Over right cover	5	11		
Over left cover	6	17		
Over heating cover	20	263		
Duration of anesthesia (min)	413 ± 231	307 ± 219	46%	< 0.0001

Data are presented as numbers or means ± S.D. [a]: Standardized difference for a covariate is the mean difference between the groups divided by the S.D., converted into a percentage

surgery, the body temperatures had increased by 0.5° C and 0.1°C from those at the start of surgery in the Under and Control groups, respectively. There was a significant difference in body temperature at the end of surgery between the Under and Control groups (p < 0.0001, Fig. 3).

As shown in Fig. 4, the incidence of hypothermia was identical between the Under (7%, 77/1060) and Control (7%, 274/4003) groups before matching (odds ratio: 1.07, 95% confidence interval: 0.82–1.39, p = 0.91). After matching, 33 and 63 patients had hypothermia in the Under and Control groups, respectively, with the incidence of hypothermia being significantly lower in the Under group (7%, 33/489) than in the Control group (13%, 63/489) (odds ratio: 0.49, 95% confidence interval: 0.31–0.76, p = 0.0013).

Discussion

In the present study, we first applied propensity score matching of the patients in the Under and Control groups. We then compared the incidence of intraoperative hypothermia between the two groups. The incidence of hypothermia was significantly lower in the Under group than in the Control group at the end of surgery, as suggested by a significantly higher body temperature at the end of surgery in the Under group compared with the Control group.

A few prospective studies have recently reported the efficacy of underbody blankets in patients undergoing cardiac or abdominal surgery [16–18]. Those reports showed that warming by underbody blankets resulted in an ~ 0.5°C higher body temperature compared with controls, which is consistent with the current results. In

Effect of forced-air warming by an underbody blanket on end-of-surgery hypothermia: A propensity...

95

Table 2 Characteristics of the patients after propensity score matching

	Under group	Control group	Standardized difference[a]	P value
Number	489	489		
Age (years)	57 ± 21	57 ± 20	0%	0.861
Male / female	262 / 227	291 / 198		0.061
Height (cm)	158 ± 18	159 ± 15	6%	0.409
Weight (kg)	55 ± 17	57 ± 17	12%	0.779
ASA-PS				0.247
1 / 2	95 / 277	78 / 271		
3 / 4 / 5	110 / 7 / 0	129 / 11 / 0		
Type of surgery				0.695
Craniotomy	4	6		
ENT	51	53		
Thoracic	34	41		
Cardiovascular	67	84		
Endovascular aortic repair	17	19		
Abdominal (Laparoscopic)	69	70		
Abdominal (No laparoscopic)	155	143		
Surface of the trunk	33	26		
Orthopedic	21	21		
Spinal	29	22		
Unclassifiable	9	4		
Type of warming method				0.659
Over full cover	32	38		
Over upper cover	112	97		
Over lower cover	172	178		
Over right cover	2	1		
Over left cover	4	6		
Over heating cover	17	20		
Duration of anesthesia (min)	403 ± 222	431 ± 347	8%	0.137

Data are presented as numbers or means ± S.D. [a]: Standardized difference for a covariate is the mean difference between the groups divided by the S.D., converted into a percentage. The absolute differences in the mean values of the numerical cofounders included in the matching were less than 15% of the standard deviations

the most recent report, however, Alparslan et al. showed that forced-air warming by underbody blankets was as efficient as that by upper body blankets in patients undergoing lower abdominal surgery [19]. The average intraoperative body temperatures of the patients using underbody and upper body blankets were 36.3°C and 36.1°C, respectively. The authors explained that greater heat loss via radiation occurred in the patients warmed by underbody blankets, because the upper frontal body was uncovered in their experimental conditions. However, their comparisons may have been statistically fallacious, because they used the unpaired t-test or Mann–Whitney U-test to compare the change in body temperature at each time point without using repeated-measures analysis of variance. Nevertheless, we agree with their implication that the patient profile and type of

surgery performed are limitations in the research on forced-air warming blankets.

In the current study, to reduce the bias caused by the lack of randomization, we applied propensity score matching to the data obtained retrospectively from the electronic medical records of patients who underwent various surgical procedures. The use of propensity scores should be considered when comparing two treatments in an observational design, particularly in cases of highly imbalanced treatment groups, a large number of confounders, or a low number of events [22–24]. Indeed, as shown in Table 1, there were many imbalances between the Under and Control groups, such as the baseline characteristics of the patients, type of surgery, and method of warming. Furthermore, the incidence of hypothermia, the primary endpoint, in each group was

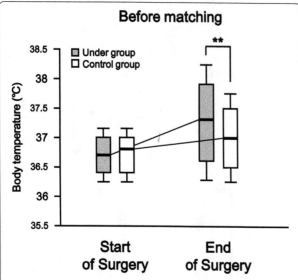

Fig. 2 Body temperatures of both groups at the start and end of surgery before propensity score matching. The box and whisker plot shows the median (bold line in box), 25th–75th percentile (top and bottom of the box), and 1.5-fold interquartile range (ends of whiskers) values. **: $P < 0.01$ vs. Control group

low (7% in both groups; Fig. 4). We recognize that the application of propensity score matching in our cohort was reasonable. As shown in Table 2, the matching was considered appropriate, because the standardized differences after matching were less than those before matching by nearly 10%, as was also described previously [24]. Only after matching did we detect a difference in the

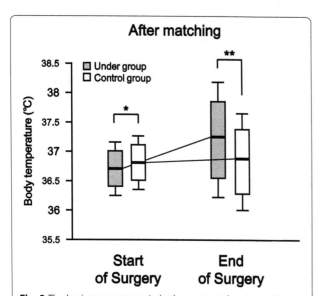

Fig. 3 The body temperatures in both groups at the start and end of surgery after propensity score matching. The box and whisker plot shows the median (bold line in box), 25th–75th percentile (top and bottom of the box), and 1.5-fold interquartile range (ends of whiskers) values. *: $P < 0.05$ vs. Control group. **: $P < 0.01$ vs. Control group

incidence of hypothermia between the matched cohorts compared with before matching (Fig. 4). In this study, we demonstrated the effects of forced-air warming using an underbody blanket.

Unexpectedly, after matching, the body temperature at the start of surgery showed a tendency to be higher in the Control group than in the Under group, although there was no significant difference between the two groups before matching (before matching: $p = 0.30$; after matching: $p = 0.04$; Figs. 2 and 3). One possible explanation for this difference is that the sex distribution changed after matching (Table 2). In the Control group, the proportions of males and females among the total patients were 51% (2054/4003) and 49% (1949/4003) before matching but 60% (291/489) and 40% (198/489) after matching, respectively. One reason for this is that the number of patients in the Control group who underwent gynecological surgery was lower before compared with after propensity score matching (data not shown). The body temperature of females may be lower than that of males [19, 25], perhaps attributed to the lower skeletal muscle mass of females, which results in a lower basal metabolic rate. However, our subgroup analysis showed no significant difference in body temperature before surgery between the male and female patients of the Control group after matching (data not shown). The underlying mechanism remains unknown under our experimental conditions.

The present study has several important limitations that should be noted. First, the cohort did not include all types of surgery, such as those lasting less than 1 h in duration. Such minor surgeries do not require temperature monitoring at the bladder. This exclusion criterion may have produced selection bias. However, if these patients were included in the analysis, the effect of warming by the underbody blanket would likely have been small. In addition, propensity score matching *per se* may introduce potential selection bias. Although we robustly matched 988 patients using a previously described method [21], the ratio of matched patients to all patients in the Control group was only 12% (489/4003). Furthermore, as described above, many of the patients who underwent gynecological surgery in the Control group were not included in the matched cohort. Thus, in the current study, selection bias may have been present. Second, the anesthesiologists and nurses changed the temperature of the forced airflow according to body temperature values during surgery. This information bias could not be minimized in our study design. In addition, propensity score matching methods ensure balance only of the measured, and not the unmeasured, confounders [24]. The variables that were not measured, such as intraoperative patient position,

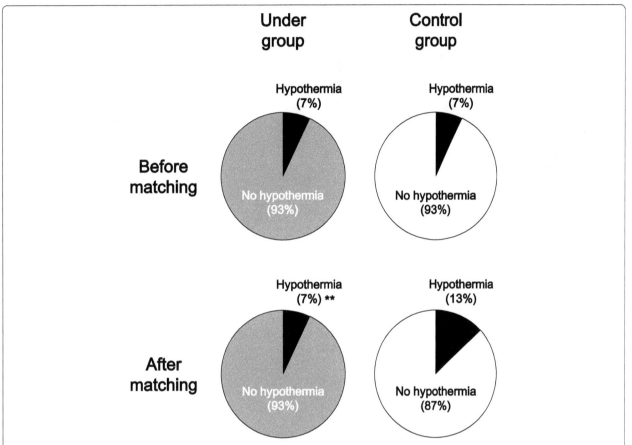

Fig. 4 The incidence of hypothermia in the Under (left panels) and Control (right panels) groups before (upper panels) and after (lower panels) propensity score matching. **: P < 0.01 vs. Control group after matching

presence of fever of unknown origin, ambient temperature, or amount of bleeding during surgery, may have influenced the interpretation of the data by introducing information bias. Taking these limitations into consideration, prospective studies with randomization to minimize confounding are needed. In our ongoing trial (UMIN Clinical Trials Registry identifier UMIN000027991), we are comparing body temperatures in female patients undergoing gynecological surgery in the lithotomy position using underbody versus upper body blankets as the warming methods (unpublished).

Conclusions

The present study suggests that underbody blankets help reduce the incidence of intra-operative hypothermia. The underbody blanket resulted in superior forced-air warming performance compared with the control warming methods.

Acknowledgements
The author (H.S.) thanks Kazuhisa Murakami, Nihon Kohden Corp., Tokyo, for his technical support in obtaining the patient data.

Authors' contributions
HS and SS designed and conducted the study. HS collected the clinical data from the patients' medical records. HS and SS analyzed and interpreted the data and wrote the draft of the manuscript. DK and J-IH helped prepare the manuscript and jointly developed the structure and arguments for the paper. NK and MY made critical revisions and contributed to writing of the manuscript. All authors approved the final manuscript.

Author details
[1]Department of Anesthesiology and Perioperative Medicine, Tohoku University School of Medicine, 2-1, Seiryo-machi, Aoba-ku, Sendai, Miyagi 980-8575, Japan. [2]Department of Anesthesia, Saitama Children's Medical Center, 1-2, Shin-toshin, Chuo-ku, Saitama City, Saitama 330-8777, Japan. [3]Department of Anesthesia, Katta General Hospital, 36 Shimoharaoki, Kuramoto, Fukuoka, Shiroishi, Miyagi 989-0231, Japan.

References
1.   Kurz A, Sessler DI, Lenhardt R. Perioperative normothermia to reduce the incidence of surgical-wound infection and shorten hospitalization. Study of Wound Infection and Temperature Group. N Engl J Med. 1996;334:1209–15.
2.   Kabbara A, Goldlust SA, Smith CE, Hagen JF, Pinchak AC. Randomized prospective comparison of forced air warming using hospital blankets versus commercial blankets in surgical patients. Anesthesiology. 2002;97:338–44.
3.   Perl T, Bräuer A, Timmermann A, Mielck F, Weyland W, Braun U. Differences among forced-air warming systems with upper body blankets are small. A randomized trial for heat transfer in volunteers. Acta Anaesthesiol Scand. 2003;47:1159–64.

4. Frank SM, Fleisher LA, Breslow MJ, Higgins MS, Olson KF, Kelly S, et al. Perioperative maintenance of normothermia reduces the incidence of morbid cardiac events. A randomized clinical trial. JAMA. 1997;277:1127–34.
5. Schmied H, Kurz A, Sessler DI, Kozek S, Reiter A. Mild hypothermia increases blood loss and transfusion requirements during total hip arthroplasty. Lancet (London, England). 1996;347:289–92.
6. Rajagopalan S, Mascha E, Na J, Sessler DI. The effects of mild perioperative hypothermia on blood loss and transfusion requirement. Anesthesiology. 2008;108:71–7.
7. Lenhardt R, Marker E, Goll V, Tschernich H, Kurz A, Sessler DI, et al. Mild intraoperative hypothermia prolongs postanesthetic recovery. Anesthesiology. 1997;87:1318–23.
8. Bush HL, Hydo LJ, Fischer E, Fantini GA, Silane MF, Barie PS. Hypothermia during elective abdominal aortic aneurysm repair: the high price of avoidable morbidity. J Vasc Surg. 1995;21:392–400.
9. Mahoney CB, Odom J. Maintaining intraoperative normothermia: a meta-analysis of outcomes with costs. AANA J. 1999;67:155–63.
10. Radauceanu DS, Dragnea D, Craig J. NICE guidelines for inadvertent peri-operative hypothermia. Anaesthesia. 2009;64:1381–2.
11. Scott AV, Stonemetz JL, Wasey JO, Johnson DJ, Rivers RJ, Koch CG, et al. Compliance with surgical care improvement project for body temperature management (SCIP Inf-10) is associated with improved clinical outcomes. Anesthesiology. 2015;123:116–25.
12. Pei L, Huang Y, Xu Y, Zheng Y, Sang X, Zhou X, et al. Effects of ambient temperature and forced-air warming on intraoperative core temperature: a factorial randomized trial. Anesthesiology. 2018;128:903–11.
13. Bräuer A, Quintel M. Forced-air warming: technology, physical background and practical aspects. Curr Opin Anaesthesiol. 2009;22:769–74.
14. Sessler DI, Moayeri A. Skin-surface warming: heat flux and central temperature. Anesthesiology. 1990;73:218–24.
15. Bräuer A, English MJM, Lorenz N, Steinmetz N, Perl T, Braun U, et al. Comparison of forced-air warming systems with lower body blankets using a copper manikin of the human body. Acta Anaesthesiol Scand. 2003;47:58–64.
16. Insler SR, Bakri MH, Nageeb F, Mascha E, Mihaljevic T, Sessler DI. An evaluation of a full-access underbody forced-air warming system during near-normothermic, on-pump cardiac surgery. Anesth Analg. 2008;106:746–50.
17. Teodorczyk JE, Heijmans JH, van Mook WNKA, Bergmans DCJJ, Roekaerts PMHJ. Effectiveness of an underbody forced warm-air blanket during coronary artery bypass surgery in the prevention of postoperative hypothermia: a prospective controlled randomized clinical trial. Open J Anesthesiol. 2012;02:65–9.
18. Pu Y, Cen G, Sun J, Gong J, Zhang Y, Zhang M, et al. Warming with an underbody warming system reduces intraoperative hypothermia in patients undergoing laparoscopic gastrointestinal surgery: a randomized controlled study. Int J Nurs Stud. 2014;51:181–9.
19. Alparslan V, Kus A, Hosten T, Ertargin M, Ozdamar D, Toker K, et al. Comparison of forced-air warming systems in prevention of intraoperative hypothermia. J Clin Monit Comput. 2018;32:343–9.
20. Kawashima Y, Takahashi S, Suzuki M, Morita K, Irita K, Iwao Y, et al. Anesthesia-related mortality and morbidity over a 5-year period in 2,363,038 patients in Japan. Acta Anaesthesiol Scand. 2003;47:809–17.
21. Connors AF, Speroff T, Dawson NV, Thomas C, Harrell FE, Wagner D, et al. The effectiveness of right heart catheterization in the initial care of critically ill patients. SUPPORT investigators. JAMA. 1996;276:889–97.
22. Rubin DB. Estimating causal effects form large data sets using propensity scores. Ann Intern Med. 1997;127:757–63.
23. Joffe MM, Rosenbaum PR. Invited commentary: propensity scores. Am J Epidemiol. 1999;150:327–33.
24. Sainani KL. Propensity scores: uses and limitations. PM&R. 2012;4:693–7.
25. Ng SF, Oo CS, Loh KH, Lim PY, Chan YH, Ong BC. A comparative study of three warming interventions to determine the most effective in maintaining perioperative normothermia. Anesth Analg. 2003;96:171–6.

14

The effects of labor on airway outcomes with Supreme™ laryngeal mask in women undergoing cesarean delivery under general anesthesia

Ming Jian Lim[1], Hon Sen Tan[1,2], Chin Wen Tan[1,2], Shi Yang Li[3], Wei Yu Yao[3], Yong Jing Yuan[4], Rehena Sultana[5] and Ban Leong Sng[1,2*] (iD)

Abstract

Background: Pregnancy is associated with higher incidence of failed endotracheal intubation and is exacerbated by labor. However, the influence of labor on airway outcomes with laryngeal mask airway (LMA) for cesarean delivery is unknown.

Methods: This is a secondary analysis of a prospective cohort study on LMA use during cesarean delivery. Healthy parturients who fasted > 4 h undergoing Category 2 or 3 cesarean delivery with Supreme™ LMA (sLMA) under general anesthesia were included. We excluded parturients with BMI > 35 kg/m^2, gastroesophageal reflux disease, or potentially difficult airway (Mallampati score of 4, upper respiratory tract or neck pathology). Anesthesia and airway management reflected clinical standard at the study center. After rapid sequence induction and cricoid pressure, sLMA was inserted as per manufacturer's recommendations. Our primary outcome was time to effective ventilation (time from when sLMA was picked up until appearance of end-tidal carbon dioxide capnography), and secondary outcomes include first-attempt insertion failure, oxygen saturation, ventilation parameters, mucosal trauma, pulmonary aspiration, and Apgar scores. Differences between labor status were tested using Student's t-test, Mann-Whitney U test, or Fisher's exact test, as appropriate. Quantitative associations between labor status and outcomes were determined using univariate logistic regression analysis.

Results: Data from 584 parturients were analyzed, with 37.8% in labor. Labor did not significantly affect time to effective ventilation (mean (SD) for labor: 16.0 (5.75) seconds; no labor: 15.3 (3.35); mean difference: -0.65 (95%CI: − 1.49 to 0.18); $p = 0.1262$). However, labor was associated with increased first-attempt insertion failure and blood on sLMA surface. No reduction in oxygen saturation or pulmonary aspiration was noted.

Conclusions: Although no significant increase in time to effective ventilation was noted, labor may increase the number of insertion attempts and oropharyngeal trauma with sLMA use for cesarean delivery in parturients at low risk of difficult airway. Future studies should investigate the effects of labor on LMA use in high risk parturients.

(Continued on next page)

* Correspondence: sng.ban.leong@singhealth.com.sg
[1]Department of Women's Anesthesia, KK Women's and Children's Hospital, 100 Bukit Timah Road, Singapore 229899, Singapore
[2]Duke-NUS Medical School, 8 College Road, Singapore 169857, Singapore

(Continued from previous page)

Keywords: Obstetrics, Mallampati score, Airway

Background

Pregnancy is associated with higher risk of failed endotracheal intubation, with an estimated incidence of 1:250 compared to 1:2000 in non-pregnant patients [1, 2]. Although recent reports from the Mothers and Babies: Reducing Risk through Audits and Confidential Enquiries (MBRRACE-UK) have shown a reduction in anesthesia-related deaths [3], hypoxia resulting from failure to intubate or ventilate is a consistent cause of maternal mortality. Airway-related mortality occurs in 2.3 per 100,000 cesarean deliveries under general anesthesia compared to 1 per 180,000 in the general surgical population [4], which may be exacerbated by declining use of general anesthesia for cesarean delivery and concomitant reduction in training and experience with endotracheal intubation in obstetrics [4, 5].

Labor has been associated with anatomical changes that increase the likelihood of difficult intubation, and Mallampati scores after labor were 1 to 2 grades higher compared to pre-labor, with a greater proportion of parturients possessing Mallampati scores of 3 or 4 [6, 7]. The Mallampati score is a common bedside airway assessment used to predict difficult intubation [8]; with scores of 3 or 4 corresponding to relative risks of 7.6 and 11.3 for difficult intubation compared to a score of 1, respectively [9]. Moreover, labor significantly decreases oropharyngeal area and volume, which may further impede endotracheal intubation [6]. These anatomical changes are attributed to laryngeal edema arising from rapid intravenous fluid administration, antidiuretic effects of oxytocin, and prolonged straining during labor [10].

Despite concerns that labor may increase the risk of difficult endotracheal intubation, to our knowledge the effects of labor on laryngeal mask airway (LMA) use during cesarean delivery have not been elucidated. This is of particular importance given the recent recommendations of the LMA as a second-line or "rescue" airway device in the event of failed endotracheal intubation [1, 2, 11–13]. In fact, obstetric airway management guidelines have specifically recommended the use of second-generation LMAs to maintain ventilation and oxygenation in the event of failed endotracheal intubation [14]. Second-generation LMAs such as Supreme™ contain a separate channel to isolate the gastrointestinal tract with high sealing pressures and reduce the risk of pulmonary aspiration if they are well positioned [15–17]. Subsequent studies have demonstrated the efficacy and safety of the Supreme™ LMA (sLMA) as an alternative to endotracheal intubation for selected parturients undergoing cesarean delivery [18–20]. However, notwithstanding the utility of the LMA as a rescue airway device, LMA use in pregnant parturients is associated with a first-attempt failure rate of 2% [18, 19], and underscores the importance of identifying perinatal factors that may increase the likelihood of LMA failure. Therefore, the objective of this study is to investigate the potential effects of labor on airway outcomes with the use of sLMA for cesarean delivery under general anesthesia. Our primary outcome is time to effective ventilation, and secondary outcomes include oxygenation and ventilation parameters, seal pressure, and oropharyngeal mucosal trauma.

Methods

This is a secondary analysis of a prospective cohort study investigating the use of sLMA during cesarean delivery [18]. With this dataset, we had previously published the association of Mallampati scores on airway outcomes with sLMA use for cesarean delivery [21]. Approval was obtained from the Institutional Review Board at the Quanzhou Women's and Children's Hospital, Fujian Province, China, (dated 11 Nov 2013) and registered with clinicaltrials.gov (NCT02026882) on 3 January 2014.

Analysis was performed on data from 584 parturients, enrolled between January 2014 to December 2014 at Quanzhou Women's and Children's Hospital. At this center, approximately 35% of parturients undergo cesarean delivery mostly due to maternal request, with the majority of cases performed under general anesthesia using the sLMA as the airway device of choice. Enrolled parturients were American Society of Anesthesiologists (ASA) physical status classification I to III, underwent Category 2 or 3 cesarean delivery under general anesthesia, and had fasted for 4 or more hours. We excluded parturients with BMI > 35 kg/m^2, underwent cesarean delivery under regional anesthesia, had known gastroesophageal reflux disease, or with potentially difficult airway defined as having Mallampati score of 4, upper respiratory tract or neck pathology. The parturients were analyzed according to the presence or absence of labor before cesarean delivery, defined as the presence of painful uterine contractions associated with cervical dilation [22].

Anesthesia and airway management reflects the clinical standard at the study center. All parturients were given intravenous ranitidine for aspiration prophylaxis, and electrocardiogram, pulse oximetry, capnography, and non-invasive blood pressure monitors were applied.

After preoxygenation for 3 min, a rapid sequence induction with intravenous propofol (2–3 mg/kg), succinylcholine (100 mg) and application of cricoid pressure by a trained anesthetic assistant was performed, followed by sLMA insertion. All sLMA were inserted using the recommended single-handed rotational technique, and were performed by three investigators (Yao, Li, and Yuan), each with more than 5 years of experience in sLMA use for cesarean delivery. sLMA size was chosen according to manufacturer's guidelines but can be changed to a more appropriate size according to the discretion of the anesthesiologist. Cricoid pressure was released upon inflation of the sLMA cuff with a manometer to 60 cmH_2O and confirmation of the ability to ventilate via auscultation of breath sounds and presence of end-tidal carbon dioxide with capnography. Airway maneuvers to assist sLMA insertion such as head-tilt or jaw thrust were permitted. The time to effective ventilation, defined as the time from when the sLMA was picked up until the appearance of end-tidal carbon dioxide capnography, and number of attempts at sLMA insertion with each attempt defined as complete insertion and removal of the sLMA, were recorded. Next, a pre-mounted #14 orogastric tube was advanced through the gastric drainage port of the sLMA. After confirmation of adequate placement by aspiration of gastric contents and auscultation of a "swoosh" over the epigastric area with injection of 5 mL of air, suctioning of the orogastric tube was performed. Lastly, sLMA seal pressure was measured by closing the adjustable pressure limiting valve while maintaining 3 L/min fresh gas flow in a closed circle circuit and observing the airway pressure at equilibrium.

Cesarean delivery was allowed to commence if the following criteria were met: presence of a square-wave capnograph, sLMA cuff pressure of 60 cmH_2O, sLMA bite block position located between the incisors, adequately-positioned orogastric tube, and seal pressure of > 20 cmH_2O. Endotracheal intubation would be performed if sLMA insertion was not successful after two attempts, took more than 1 min, or desaturation occurred (oxygen saturation $< 92\%$). All parturients were positioned in left lateral tilt using a wedge. Rocuronium (0.5 mg/kg) was given to maintain muscle relaxation, and anesthesia was maintained with 1.5 to 2% sevoflurane and 50% mix of nitrous oxide in oxygen. Mechanical ventilation was instituted with a tidal volume of 6 to 10 ml/kg and respiratory rate of 10 to 16 breaths/min. The incidence of airway complications, defined as airway obstruction, inadequate oxygenation or ventilation, bronchospasm, laryngospasm and clinical signs of pulmonary aspiration including hypoxemia, auscultation of wheezing or crepitations, and postoperative dyspnea were recorded. The obstetricians were advised to avoid excessive fundal pressure during delivery of the fetus. Upon completion of surgery, the orogastric tube was suctioned and removed, and the sLMA was withdrawn and inspected for the presence of blood. An independent assessor reviewed the patient before discharge from the post-anesthesia care unit to record the incidence of sore throat and voice hoarseness.

The primary airway outcome is time to effective ventilation and secondary outcomes include first-attempt sLMA insertion failure, oropharyngeal leak pressure, peak airway pressure, lowest oxygen saturation during sLMA insertion, volume and pH of gastric aspirate, pH of the sLMA laryngeal surface.

Statistical analysis

All demographic, anesthetic, and clinical were summarized based on parturient's labor status. Categorical data were summarized as frequency with the corresponding proportion, while continuous variables were presented as mean (standard deviation (SD)) or median (interquartile range (IQR)), as appropriate. Differences between labor status for continuous data were tested using Student's t-test or Mann-Whitney U test, whichever appropriate, while categorical data was tested using the Fisher's exact test. Univariate logistic regression analysis was used to express quantitative association between labor status and other factors. Associations from logistic regression analysis were expressed as odds ratios (OR) with 95% confidence intervals (95%CI). Time to effective ventilation (primary outcome), oropharyngeal leak pressure, peak airway pressure, lowest oxygen saturation during sLMA insertion, volume and pH of gastric aspirate, and pH of the sLMA laryngeal surface were treated as continuous data. First-attempt sLMA insertion failure was treated as binary data. Significance level was set at $p < 0.05$ and all tests were two-sided. SAS 9.4 software (SAS Institute Inc., Cary, NC, USA) was used for all analysis. A post-hoc power calculation showed that we had 95% power to detect a difference of 2 s in time to effective ventilation with SD of 5, allocation ratio as 1:1, an alpha error of 0.05 and two-sided significance.

Results

Data from all 584 parturients enrolled in the prospective cohort study were analyzed, of whom 221 (37.8%) were in labor and 363 (62.2%) were not in labor. There was no withdrawal or dropout. Parturient, obstetric, fetal, and surgical characteristics are summarized in Table 1. Labor was associated with significantly lower maternal weight, gestational age, and fetal weight. In addition, labor was associated with increased Category 2 cesarean delivery and longer surgical duration. Of note, there was no significant association between labor status and Mallampati scores.

Table 1 Parturient, fetal and surgical characteristics, and univariate associations with labor status

Characteristics	Labor Status		Univariate analysis	
	Labor **N** = 221	No Labor **N** = 363	Unadjusted OR (95% CI)	P - value
Age (years), mean (SD)	28.5 (4.19)	29.1 (4.10)	0.97 (0.93 to 1.01)	0.1136
Weight (kg), mean (SD)	66.7 (7.84)	69.8 (9.88)	0.96 (0.95 to 0.99)	0.0001
Height (m), mean (SD)	1.6 (0.12)	1.6 (0.07)	0.71 (0.11 to 4.48)	0.7109
ASA status, mean (SD)	1.8 (0.44)	1.8 (0.44)	1.04 (0.71 to 1.52)	0.8571
Mallampati score, mean (SD)	1.7 (0.67)	1.8 (0.66)	0.86 (0.66 to 1.10)	0.2257
Baseline SBP (mmHg), mean (SD)	123.2 (14.44)	122.1 (11.88)	1.01 (0.99 to 1.02)	0.3151
Duration of surgery (min), mean (SD)	30.8 (9.96)	28.7 (9.01)	1.02 (1.01 to 1.04)	0.0101
Cesarean, n (%)				< 0.0001
Category 2	169 (76.5)	24 (6.6)	Reference	–
Category 3	52 (23.5)	339 (93.4)	45.91 (27.36 to 77.04)	–
Gestation (weeks), mean (SD)	37.1 (2.52)	38.4 (1.15)	0.67 (0.60 to 0.75)	< 0.0001
Fetal weight (g), mean (SD)	2766 (578)	3167 (447)	0.998 (0.998 to 0.999)	< 0.0001

Abbreviations: *ASA* American Society of Anesthesiologists, *SBP* Systolic blood pressure

Airway outcomes with sLMA insertion were summarized in Table 2. Laboring parturients had mean time to effective ventilation of 16.0 (SD 5.75) seconds with sLMA insertion, compared to 15.3 (SD 3.35) seconds in non-laboring parturients. Based on univariate analysis, presence of labor was not associated with significant change in our primary outcome of time to effective ventilation, with a mean reduction of 0.65 s (95%CI – 1.49 to 0.18, *p* = 0.1262).

However, labor was associated with increased first-attempt sLMA insertion failure, although all sLMA insertions were successful with a maximum of two attempts. In addition, laboring parturients were found to have significantly lower seal and peak airway pressures, decreased minimum and maximum tidal volumes, lower gastric aspirate volume, lower sLMA laryngeal surface pH, and increased incidence of blood on sLMA. There was no significant change in lowest oxygen saturation

Table 2 Airway outcomes with sLMA insertion and univariate associations with labor status

Continuous variables	Labor Status		Univariate analysis	
	Labor **N** = 221	No Labor **N** = 363	Mean difference (95% CI)	*p*-value
Time to effective ventilation (s), mean (SD)	16.0 (5.75)	15.3 (3.35)	-0.65 (−1.49 to 0.18)	0.1262
Seal pressure (cmH$_2$O), mean (SD)	26.8 (3.44)	27.5 (3.87)	0.79 (0.19 to 1.4)	0.0104
Peak airway pressure (cmH$_2$O), mean (SD)	17.3 (3.76)	18.9 (4.03)	1.54 (0.89 to 2.19)	< 0.0001
Minimum tidal volume (ml), mean (SD)	465.0 (45.62)	484.2 (57.12)	19.17 (10.75 to 27.6)	< 0.0001
Maximum tidal volume (ml), mean (SD)	477.9 (42.61)	501.1 (52.63)	23.21 (15.39 to 31.03)	< 0.0001
Lowest SpO$_2$ (%), mean (SD)	98.6 (1.10)	98.5 (1.14)	−0.10 (−0.29 to 0.09)	0.3012
Gastric aspirate volume (mL), mean (SD)	12.0 (7.16)	15.5 (17.12)	3.53 (1.53 to 5.54)	0.0006
pH of gastric aspirate, mean (SD)	2.3 (0.62)	2.4 (0.95)	0.11 (−0.02 to 0.24)	0.0851
pH of sLMA laryngeal surface, mean (SD)	7.0 (0.55)	7.1 (0.39)	0.08 (0.00 to 0.16)	0.0559
Binary variables	**Labor** **N = 221**	**No Labor** **N = 363**	**Unadjusted odds ratio** **(95%CI)**	***p*-value**
First-attempt sLMA insertion failure, n (%)	9 (4.07)	1 (0.28)	15.37 (1.93 to 122.14)	0.0098
Blood on sLMA, n (%)	7 (3.17)	1 (0.28)	11.84 (1.45 to 96.82)	0.0212
Sore throat, n (%)	14 (6.33)	24 (6.61)	0.96 (0.48 to 1.89)	0.8959
Voice hoarseness, n (%)	2 (0.90)	2 (0.55)	1.65 (0.23 to 11.79)	0.6185

Table 3 Maternal and fetal outcomes, and univariate associations with labor status

Fetal outcomes	Labor Status		Univariate analysis	
	Labor $N = 221$	No Labor $N = 363$	Unadjusted odds ratio (95% CI)	*p*-value
Venous cord pH, mean (SD)	7.3 (0.05)	7.3 (0.06)	0.08 (0.00 to 1.80)	0.1110
1-min fetal Apgar, mean (SD)	8.7 (1.47)	9.4 (0.76)	0.52 (0.43 to 0.63)	< 0.0001
5-min fetal Apgar, mean (SD)	9.4 (1.05)	9.9 (0.30)	0.24 (0.16 to 0.34)	< 0.0001
Patient satisfaction (0–100%), mean (SD)	84.3 (9.75)	87.2 (7.64)	0.96 (0.48 to 1.89)	0.0001

and incidence of sore throat or voice hoarseness. No episodes of bronchospasm, laryngospasm, or pulmonary aspiration were noted in either group.

Maternal and fetal outcomes are summarized in Table 3. Presence of labor was associated with lower 1- and 5-min Apgar scores, and reduced patient satisfaction. No significant change in umbilical venous cord pH was noted.

Discussion

In our study cohort of 584 parturients, 37.8% were in labor while 62.2% were not in labor. Labor was not associated with a significant difference in time to effective ventilation. However, labor was associated with significantly increased incidence of first-attempt sLMA insertion failure, lower seal pressure, lower peak airway pressure, and decreased maximum and minimum tidal volumes, albeit without significant reduction in oxygen saturation. No episodes of pulmonary aspiration was noted. Labor also increased the incidence of blood on the sLMA, but without corresponding change in sore throat or voice hoarseness. In addition, 1- and 5-min Apgar scores were reduced, but with no significant change in umbilical venous cord pH.

To our knowledge, this is the first study that investigated the effects of labor on airway outcomes during sLMA use for cesarean delivery. We noted that laboring parturients had significantly higher first-attempt sLMA insertion failure (4.1%) compared to non-laboring parturients (0.3%), but without concomitant increase in time to effective ventilation or desaturation. Nonetheless, the first-attempt insertion failure rate in laboring parturients was double the incidence of 2% reported by other studies that did not account for labor status [19, 23]. Higher first attempt insertion failure rate will likely increase the time to establishment of anesthesia for cesarean delivery which was not accounted for in other studies [24, 25]. Furthermore, successful sLMA insertion was achieved after a maximum of two attempts in our study population, but we should be cognizant that high risk parturients with Mallampati score of 4, upper respiratory tract or neck pathology were excluded from our study. Hence, the effects of labor on time to effective ventilation and

first-attempt insertion failure in high-risk difficult obstetric airway should be investigated in future studies.

Labor was associated with significant reduction in seal pressure, peak airway pressure, and minimum and maximum tidal volumes. However, the reduction in tidal volumes are unlikely to be due to the reduction in sLMA seal pressure, given the clinically insignificant mean difference of 0.8 cmH$_2$O, and that peak airway pressures did not exceed seal pressures in either group. Instead, the observed difference in tidal volumes may be due to the lower maternal weight in the laboring group, since tidal volumes could be adjusted according to body weight.

We did not find a significant change in Mallampati scores in laboring parturients, in contrast to other studies where Mallampati scores were found to increase 1 to 2 grades in laboring parturients [6, 7]. However, Boutonnet et al. reported that Mallampati scores remain unchanged for 37% of parturients in labor [7], and our study may not be adequately powered to detect a significant change in Mallampati scores. Nonetheless, we have previously shown that Mallampati scores of 3 or 4 did not significantly affect time to effective ventilation, first attempt failure rate, or sLMA seal pressure compared to parturients with Mallampati scores of 1 or 2 undergoing cesarean delivery [21].

The higher incidence of blood on the sLMA suggests that labor increases the risk of oropharyngeal trauma during sLMA insertion, but without corresponding increase in the incidence of sore throat or voice hoarseness. The increase in oropharyngeal trauma may be attributed to fluid accumulation and increased airway edema that occur during labor [6, 26] and possibly associated with the increased number of sLMA insertion attempts in laboring parturients.

Interestingly, gastric aspirate volume was significantly reduced in laboring parturients. This difference may reflect a change in gastric emptying time. Traditionally, pregnancy and labor has been hypothesized to impair gastric motility and emptying, but this has been challenged recently [27], with guidelines even encouraging fluid intake during labor [28]. In early labor, the rate of gastric emptying has been shown to remain unchanged or increase, while advanced labor is associated with delayed gastric emptying [29]. Information on cervical dilation was not collected in this study, and hence we are unable to comment on the stage of labor at the time of cesarean delivery. Nonetheless, the use of LMA in pregnancy raises concern of exacerbating the risk of gastric regurgitation and pulmonary aspiration. Although this study was not powered to investigate the risk of pulmonary aspiration, no episodes of clinical aspiration were detected. Furthermore, the sLMA surface pH, being a surrogate indicator of possible gastric regurgitation, did not reflect that of gastric content.

The use of sLMA in laboring parturients was associated with reduced 1- and 5-min Apgar scores. Of note, the lack of significant reduction in maternal oxygen saturation during sLMA insertion suggests that maternal hypoxemia is unlikely to be the cause of reduced Apgar scores. Instead, the reduction in Apgar scores may be related to the clinical indication prompting urgent cesarean delivery, as demonstrated by the higher proportion of Category 2 cesarean deliveries in laboring parturients. Nonetheless, labor was not associated with significant change in umbilical venous pH, which is arguably a more objective assessment of fetal status, due to the subjectivity of the Apgar score [30].

We acknowledge several limitations with our study. The cesarean delivery rate at the study center is 35%, and sLMA is used for over 2000 deliveries annually. Hence, familiarity with the use of sLMA could have influenced the time to effective ventilation and first-attempt insertion success rate, and these findings may not be applicable to other centers. Cricoid pressure was applied by anesthetic assistants according to routine hospital practice, who were trained to be consistent in this technique, however, the amount of cricoid pressure was not directly measured. In addition, there was no reliable method of blinding the anesthesiologists and the healthcare team on the labor status of the study parturients, which may have influenced our results. The use of sLMA in parturients undergoing general anesthesia raises concerns of gastric regurgitation and pulmonary aspiration. Although we did not detect any clinical signs of pulmonary aspiration or regurgitation, this study was not powered to detect these outcomes. Finally, we excluded parturients with high risk of difficult airway, hence our results may not apply to these parturients.

Conclusions
In summary, our study found that labor is not associated with significant change in time to effective ventilation when sLMA was used in general anesthesia for cesarean delivery. However, laboring parturients had increased incidence of first-attempt sLMA insertion failure and oropharyngeal trauma, compared to non-laboring parturients. No reduction in oxygen saturation or episodes of pulmonary aspiration were noted. Further research is needed to determine the effects of labor on sLMA use in parturients at higher risk of difficult airway.

Abbreviations
ASA: American Society of Anesthesiologists; CI: Confidence intervals; IQR: Inter-quartile range; MBRRACE-UK: Mothers and Babies: Reducing Risk through Audits and Confidential Enquiries; OR: Odds ratio; LMA: Laryngeal mask airway; sLMA: Supreme™ LMA; SD: Standard deviation

Acknowledgements
We would like to thank Ms. Agnes Teo (Senior Clinical Research Coordinator) for her administrative and study coordination support.

Authors' contributions
MJL: data analysis, revising the article and final approval of the version to be submitted. HST: data analysis, revising the article and final approval of the version to be submitted. CWT: data analysis, revising the article and final approval of the version to be submitted. SYL: study design, data collection, patient recruitment and final approval of the version to be submitted. WYY: data collection, patient recruitment and final approval of the version to be submitted. YJY: data collection, patient recruitment and final approval of the version to be submitted. RS: data analysis, revising the article and final approval of the version to be submitted. BLS: study design, data collection, data analysis, revising the article critically for important intellectual content and final approval of the version to be submitted. All authors read and approved the final manuscript.

Author details
[1]Department of Women's Anesthesia, KK Women's and Children's Hospital, 100 Bukit Timah Road, Singapore 229899, Singapore. [2]Duke-NUS Medical School, 8 College Road, Singapore 169857, Singapore. [3]Department of Anesthesiology and Perioperative Medicine, Quanzhou Macare Women's Hospital, Quanzhou, Fujian Province, China. [4]Department of Anesthesiology, Qinghai University Affiliated Hospital, Xining, Qinghai Province, China. [5]Centre for Quantitative Medicine, Duke-NUS Medical School, 8 College Road, Singapore 169857, Singapore.

References
1. Hawthorne L, Wilson R, Lyons G, Dresner M. Failed intubation revisited: 17-yr experience in a teaching maternity unit. Br J Anaesth. 1996;76(5):680–4.
2. Rahman K, Jenkins JG. Failed tracheal intubation in obstetrics: no more frequent but still managed badly. Anaesthesia. 2005;60(2):168–71.
3. Knight M, Bunch K, Tuffnell D, Shakespeare J, Kotnis R, Kenyon S, Kurinczuk JJ. MBRRACE-UK. Saving Lives, Improving Mothers' Care - Lessons learned to inform maternity care from the UK and Ireland Confidential Enquiries into Maternal Deaths and Morbidity 2015–17. Oxford: National Perinatal Epidemiology Unit, University of Oxford; 2019.
4. Delgado C, Ring L, Mushambi M. General anaesthesia in obstetrics. BJA Education. 2020;20(6):201–7.
5. Johnson RV, Lyons GR, Wilson RC, Robinson AP. Training in obstetric general anaesthesia: a vanishing art? Anaesthesia. 2000;55(2):179–83.
6. Kodali BS, Chandrasekhar S, Bulich LN, Topulos GP, Datta S. Airway changes during labor and delivery. Anesthesiology. 2008;108(3):357–62.
7. Boutonnet M, Faitot V, Katz A, Salomon L, Keita H. Mallampati class changes during pregnancy, labour, and after delivery: can these be predicted? Br J Anaesth. 2010;104(1):67–70.
8. Roth D, Pace NL, Lee A, Hovhannisyan K, Warenits AM, Arrich J, Herkner H. Airway physical examination tests for detection of difficult airway management in apparently normal adult patients. Cochrane Database Syst Rev. 2018;5:CD008874.
9. Rocke DA, Murray WB, Rout CC, Gouws E. Relative risk analysis of factors associated with difficult intubation in obstetric anesthesia. Anesthesiology. 1992;77(1):67–73.
10. Mackenzie AI. Laryngeal oedema complicating obstetric anaesthesia: three cases. Anaesthesia. 1978;33(3):271.

11. Barnardo PD, Jenkins JG. Failed tracheal intubation in obstetrics: a 6-year review in a UK region. Anaesthesia. 2000;55(7):690–4.

12. McDonnell NJ, Paech MJ, Clavisi OM, Scott KL. Difficult and failed intubation in obstetric anaesthesia: an observational study of airway management and complications associated with general anaesthesia for caesarean section. Int J Obstet Anesth. 2008;17(4):292–7.

13. Quinn AC, Milne D, Columb M, Gorton H, Knight M. Failed tracheal intubation in obstetric anaesthesia: 2 yr national case-control study in the UK. Br J Anaesth. 2013;110(1):74–80.

14. Mushambi MC, Kinsella SM, Popat M, Swales H, Ramaswamy KK, Winton AL, Quinn AC, Obstetric Anaesthetists A, Difficult Airway S. Obstetric Anaesthetists' Association and Difficult Airway society guidelines for the management of difficult and failed tracheal intubation in obstetrics. Anaesthesia. 2015;70(11):1286–306.

15. Bercker S, Schmidbauer W, Volk T, Bogusch G, Bubser HP, Hensel M, Kerner T. A comparison of seal in seven supraglottic airway devices using a cadaver model of elevated esophageal pressure. Anesthesia Analgesia. 2008; 106(2):445–8 table of contents.

16. Sorbello M. Evolution of supraglottic airway devices: the Darwinian perspective. Minerva Anestesiol. 2018;84(3):297–300.

17. Sorbello M. Expanding the burdens of airway management: not only endotracheal tubes. Minerva Anestesiol. 2019;85:4–6.

18. Li SY, Yao WY, Yuan YJ, Tay WS, Han N-LR, Sultana R, Assam PN, Sia AT-H, Sng BL. Supreme™ laryngeal mask airway use in general anesthesia for category 2 and 3 Cesarean delivery: a prospective cohort study. BMC Anesthesiol. 2017;17:169.

19. Yao WY, Li SY, Sng BL, Lim Y, Sia AT. The LMA supreme in 700 parturients undergoing cesarean delivery: an observational study. Can J Anaesth. 2012; 59(7):648–54.

20. Yao WY, Li SY, Yuan YJ, Tan HS, Han NR, Sultana R, Assam PN, Sia AT, Sng BL. Comparison of supreme laryngeal mask airway versus endotracheal intubation for airway management during general anesthesia for cesarean section: a randomized controlled trial. BMC Anesthesiol. 2019;19(1):123.

21. Tan HS, Li SY, Yao WY, Yuan YJ, Sultana R, Han NR, Sia ATH, Sng BL. Association of Mallampati scoring on airway outcomes in women undergoing general anesthesia with supreme laryngeal mask airway in cesarean section. BMC Anesthesiol. 2019;19(1):122.

22. World Health Organization (WHO) - WHO recommendation on definitions of the latent and active first stages of labour. [https://extranet.who.int/rhl/topics/preconception-pregnancy-childbirth-and-postpartum-care/care-during-childbirth/care-during-labour-1st-stage/who-recommendation-definitions-latent-and-active-first-stages-labour-0]. Accessed 12 July 2020.

23. Han TH, Brimacombe J, Lee EJ, Yang HS. The laryngeal mask airway is effective (and probably safe) in selected healthy parturients for elective cesarean section: a prospective study of 1067 cases. Can J Anaesth. 2001; 48(11):1117–21.

24. Krom AJ, Cohen Y, Miller JP, Ezri T, Halpern SH, Ginosar Y. Choice of anaesthesia for category-1 caesarean section in women with anticipated difficult tracheal intubation: the use of decision analysis. Anaesthesia. 2017; 72(2):156–71.

25. Sorbello M, Micaglio M. Category-1 caesarean section, airways and Julius Caesar. Anaesthesia. 2017;72(9):1153–4.

26. Pilkington S, Carli F, Dakin MJ, Romney M, De Witt KA, Dore CJ, Cormack RS. Increase in Mallampati score during pregnancy. Br J Anaesth. 1995;74(6): 638–42.

27. Bataille A, Rousset J, Marret E, Bonnet F. Ultrasonographic evaluation of gastric content during labour under epidural analgesia: a prospective cohort study. Br J Anaesth. 2014;112(4):703–7.

28. Smith I, Kranke P, Murat I, Smith A, O'Sullivan G, Soreide E, Spies C, in't Veld B, European Society of A. Perioperative fasting in adults and children: guidelines from the European Society of Anaesthesiology. Eur J Anaesthesiol. 2011;28(8):556–69.

29. O'Sullivan G, Scrutton M. NPO during labor. Is there any scientific validation? Anesthesiol Clin North Am. 2003;21(1):87–98.

30. Allanson ER, Waqar T, White C, Tuncalp O, Dickinson JE. Umbilical lactate as a measure of acidosis and predictor of neonatal risk: a systematic review. BJOG. 2017;124(4):584–94.

15

Comparison of videolaryngoscope-guided versus standard digital insertion techniques of the ProSeal™ laryngeal mask airway

Ulku Ozgul[1]* , Feray Akgul Erdil[1], Mehmet Ali Erdogan[1], Zekine Begec[1], Cemil Colak[2], Aytac Yucel[1] and Mahmut Durmus[1]

Abstract

Background: This study were designed to investigate the usefulness of the videolaryngoscope-guided insertion technique compared with the standard digital technique for the insertion success rate and insertion conditions of the Proseal™ laryngeal mask airway (PLMA).

Methods: Prospective, one hundred and nineteen patients (ASA I–II, aged 18–65 yr) were randomly divided for PLMA insertion using the videolaryngoscope-guided technique or the standard digital technique. The PLMA was inserted according to the manufacturer's instructions in the standard digital technique group. The videolaryngoscope-guided technique was performed a C-MAC® videolaryngoscope with D-Blade, under gentle videolaryngoscope guidance, the epiglottis was lifted, and the PLMA was advanced until the tip of the distal cuff reached the oesophagus inlet. The number of insertion attempts, insertion time, oropharyngeal leak pressure, leak volume, fiberoptic bronchoscopic view, peak inspiratory pressure, ease of gastric tube placement, hemodynamic changes, visible blood on PLMA and postoperative airway morbidity were recorded.

Results: The first-attempt success rate (the primary outcome) was higher in the videolaryngoscope-guided technique than in the standard digital technique ($p = 0.029$). The effect size values with 95% confidence interval were 0.19 (0.01–0.36) for the first and second attempts, 0.09 (− 0.08–0.27) for the first and third attempts, and not computed for the second and third attempts by the groups, respectively.

Conclusion: Videolaryngoscope-guided insertion technique can be a help in case of difficult positioning of a PLMA and can improve the PLMA performance in some conditions. We suggest that the videolaryngoscope-guided technique may be a useful technique if the digital technique fails.

Keywords: Equipment, Proseal laryngeal mask airway, Insertion technique, Video-laryngoscopy

* Correspondence: ulku.ozgul@inonu.edu.tr
[1]School of Medicine, Department of Anesthesiology and Reanimation, Inonu University, Malatya, Turkey

Background

The ProSeal™ laryngeal mask airway (PLMA; Teleflex Medical Athlone, Co. Westmeath, Ireland) is a laryngeal mask device with a double cuff to improve the seal and incorporates a drainage tube to prevent a risk of aspiration and gastric insufflation. The PLMA is inserted via digital manipulation, similar to how the classic™ laryngeal mask airway (cLMA) is inserted, or with an introducer tool according to the manufacturer's recommendations. Although cLMA insertion success on the first attempt with this technique is high, the PLMA insertion success rate is lower than that of the cLMA (91% vs 82%). Downfolded of the epiglottis during device insertion, the distal cuff folded over backwards, impaction at the back of the mouth, and failure of the distal cuff to reach its correct position in the hypopharynx can cause failed and/or delayed insertion with these techniques [1–3].

Many techniques have been described to facilitate LMA insertion, and these techniques have improved insertion conditions and insertion success rate [4–9]. It was first reported by Lee that the laryngoscope can improve the placement of LMA in an adult [10]. Then, direct laryngoscopy alone or laryngoscope-assisted guided techniques were used for this purpose [4, 8, 11–14]. These methods do have theoretical disadvantages, such as haemodynamic and airway stimulation and pharyngeal or oesophageal trauma [4, 8].

The C-MAC® videolaryngoscope (Karl Storz, Tuttlingen, Germany) provides several advantages for airway management because it improves the laryngeal view without the need for aligning all axes and ensures high-quality images with stable hemodynamic status during laryngoscopy [15, 16]. Recently, the Glidescope™/gastric tube-guided technique was used to facilitate difficult PLMA positioning [17].

We hypothesized that the C-MAC® videolaryngoscope-guided PLMA insertion technique would provide a better success rate for PLMA insertion than that of the standard digital technique. The purpose of the present study was to compare the insertion success rate and insertion conditions of the PLMA between the videolaryngoscope-guided insertion technique and the standard digital technique.

Methods

The prospective, randomized controlled study adheres to CONSORT guideline. This study was performed after approval of the local ethics committee (Malatya Clinical Research Ethics Committee, 2019/36, February 20, 2019) and written informed consent from the patients.

The study was registered prior to patient enrolment at clinicaltrials.gov (identifier: NCT03852589, principal investigator: Ulku Ozgul, date of registration: February 22, 2019). We enrolled 119 patients with an American Society of Anesthesiologists (ASA) physical status of I-II, who were aged between 18 and 65 years and were scheduled for elective surgery in the supine position under general anaesthesia using the PLMA for airway management between March 2019 and April 2019. Patients with increased aspiration risk, body mass index > 35 kg/m^2, a known or predicted difficult airway (Mallampati score > 2 or mouth opening < 3 cm), a disease related to the cervical spine, pre-existing sore throat or hoarseness or those with anticipated difficult airway were excluded.

Before anesthesia induction, patients were premedicated with 0.02 mg/kg i.v. midazolam. In the operating room, standard anesthetic monitoring was applied with electrocardiogram, non-invasive blood pressure, and peripheral oxygen saturation monitoring. All patients underwent a standard general anesthesia technique without the use of neuromuscular blocking agent after 3 min of preoxygenation with a face mask. Induction of anesthesia was carried out with remifentanil 2 μg/kg over 60 s and propofol 2 mg/kg mixed with 40 mg lidocaine over 30 s. The patients were ventilated with a facemask until conditions were suitable for PLMA insertion (loss of eyelash reflex, jaw relaxation, and the absence of movement). Additional boluses of 0.5 mg/kg i.v. propofol were given as required until an adequate level of anesthesia was achieved for PLMA placement. The PLMA was checked for leaks, and the back surface was lubricated with a water-soluble gel and sixty seconds after induction, the PLMA was inserted by an experienced anesthetist. Patients were not aware of the groups allocated. The data during anesthesia and postoperative period were collected by blinded observers.

Using a web-based randomization generation sequence from random allocation rule, the patients were randomly divided into two groups of 60 each [18]. The C-MAC® videolaryngoscope-guided insertion group was named Group V, and the standard digital insertion group was named Group D. All interventions were performed using a midline approach on patients in the sniffing position with the cuff fully deflated. The size of the PLMA was determined according to the patient's weight: size 3 for ≤50 kg, size 4 for 50–70 kg, size 5 for 70–100 kg.

The videolaryngoscope-guided technique was performed a C-MAC® videolaryngoscope with D-Blade as follows. Under gentle videolaryngoscope guidance, the epiglottis was lifted, and the PLMA was advanced until the tip of the distal cuff reached the oesophagus inlet.

The standard digital technique was performed according to the manufacturer's instructions [19]. In Group D, the PLMA was pressed with the index finger and forwarded around the palatopharyngeal curve until the resistance was felt.

After the PLMA was inserted, the cuff was inflated with air based on the amount of air proposed by the manufacturing company. With the cuff manometer (VBM Medizintechnik, Sulz, Germany), the maximum pressure was set to 60 cmH$_2$O. Effective ventilation was confirmed using chest expansion and square wave capnography. Then, it was fixed according to the manufacturer's recommended [19].

A well-lubricated gastric tube (14 French) was inserted along the drainage tube. Correct gastric tube placement was evaluated by fluid suction or air injected by epigastric stethoscopy.

A maximum of three attempts were allowed for the insertion of PLMA. If insertion failed after these attempts, alternative techniques were used, and the patient was excluded. Upon failed PLMA passage into the pharynx, PLMA malposition (air leakage despite cuff inflation), or ineffective ventilation (maximum expired tidal volume < 6 ml/kg), the trial was defined as failed insertion.

After successful PLMA insertion, anesthesia was maintained with sevoflurane 1.5 to 2%, using a 50:50 mixture of oxygen and air and remifentanil infusion (0.05–0.2 µg/kg /min). Patients were ventilated in synchronized intermittent mandatory ventilation mode until the end of the operation.

The heart rate, mean arterial blood pressure and peripheric oxygen saturation levels were recorded prior to anesthesia induction (t0); immediately after induction (t1); immediately after insertion of the PLMA (t2); and at 3 min (t3), 5 min (t4), and 10 min (t5) after PLMA insertion.

The incidence of postoperative airway morbidity during PLMA insertion and anesthesia, such as desaturation, airway obstruction, coughing, laryngospasm, bronchospasm, and trauma of the mouth, lip and tongue, were recorded. Any visible blood staining on the videolaryngoscope blade or PLMA was documented at removal.

At the end of the operation, the PLMA was removed when patients were able to sufficient spontaneous respiration and obey comments. After patients were taken to the recovery unit, sore throat, dysphagia, and dysphonia were noted within the postoperative period of 1 to 24 h. Symptoms were graded by the patient as mild, moderate or severe. Trained observers collected the data at 1 h and 24 h postoperatively.

The primary outcome was the first-attempt insertion success rate. The number of insertion attempts was recorded.

Secondary outcomes were insertion time, oropharyngeal leak pressure (OLP), leak volume, fibreoptic bronchoscopic view, peak inspiratory pressure, haemodynamic changes and postoperative airway morbidity.

When the OLP was measured, the pressure-limiting valve was set to 40 cmH$_2$O, the expiratory valve of the circle system was fixed at a gas flow of 3 L/min and the ventilator was placed in manual mode. For measuring OLP, the ventilator pressure gauge and spirometer were used and defined as the point at which the steady state of airway pressure was reached. Oropharyngeal leak

pressure was detected by both an audible noise that could be heard over the mouth and manometric stability; the leak was equilibrated with fresh gas flow [20].

Leak volume was evaluated by the difference between the inspiratory and expiratory tidal volumes and obtained from the anesthesia machine's spirometry measurements during mechanical ventilation. The leak volume was measured three times, and its average was recorded. Peak inspiratory pressures were noted.

Insertion time was recorded as the time from picking up the device (or videolaryngoscope blade) until the appearance of the first square capnography wave.

The anatomical position of the PLMA was assessed with a fibreoptic bronchoscope (11302BD2, diameter 3.7 mm; length 65 cm; Karl Storz, Tuttlingen, Germany) by a blinded observer. The scoring used was that described by Brimacombe and Berry in our study as follows: 4 = only vocal cords visible; 3 = vocal cords plus posterior epiglottis visible; 2 = vocal cords plus anterior epiglottis visible; and 1 = vocal cords invisible [21].

The insertion of the orogastric tube was graded using a subjective scale of 1–3: 1 = easy; 2 = difficult; 3 = impossible to insert the device.

The minimum sample size required to detect a significant difference of the first attempt between the groups required at least 56 in each group (112 in total), considering type I error (alpha) of 0.05, power (1-beta) of 0.8, effect size of 0.6 and a two-sided alternative hypothesis [4].

The data were expressed as the mean (standard deviation, SD), median (min-max) or frequency with percentage depending upon the overall variable distribution. Normality was assessed using the Shapiro-Wilk test. The qualitative data were analysed with Pearson's chi-square test, Yate's corrected chi-square test and Fisher's exact test where appropriate. The quantitative data were analysed by independent samples t-test and Mann Whitney U test as appropriate. The normally distributed data for repeated observations were compared by repeated measures analysis of variance (rANOVA) accompanied by Bonferroni test. $P < 0.05$ values were considered significant. IBM SPSS Statistics for Windows, Version 25.0. Armonk, NY: IBM Corp. was used for statistical analyses.

Results

One hundred and twenty patients were recruited for the study. One patient was excluded from the study due to failed PLMA insertion in Group D. A total of 119 patients were included in the statistical analysis (Fig. 1).

Patient characteristics were shown in Table 1. The first-attempt success rate was higher in Group V than in Group D ($p = 0.029$). The effect size values with 95% confidence interval were 0.19 (0.01–0.36) for the first and second attempts, 0.09 (– 0.08–0.27) for the first and

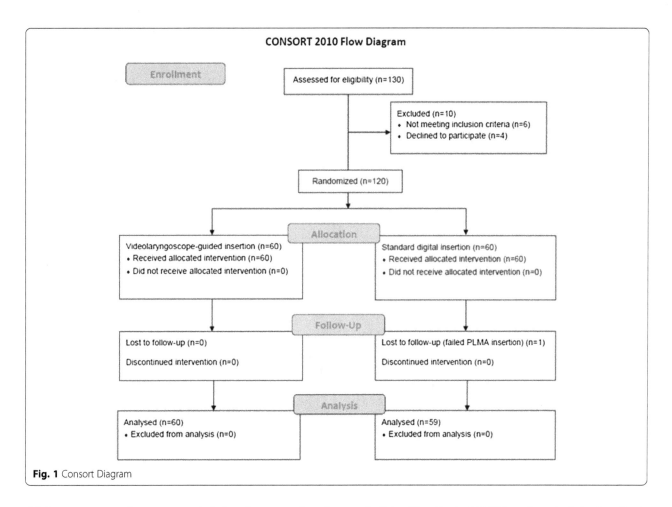

Fig. 1 Consort Diagram

third attempts, and not computed for the second and third attempts by the groups, respectively.

The fibreoptic position scores were better in Group V than in Group D ($p < 0.001$). In Group V, the fibreoptic view was found to be Brimacombe's grade 4 in 45 patients (75%) and grade 3 in 15 patients (25%). There were no grade 2 or grade 1 in the patients. In Group D, the fibreoptic view was found to be Brimacombe's grade 4 in 15 patients (25.4%), grade 3 in 16 patients (27.1%), grade 2 in 22 patients (37.2%) and grade 1 in 6 patients (10.1%).

The PLMA insertion time was longer in Group V than in Group D ($p < 0.001$). There were no differences in oropharyngeal leak pressures between the groups. The peak inspiratory pressure was lower in Group V than in Group D ($p = 0.004$). Orogastric tube insertion was more successful in Group V compared to Group D ($p < 0.001$) (Table 2).

Table 1 Patients characteristics. Data expressed as frequency (%), mean ± SD

Variables	Group V (n = 60)	Group D (n = 59)	P value
Age (y)	38.13 ± 11.45	38.16 ± 13.58	0.987
Weight (kg)	75.33 ± 11.84	74.22 ± 13.03	0.627
Height (cm)	170.45 ± 9.29	167.93 ± 8.42	0.125
BMI (kg/m^2)	25.95 ± 3.8	26.31 ± 4.02	0.618
Gender (M:F)	37 /23	29 /30	0.190
ASA (I:II)	43 / 17	41 /18	0.797
Mallampati (I:II)	53 / 7	47 /12	0.200
Duration of Anesthesia (min)	96.83 ± 27.31	87.13 ± 33.73	0.087
Size of PLMA (3/4/5)	2/44/14	6/32/21	0.071

Group V, videolaryngoscope-guided group; Group D, standard digital group; M, male; F, female; BMI, body mass index; ASA, American Society of Anesthesiologists; PLMA, Proseal™ laryngeal mask airway

Table 2 Comparative data of PLMA insertions. Data are mean ± standard deviation, frequencies or median (min-max)

Variables	Group V (n = 60)	Group D (n = 59)	P value	Effect size with 95% C.I.
Insertion success (n)				
First attempt	60	53 (89.8%)		0.19 (0.01–0.36)[a]
Second attempt	0	4 (6.7%)	0.029	0.09 (−0.08–0.27)[b]
Third attempt	0	1 (1.6%)		NaN[c]
Overall	60/60 (100%)	59/60 (98.3%)		
Insertion time (sec)	38.36 ± 6.44	28.59 ± 9.44	< 0.001	
Oropharyngeal leak pressure (cmH$_2$O)	30.28 ± 8.3	29.86 ± 6.91	0.764	
Leak volume (L)	0.13 ± 0.15	0.19 ± 0.26	0.143	
Fibreoptic score	4 (3–4)	3 (1–4)	< 0.001	
Peak inspiratuar pressure (cmH$_2$O)	11.21 ± 2.94	13.01 ± 3.73	0.004	
Orogastric tube insertion				
easy / difficult / impossible	60/0/0	46/11/2	< 0.001	

Group V, videolaryngoscope-guided group; Group D, standard digital group; [a] First and second attempts by the groups (2 × 2 crossstab); [b] First and third attempts by the groups (2 × 2 crossstab); [c] second and third attempts by the groups (2 × 2 crossstab) can not be computed

The haemodynamic parameters (heart rate and mean arterial pressure) were similar at all measurement times between the two groups (Table 3). The HR and MA*P* values in immediately after induction and at 1 min, 3 min, 5 min and 10 min after intubation were lower compared with the baseline values between the two groups.

Postoperative airway morbidity was similar between the two groups. Postoperative sore throat was observed in 7 patients in Group V and 4 patients in Group D at 1 h and in 2 patients in Group V and 2 patients in Group D at 24 h, and there were no differences between the groups in the incidence of sore throat. Postoperative dysphagia developed in two patients in Group V and two patients in Group D, and there was no difference between the groups. Postoperative dysphonia was not

observed in any patients. The visible blood on the PLMA after tube removal was observed in two patients in Group V and 5 patients in Group D, and there was no statistically significant difference (Table 4).

Discussion

We found that the first-attempt success rate of the PLMA with the videolaryngoscope-guided insertion technique was superior. Additionally, fibreoptic scoring, orogastric tube placement success and peak inspiratory pressure were better in the videolaryngoscope-guided technique than in the standard digital technique.

It was reported that second-generation SADs (i-gel, PLMA, LMA Supreme) have reliable first-time placement, high seal pressure, separation of gastrointestinal

Table 3 Hemodynamic parametres. Data are mean ± standard deviation

Variables	Group V (n = 60)	Group D (n = 59)	P value
Heart rate (beat/min)			
Baseline	78.18 ± 12.47	81.33 ± 12.59	0.17
After induction immediately	71.26 ± 9.85	71.25 ± 10.39	0.995
After intubation 1 min	68.41 ± 9.17	69.11 ± 10.28	0.695
After intubation 3 min	67.5 ± 9.01	69.13 ± 9.22	0.33
After intubation 5 min	67.63 ± 8.91	70.64 ± 10.22	0.089
After intubation 10 min	66.75 ± 10.67	70.2 ± 9.74	0.068
Mean Arterial Pressure (mmHg)			
Baseline	99.35 ± 10.09	101.15 ± 13.38	0.408
After induction immediately	69.55 ± 9.51	70.47 ± 10.51	0.616
After intubation 1 min	68.98 ± 8.78	67.71 ± 5.67	0.351
After intubation 3 min	68.8 ± 7.7	68.69 ± 6.94	0.938
After intubation 5 min	71.28 ± 8.84	71.38 ± 9.17	0.949
After intubation 10 min	72.63 ± 9.2	74.27 ± 9.56	0.343

Group V, videolaryngoscope-guided group; Group D, standard digital group

Table 4 Complications after removal of PLMA. Data are presented as frequencies

Variables	Group V (n = 60)	Group D (n = 59)	P value
Sore throat mild/moderate/severe (n)			
Postoperative 1 h	7/0/0	4/0/0	0.55
Postoperative 24 h	2/0/0	2/0/0	0.99
Dysphagia mild/moderate/severe (n)			
Postoperative 1 h	2/0/0	2/0/0	0.99
Postoperative 24 h	0/0/0	0/0/0	
Dysphonia mild/moderate/severe (n)			
Postoperative 1 h	0/0/0	0/0/0	
Postoperative 24 h	0/0/0	0/0/0	
Visible blood on PLMA (n)	2	5	0.27

Group V, videolaryngoscope-guided group; Group D, standard digital group

and respiratory tracts and are recommended to intubation fail for airway rescue as well by Difficult Airway Society guideline [22]. Successful placement is most likely on the first attempt. Repeated attempts at inserting a SAD increases the probability of airway trauma and may delay the decision to accept failure. Many studies demonstrated that in cases of failed conventional insertion of SADs, PLMA manufacturer's introducer, 90° rotational technique, laryngoscope/videolaryngoscope-assisted or catheter-assisted techniques had the high success rate [9]. So, we designed the study to compare with the videolaryngoscope asisted and digital technique.

There are contradictory results of LMA insertion using direct laryngoscopy or laryngoscope-assisted guided techniques. Kim et al. showed that the rate of success at the first attempt was similar between standard digital and laryngoscope-guided insertion [14]. However, many other studies that used different LMA types indicated that the laryngoscope-guided insertion technique is more successful than were the digital or rotational techniques [8, 11, 14, 15, 23]. Additionally, the laryngoscope-guided, gum elastic bougie-guided technique was superior to the digital and introducer technique [4]. The success rate on the first attempt was also higher in the videolaryngoscope-guided technique in our study. A possible reason for the higher insertion success rate in the videolaryngoscope-guided technique was the ability to direct the distal cuff around the back of the mouth and into the hypopharynx, which improves the functional and anatomical optimization. The success rate in the present study for the standard digital technique was similar to that in previous studies [2–4].

At the suitable depth of anesthesia, spontaneous breathing may be easily inhibited by opioids and hypnotic drugs without neuromuscular blockers. No using neuromuscular blocking agent prevents the undesirable side effects of these agents, such as prolonged neuromuscular block, and may lead to the need of

neuromuscular antagonist [9, 24]. So, we did not prefer a neuromuscular blocking agent.

Laryngeal mask airway placement can assesed using fibreoptic laryngoscopy [13]. Positioning can be confirmed by fibreoptic evaluation, on which vocal cords were clearly seen, often with the posterior part of epiglottis visible (but not the tip) and with the cuff optimally placed on the midline. Fibreoptic scoring was used in previous studies; however, different results were reported. Campbell et al. found that 91.5% of direct laryngoscopy patients had an ideal LMA insertion position; however, an ideal fibreoptic position was observed in 42% of patients in the standard digital group. Our results are consistent with those of Campbell et al. [13]. Videolaryngoscopy provides visualization of the epiglottis and can prevent downfolding of the epiglottis, distal cuff misplacement and backward folding, as well as proximal LMA cuff displacement during LMA placement. Therefore, video laryngoscopy may improve insertion conditions and prevent airway gas leaks, airway obstruction and impaired gas exchange [25].

The oropharyngeal leak test is usually administered to quantify the seal with the airway for using an LMA [19]. The double-cuff design of the PLMA provides an excellent sealing effect for positive pressure ventilation compared to cLMA [2, 3]. Kim et al. reported that the OLP (21.4 ± 8.6 cmH$_2$O) was higher in the laryngoscope-guided technique that used cLMA [13]. Our OLP value was 30 cmH$_2$O in the videolaryngoscope-guided technique and was different from their finding. A possible reason for the higher OLP was that the PLMA device was used in our study. The results of our OLP value were similar to that in studies that used the PLMA [4].

It was reported that LMA placement using the standard digital technique prevents airway trauma and avoids haemodynamic changes [2, 26]. In our study, haemodynamic parameters and incidence of postoperative airway morbidity were similar in both groups. The reason for these results may be the use of C-MAC® videolaryngo-scopy, the incorporation of gently lifting the epiglottis. Many studies have indicated that videolaryngoscopy leads to fewer haemodynamic responses than does direct laryngoscopy during endotracheal intubation [17, 27]. The C-MAC® videolaryngoscope may be also less traumatic than direct laryngoscopy [28]. Additionally, the studies with laryngoscope-guided insertion of an LMA did not present significant differences in haemodynamic parameters compared to the standard digital technique [8, 14, 23].

The insertion time was longer (by approximately 10 s) in the videolaryngoscope-guided insertion group than in the standard digital insertion group (38 vs 28 s) in the present study. Several studies determined that the insertion time with direct laryngoscopy or laryngoscope-assisted guided techniques was longer than the time required for the standard digital technique [7, 14]. Our results are also similar to these. The result may be related to the videolaryngoscope-guided insertion group requiring extra time for laryngoscope insertion. However, the difference is not clinically important, as emphasized in previous studies [7, 28].

Correct positioning of the PLMA can be detected by correct orogastric tube insertion. Smooth passage of a drainage tube into the stomach shows that the distal cuff of the PLMA is not folded, and the lumen is aligned with the oesophagus [25, 28]. When the PLMA does not achieve an ideal position, it allows venting of air during positive pressure ventilation. Orogastric tube insertion success in our study showed superiority of the videolaryngoscope-guided insertion technique over the standard digital technique. This finding may prove that PLMA insertion significantly improves the ideal positioning.

There are some limitations in the present study. First, all interventions were by the same, more experience anesthetist, and the results may not be applicable to less experienced practitioners. Second, skill acquisition of the C-MAC videolaryngoscope requires a brief period of learning and regular practice. Third, all patients had Mallampati scores I or II, so our results may not conform to patients who had potentially difficult airways. Finally, the anesthetist who performed PLMA insertion was not blinded, which may lead to bias. However, other observers who collected data were blinded.

Conclusion

The standard digital insertion technique has successful insertion rate with easy, time saving, cheap, be used everywhere and simple training. Videolaryngoscope-guided insertion technique can be a help in case of difficult positioning of a PLMA and can improve the PLMA performance in some conditions. We suggest that the videolaryngoscope-guided technique may be a useful technique if the digital technique fails.

Abbreviations
ASA: American Society of Anesthesiologists; cLMA: classic™ laryngeal mask airway; OLP: oropharyngeal leak pressure; PLMA: Proseal™ laryngeal mask airway

Acknowledgements
None.

Authors' contributions
UO and FAE were resposible for conceived, designed this study and collected the data. MAE and MD were responsible for study execution and manuscript writing. CÇ was responsible for data analysis. ZB and AY were responsible interpretation of results and manuscript writing. All authors have read and approved the final version of the manuscript.

Author details
[1]School of Medicine, Department of Anesthesiology and Reanimation, Inonu University, Malatya, Turkey. [2]School of Medicine, Department of Biostatistics, and Medical Informatics, Inonu University, Malatya, Turkey.

References
1. Brimacombe J, Keller C. The ProSeal laryngeal mask airway: a randomized, crossover study with the standard laryngeal mask airway in paralyzed, anesthetized patients. Anesthesiology. 2000;93:104–9.
2. Keller C, Brimacombe J. Mucosal pressure and oropharyngeal leak pressure with the ProSeal versus laryngeal mask airway in anaesthetized paralysed patients. Br J Anaesth. 2000;85:262–6.
3. Brimacombe J, Keller C, Fullekrug B, Agrò F, Rosenblatt W, Dierdorf SF, et al. A multicenter study comparing the ProSeal and classic laryngeal mask airway in anesthetized, nonparalyzed patients. Anesthesiology. 2002;96:289–95.
4. Brimacombe J, Keller C, Judd DV. Gum elastic bougie-guided insertion of the ProSeal laryngeal mask airway is superior to the digital and introducer tool techniques. Anesthesiology. 2004;100:25–9.
5. Hwang JW, Park HP, Lim YJ, Do SH, Lee SC, Jeon YT. Comparison of two insertion techniques of ProSeal laryngeal mask airway: standard versus 90-degree rotation. Anesthesiology. 2009;110:905–7.
6. Chen HS, Yang SC, Chien CC, Spielberger J, Hung KC, Chung KC. Insertion of the ProSeal™ laryngeal mask airway is more successful with the flexi-slip™ stylet than with the introducer. Can J Anesth. 2011;58:617–23.
7. El Beheiry H, Wong J, Nair G, Chinnappa V, Arora G, Morales E, et al. Improved esophageal patency when inserting the ProSeal laryngeal mask airway with an Eschmann tracheal tube introducer. Can J Anesth. 2009;56:725–32.
8. Koay CK, Yoong CS, Kok P. A randomized trial comparing two laryngeal mask airway insertion techniques. Anaesth Intensive Care. 2001;29:613–5.
9. Sorbello M, Petrini F. Supraglottic airway devices: the search for the best insertion technique or the time to change our point of view? Turk J Anaesthesiol Reanim. 2017;45:76–82.
10. Lee JJ. Laryngeal mask and trauma to uvula. Anaesthesia. 1989;44:1014–5.
11. Nalini KB, Shivakumar S, Archana S, Sandhya Rani DC, Mohan CV. Comparison of three insertion techniques of ProSeal laryngeal mask airway: a randomized clinical trial. J Anaesthesiol Clin Pharmacol. 2016;32:510–4.
12. Chandan SN, Sharma SM, Raveendra US, Rajendra Prasad B. Fiberoptic assessment of laryngeal mask airway placement: a comparison of blind insertion and insertion with the use of a laryngoscope. J Maxillofac Oral Surg. 2009;8:95–8.
13. Campbell RL, Biddle C, Assudmi N, Campbell JR, Hotchkiss M. Fiberoptic assessment of laryngeal mask airway placement: blind insertion versus direct visual epiglottoscopy. J Maxillofac Oral Surg. 2004;62:1108–13.
14. Kim GW, Kim JY, Kim SJ, Moon YR, Park EJ, Park SY. Conditions for laryngeal mask airway placement in terms of oropharyngeal leak pressure: a comparison between blind insertion and laryngoscope-guided insertion. BMC Anesthesiol. 2019;19:4.
15. Xue FS, Li HX, Liu YY, Yang GZ. Current evidence for the use of C-MAC videolaryngoscope in adult airway management: a review of the literature. Ther Clin Risk Manag. 2017;13:831–41.

16. Rajan S, Kadapamannil D, Barua K, Tosh P, Paul J, Kumar L. Ease of intubation and hemodynamic responses to nasotracheal intubation using C-MAC videolaryngoscope with D blade: a comparison with use of traditional Macintosh laryngoscope. J Anaesthesiol Clin Pharmacol. 2018;34:381–5.

17. Micaglio M, Parotto M, Trevisanuto D, Zanardo V, Ori C. Glidescope/gastric-tube guided technique: a back-up approach for ProSeal LMA insertion. Can J Anesth. 2006;53:1063–4.

18. Arslan AK, Colak C. RAY: randomization procedures software, biostatapps. inonu.edu.tr/RAY/

19. LMA. LMA Proseal™ Instruction Manual, 1st ed. San Diego: LMA North America Inc; 2000.

20. Keller C, Brimacombe JR, Keller K, Morris R. Comparison of four methods for assessing airway sealing pressure with the laryngeal mask airway in adult patients. Br J Anaesth. 1999;82:286–7.

21. Brimacombe J, Berry A. A proposed fiber-optic scoring system to standardize the assessment of laryngeal mask airway position. Anesth Analg. 1993;76:457.

22. Frerk C, Mitchell VS, McNarry AF, Mendonca C, Bhagrath R, Patel A, et al. Difficult Airway Society 2015 guidelines for management of unanticipated difficult intubation in adults. Br J Anaesth. 2015;115:827–48.

23. Choo CY, Koay CK, Yoong CS. A randomised controlled trial comparing two insertion techniques for the laryngeal mask airway flexible™ in patients undergoing dental surgery. Anaesthesia. 2012;67:986–90.

24. Chen BZ, Tan L, Zhang L, Shang YC. Is muscle relaxant necessary in patients undergoing laparoscopic gynecological surgery with a ProSeal LMA™? J Clin Anesth. 2013;25:32–5.

25. van Zundert AAJ, Wyssusek KH, Pelecanos A, Roets M, Kumar CM. A prospective randomized comparison of airway seal using the novel vision-guided insertion of LMA-Supreme® and LMA-Protector®. J Clin Monit Comput. 2019; https://doi.org/10.1007/s10877-019-00301-3. [Epub ahead of print].

26. Wilson IG, Fell D, Robinson SL, Smith G. Cardiovascular responses to insertion of the laryngeal mask. Anaesthesia. 1992;47:300–2.

27. Maassen RL, Pieters BM, Maathuis B, Serroyen J, Marcus MA, Wouters P, et al. Endotracheal intubation using videolaryngoscopy causes less cardiovascular response compared to classic direct laryngoscopy, in cardiac patients according a standard hospital protocol. Acta Anaesthesiol Belg. 2012;63:181–6.

28. Hernandez MR, Klock PA Jr, Ovassapian A. Evolution of the extraglottic airway: a review of its history, applications, and practical tips for success. Anesth Analg. 2012;114:349–68.

16

Feasibility of laryngeal mask anesthesia combined with nerve block in adult patients undergoing internal fixation of rib fractures

Jun Cao[†], Xiaoyun Gao[†], Xiaoli Zhang, Jing Li and Junfeng Zhang[*] (iD)

Abstract

Background: The laryngeal mask airway (LMA) is occasionally used in internal fixation of rib fractures. We evaluated the feasibility of general anesthesia with an LMA associated to a thoracic paravertebral block (TPB) and/or an erector spinae plane block (ESPB) for internal fixation of rib fractures.

Methods: Twenty patients undergoing unilateral rib fracture fixation surgery were enrolled. Each patient received general anesthesia with an LMA combined with TPB and/or ESPB, which provided a successful blocking effect. All patients received postoperative continuous analgesia (PCA) with 500 mg of tramadol and 16 mg of lornoxicam, and intravenous injection of 50 mg of flurbiprofen twice a day. Our primary outcomes including the partial pressure of arterial oxygen (PaO_2) and arterial carbon dioxide ($PaCO_2$) were measured preoperatively and on the first day after surgery. Secondary outcomes including the vital signs, ventilation parameters, postoperative numerical rating scale (NRS) pain scores, the incidence of postoperative nausea and vomiting (PONV), perioperative reflux and aspiration, and nerve block-related complications were also evaluated.

Results: Thirteen men and seven women (age 35–70 years) were enrolled. Six (30%) had a flail chest, nine (45%) had hemothorax and/or pneumothorax, and two (10%) had pulmonary contusions. The postoperative PaO_2 was higher than the preoperative value (91.2 ± 16.0 vs. 83.7 ± 15.9 mmHg, $p = 0.004$). The preoperative and postoperative $PaCO_2$ were 42.1 ± 3.7 and 43.2 ± 3.7 mmHg ($p = 0.165$), respectively. Vital signs and spontaneous breathing were stable during the surgery. The end-tidal carbon dioxide concentrations ($EtCO_2$) remained within an acceptable range (≤ 63 mmHg in all cases). NRS at T1, T2, and T3 were 3(2,4), 1(1,3), and 0(0,1), respectively. None had PONV, regurgitation, aspiration, and nerve block-related complications.

Conclusions: The technique of laryngeal mask anesthesia combined with a nerve block was feasible for internal fixation of rib fractures.

Keywords: Laryngeal mask anesthesia, Rib fractures, Thoracic paravertebral block, Erector spinae plane block

* Correspondence: zhangjunfeng@sjtu.edu.cn
[†]Jun Cao and Xiaoyun Gao contributed equally to this work.
Department of Anesthesiology, Shanghai Jiao Tong University Affiliated Sixth People's Hospital, No. 600, Yishan Rd., Shanghai, China

Background

Rib fracture is one of the most common injuries following blunt trauma, occurring in approximately 10% of all trauma patients. Surgical stabilization of rib fractures has been shown to be beneficial in those patients with flail chest and multiple severe displaced fractures [1]. In the past, general anesthesia with endotracheal intubation (ETI) was considered mandatory for rib fracture surgery. However, it might cause ventilator-induced lung injury (VILI) [2] and the patients might also have delayed awakening or even need re-intubation owing to residual general anesthetics [3]. Currently, the enhanced recovery after surgery (ERAS) protocol is well established as a standard of care for several surgeries. LMA anesthesia combined with a nerve block could offer an enhanced recovery owing to the possibility of a fast and coughless extubation and effective postoperative analgesia with less opioid [4]. Therefore, we designed this prospective observational study to evaluate the feasibility of general anesthesia with an LMA associated to regional anesthesia in elderly patients undergoing internal fixation of rib fractures.

Methods

Participants

This prospective, observational study was approved by the Ethics Committee of Shanghai Sixth People's Hospital (2019–53) and was registered at www.chictr.org.cn (ChiCTR1900023763). For this study, 20 patients who were scheduled for surgical reduction and fixation of unilateral isolated rib fractures from June to August 2019 were enrolled. Signed informed consent was obtained from all patients. The inclusion criteria were American Society of Anesthesiologists physical status I and II, age 18–70 years, body mass index (BMI) < 30, preoperative $PaO_2 > 60$ mmHg, and preoperative $PaCO_2 < 50$ mmHg. The exclusion criteria were difficult airway, esophageal reflux, myasthenia gravis, abnormal coagulation system,

gastric ulcer or hemorrhage, allergy to anesthesia-related drugs, asthma or chronic obstructive emphysema, major thoracic vascular injuries, and pregnancy.

Procedures

Non-invasive blood pressure monitoring, pulse oxygen saturation (SpO_2) monitoring, and electrocardiography were performed on the patients admitted into the operating room.

The ultrasound-guided thoracic paravertebral block (TPB) was performed on the patients who were placed in the lateral decubitus position by using the S-Nerve™ Ultrasound System (Fujifilm SonoSite Inc. Bothell, WA, USA). The transversal inferior articular process (IAP) in-plane approach was applied. A convex array probe (5–2 MHz; C60x; Fujifilm SonoSite Inc. Bothell, WA, USA) was used to visualize the vertebral lamina, internal intercostal membrane, and parietal pleura (Fig. 1a). A 22-gauge, 8-cm puncture needle (KDL medical apparatus and instruments Co. Wenzhou, China) was inserted into the thoracic paravertebral space (TPVS) from the lateral side. Ropivacaine 0.375% (20–30 ml) was injected with no air or blood aspiration.

The injection points of TPVS were selected according to the fractured rib segments requiring surgery (hereinafter referred to as "surgical segments"). If the surgical segments had less than five sequential ribs, 20 ml of ropivacaine was injected into the TPVS of the second fractured rib, referred to as a single-level block; else, 15 ml of ropivacaine was injected into the TPVS of the second and fifth fractured ribs, referred to as a double-level block. We adopted a two-person mode in TPB: one physician operated the ultrasound probe and needle while the other performed the injection and aspiration. Color Doppler ultrasound was initially used to ensure that there were no vessels in the pathway of the needle insertion while approaching the TPVS.

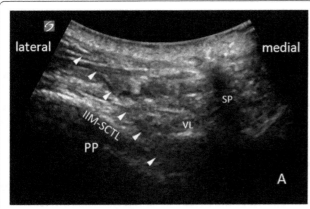
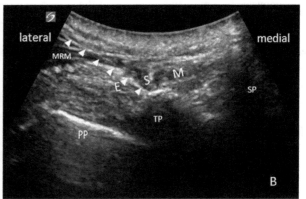

FIG. 1 Ultrasound-guided transversal in-plane approach. A, Thoracic paravertebral block. B, Erector spinae plane block. Arrowheads indicate the needle position. PP, Parietal Pleura; VL, Vertebral Lamina; TP, Transverse Process; SP, Spinae Process; IIM-SCTL, Internal Intercostal Membrane, and Superior Costotransverse Ligament; ESM, Erector Spinae Muscle; MRM, Musculus Rhomboideus Major

In the case of posterior rib fractures, ESPB was performed to enhance the regional effect of the patient's back and to supply more effective analgesia of posterior rib fractures as well [5]. Ropivacaine 0.375% (20 ml) was injected between the fifth thoracic vertebral transverse process and erector spinae muscle (ESM) on the operative side using the transversal in-plane approach under ultrasound guidance (Fig. 1b).

The effect of the regional block was evaluated 15 min after nerve blockade, and the dermatomes of sensory loss were measured by acupuncture and rubbing with alcohol gauze. If the patient felt no pain during deep-breathing and vigorous coughing, and the range of reduction area of cold or pinprick sensation covered the incision, we considered the regional effect to be satisfactory. The patient was then given LMA anesthesia and was included in this study. Otherwise, the patient was administered ETI anesthesia and excluded from the observational analysis.

Anesthesia was induced with 0.1 µg/kg sufentanil, 3 mg/kg propofol, and 0.3 mg/kg rocuronium successively. LMA Supreme™ (Teleflex Medical Co. Westmeath, Ireland) was inserted in an accurate position. Mechanical ventilation was initiated with a pressure control ventilation-volume guaranteed mode, at 6 ml/kg and a respiratory rate (RR) of 12 breaths/min. The inspiratory to expiratory ratio was 1:2. A 14# gastric tube was placed for drainage of the fluid and/or gas that might escape into the stomach during positive pressure ventilation.

During the surgery, anesthesia was maintained with sevoflurane at 0.7–1.2 age-adjusted minimum alveolar concentration (MAC) in 50% oxygen in air mixture depending on the hemodynamic responses to surgical intervention. Spontaneous breathing was maintained after recovery. A supplementary dose of 0.03 µg/kg sufentanil was allowed if the HR was 20% faster than the basic value, or RR was more than 20 breaths/min for surgical stimulation. Phenylephrine and atropine were injected if necessary. Sevoflurane inhalation was withdrawn and 50 mg of flurbiprofen was infused intravenously at 15 min before the end of the surgery. The muscle relaxant antagonist and neuromuscular blockade monitoring were not used in this study and all patients were allowed to recover on their own. The case was converted to ETI anesthesia if one of the following occurred during the surgery: 1. The surgical field was difficult to expose because of muscular tension 2. The LMA could not be placed in the correct position after three attempts 3. Hemodynamic instability occurred 4. SpO_2 was less than 90% or $EtCO_2$ was more than 70 mmHg.

PCA (infusion rate 2 ml/h, total volume 100 ml) containing 500 mg of tramadol and 16 mg of lornoxicam was routinely administered to all patients. A dosage of 50 mg of flurbiprofen was infused intravenously twice a day. If the patient's NRS was > 4, an analgesia rescue of 50 mg of pethidine was administered intramuscularly.

Data collection

The primary outcomes including PaO_2 and $PaCO_2$ were measured preoperatively and on the first day after surgery.

Secondary outcomes included:

1. vital signs during the anesthesia, tidal volume (Vt), RR, and $EtCO_2$ during spontaneous breathing;
2. postoperative time to removal of the LMA and the events of agitation or hoarseness in the post-anesthesia care unit;
3. NRS pain scores assessed at 6 (T1), 12 (T2), and 24 (T3) hours after surgery;
4. incidence of PONV within 48 h after surgery, the perioperative complications such as regurgitation, aspiration, and injuries relating to the nerve block;
5. dosages of sufentanil;
6. the number of cases that were converted to ETI during the operation.

Statistical analysis

All statistical analyses were performed using SPSS 19.0 software. The sample size was calculated based on the change of PaO_2. Seventeen patients were required to detect a mean difference of 10 mmHg and standard deviation of 10 mmHg, power of 0.8, and α-value of 0.05. Taking into consideration a potential dropout rate of 15%, we aimed to enroll 20 patients in the study. The values of arterial blood gas analysis, vital signs, ventilation parameters, postoperative extubation time, and NRS pain scores were presented as the mean ± standard deviation, median (interquartile range: min, max), or range (min-max), whichever applicable. Categorical variables such as incidence of PONV, perioperative reflux, aspiration, and nerve block-related complications were expressed as quantitative values or percentages. The results of arterial blood gas analysis measured pre- and postoperatively, were compared using Student's t-test. The significance level was considered as $p < 0.05$.

Results

Twenty patients were enrolled in this study, and their characteristics are listed in Table 1. Of the 20 patients, eight (40%) received single-level TPB, while the remaining 12 (60%) received double-level TPB. Moreover, 13 (65%) patients additionally received ESPB. All patients achieved satisfactory blockade and received LMA anesthesia. No patient required ETI anesthesia owing to the poor position of the LMA or insufficient ventilation. A flow chart of patients recruited for the study is depicted in Fig. 2.

The postoperative PaO_2 was significantly improved compared to the preoperative value (91.2 ± 16.0 vs. 83.7 ± 15.9 mmHg, $p = 0.004$). Nevertheless, there was no significant difference between preoperative and postoperative $PaCO_2$ (42.1 ± 3.7 vs. 43.2 ± 3.7 mmHg, $p = 0.165$).

Table 1 Demographics and clinical characteristics of the patients

Variable	N	Mean	%
Sex (male/female)	13/7		
Age(y)	35–70	54.15 ± 8.67	
BMI (kg/m^2)	19.1–29.7	24.29 ± 2.75	
Flail chest	6		30
Hemothorax and/or pneumothorax	10		50
Atelectasis	5		25
Pulmonary contusion	2		10
Thoracic drainage placed in surgery	9		45
Duration of surgery (min)		70 ± 21	

In most patients, the mean arterial pressure was stable, except for eight (40%) patients, whose MAPs were less than 60 mmHg transiently and were treated by phenylephrine. Patients' SpO_2 before anesthesia was 98% (93.25, 98) % and remained above 95% [99% (98, 100) %] during the operation, except for one patient whose SpO_2 declined from 100 to 87% transiently but recovered to 98% within 5 min. The duration from LMA insertion to spontaneous breathing recovery was 27.3 ± 19.4 min. Vt, RR, and $EtCO_2$ during spontaneous breathing were in the range of 205–875 ml, 7–23 breaths/min, 36–63 mmHg, respectively, except for one patient whose $EtCO_2$ exceeded 60 mmHg, ranging from 57 mmHg to 63 mmHg. The time to removal of LMA was 6 ± 3 min.

The postoperative NRS scores at T1, T2, and T3 were 3(2,4), 1(1,3), and 0(0,1), respectively. In this study, the highest score was 5 in four patients (20%). Two patients had a score of 5 at 6 h and the other two at 12 h after surgery. All four patients received one intramuscular injection of 50 mg pethidine for rescue analgesia, and pain was relieved. PONV did not occur within 48 h after surgery in all cases.

Sufentanil was administered at a dose of 9.9 ± 3.4 µg. None of the patients developed agitation or sore throat after anesthesia. Perioperative regurgitation, aspiration, and nerve block-related complications were not observed in any of the patients.

Discussion

In this study, we found that LMA anesthesia combined with nerve blocks such as TPB and ESPB could offer satisfactory

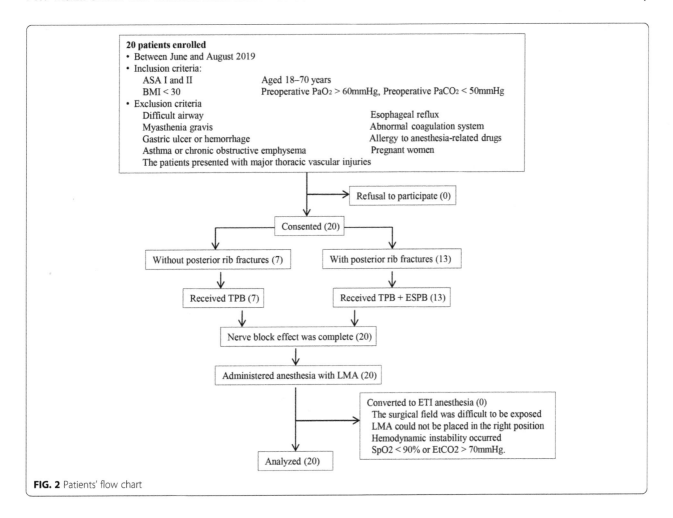

FIG. 2 Patients' flow chart

analgesia, stable hemodynamic function, good oxygenation, acceptable $EtCO_2$, and thereby a smooth recovery.

Although thoracic epidural anesthesia is a gold standard for thoracic analgesia, it can frequently induce hypotension. It is also associated with serious complications such as epidural hematoma and neuropathy [6]. Therefore, various nerve blocks can be used as alternatives to epidural anesthesia, such as the serratus anterior plane block (SAPB), intercostal nerve block (INB), and ESPB. Nevertheless, there are some limitations to the above-mentioned methods. In SAPB, the local anesthetic agent is distributed along the midaxillary line near the surgical incision, which may impede the surgeon from transecting the muscular layers. INB requires multiple injections, subjecting the patient to more pain and increases the risk of inadvertent intercostal vessel or pleural puncture. As ESPB is administered in the intermuscular space, the incidence of a complete block is about 1/3 [7]. As TPB can provide a reliable effect equivalent to that obtained with unilateral epidural anesthesia with lesser hemodynamic depression, we chose TPB for method of regional anesthesia in our study. Meanwhile, all patients maintained steady hemodynamic function with occasional administration of phenylephrine.

The intercostal (IC) and paralaminar (PL) approaches are commonly used in TPB. Yasuko Taketa et al. [8] considered that a single injection of 20 ml 0.375% ropivacaine via the PL approach could acquire 4–5 dermatomes of sensory blockade. They found that the blocked dermatomes of sensory loss were more in the PL group than in the IC group. The average number of blocked dermatomes was three in the IC group and four in the PL group. In addition, the PL approach was regarded as a better choice to block the dorsal ramus of the thoracic nerves [9]. The TPB through a PL approach may obtain a wider block effect compared to the IC approach and should be applied preferentially. Our approach regarding the TPB is the similar to Taketa's PL approach and is also consistent with the transversal IAP approach described by Krediet et al. [10] Moreover, we chose the TPVS of the second fractured rib for injection when the surgical segments were not more than four sequential ribs because we found that the area of blockade in the caudal direction was more extensive than that in the cephalic direction.

In thoracic surgery, postoperative pulmonary complications (PPCs) are problems that should be addressed. Recruitment maneuver and airway suction might be beneficial to patients during ETI anesthesia. The leak pressure of the LMA Supreme™ was 27.1 ± 5.2 cmH$_2$O according to Russo's study [11]. Thus, the LMA Supreme™ could settle for recruitment maneuver during anesthesia. Early extubation and good analgesia in our study promoted patients to have enough strength to cough and expectorate postoperatively, also beneficial to

lung recruitment. In particular, the early recovery of spontaneous breathing reduced PPCs including pneumonia and acute respiratory distress syndrome [12]. Positive pressure ventilation not only changes the pressure gradient of the thoracic cavity and interferes with the distribution of intrapulmonary ventilation, but also leads to an imbalance in the ventilation/perfusion (V/Q) ratio with excessive or inadequate tidal volume. Barotrauma and volume injury caused by mechanical ventilation can also cause VILI. The information above indicates that the spontaneous breathing might be beneficial to lung protection [12, 13]. In our study, the postoperative PaO_2 was improved compared to the preoperative values.

The patients showed various degrees of carbon dioxide retention during spontaneous breathing. The $EtCO_2$ of most patients was below 50 mmHg at the end of surgery. The highest $EtCO_2$ value in our study was 63 mmHg and occurred in a male patient whose final $EtCO_2$ was 58 mmHg at the end of the surgery. After extubation all patients were fully awake and their $PaCO_2$ was normal on the second day after surgery. The concept of permissive hypercapnia has been accepted for a long time. O'Toole et al. [14] believed that hypercapnia could produce an anti-inflammatory effect by inhibiting nuclear factor-kappa B (NF-κB). Other scholars thought that hypercapnia had a protective effect on VILI [15, 16]. Hypercapnia can also improve pulmonary compliance by a non-surfactant mechanism and enhance pulmonary vascular resistance by strengthening hypoxic pulmonary vasoconstriction to decrease the pulmonary shunt [17].

Most patients with rib fractures experienced dyspnea. The satisfactory effect of TPB could improve patient oxygenation, as respiratory amplitude increases when the patients do not feel pain [18]. The patients' Vt and RR during spontaneous breathing can meet the needs of intraoperative oxygenation, even in LMA anesthesia with 50% oxygen. Koo et al. concluded that an oxygen concentration of 50% could decrease the risk of atelectasis caused by high oxygen concentration [19]. Our results showed that all patients maintained their SpO_2 at good level during the operation, including three patients whose preoperative SpO_2 was lower than 93%. The minimum SpO_2 was 87% and occurred transiently in one case. Preoperative chest computed tomography showed a large amount of pleural effusion, incomplete atelectasis, and consolidation of the inferior lobe on the injured thorax. The decline in SpO_2 was attributed to a notable decrease in tidal volume caused by sufentanil. However, it increased to 98% in a few minutes and remained at 100% until the end of surgery.

The serratus anterior and latissimus dorsi muscles were innervated by the long thoracic and thoracodorsal nerves, respectively. TPB cannot paralyze these muscles. We found that one effective dose (ED_{95}) of rocuronium could weaken muscle twitching when the surgeons transected the muscles using a high-frequency electrotome. Murphy et al. [3] pointed out that the residual effect of muscle relaxants was one of the causes of postoperative respiratory failure, and critical respiratory events observed in 18.0% of patients undergoing thoracic surgeries. Althausen et al. reported that the incidence of re-intubation after surgical stabilization of the flail chest was 4.55% (1/22) [20]. The half dosage of muscular relaxants for ETI anesthesia in our study facilitated the patients to recover spontaneous breathing during surgery. Therefore, the patients were not monitored for neuromuscular blockade or administer muscle relaxant antagonists. Since SpO_2 was maintained above 96% during spontaneous respiration at 40% oxygen concentration, each patient was extubated with the confirmation of consciousness, blinking, good swallowing function, and fist clenching in the post-anesthesia care unit. Besides, the patients maintained a good level of cough strength after extubation and did not need re-intubation.

In our study, the analgesic effect of the nerve block was sufficient and maintained for approximately six hours after the operation. This was consistent with the duration of postoperative analgesia of TPB (303.97 ± 76.08 min) reported by Das et al. [21] Due to the PCA and intravenous infusion of flurbiprofen, most patients felt an acceptable level of pain. This indicated that the multi-mode analgesia protocol was effective and necessary for postoperative analgesia. This result also suggests that better postoperative analgesia can be achieved by TPB catheterization in a future study, as reported by Ge et al. [22].

There were several limitations to this study. Owing to the small sample size, the capacity to evaluate potential risks such as regurgitation, aspiration, and nerve block related complications was limited. Patient selection and lack of a control group also contribute to the limitations. Since the initial focus was on whether the anesthetic technique could meet the needs of rib surgery, we excluded patients with complicated extubation conditions such as respiratory failure, obesity, difficult airway, myasthenia gravis, asthma, and chronic obstructive emphysema. Although early extubation occurred and PPCs such as pneumonia and acute respiratory distress syndrome were not observed, these findings are not sufficient to declare superiority when compared with ETI anesthesia. The results in our study might provide a basis for further randomized controlled trials to assess the safety and effectiveness of this anesthesia technique.

Conclusion

We demonstrated that LMA anesthesia combined with nerve blocks could be feasibly applied in our selective patient population undergoing internal fixation of rib fractures. This practice could provide stable hemodynamic

and respiratory function, and the advantage of a smooth recovery. Our protocol could represent a draft of an ERAS anesthetic protocol for this type of surgery.

Abbreviations
LMA: Laryngeal mask airway; TPB: Thoracic paravertebral block; ESPB: Erector spinae plane block; HR: Heart rate; BP: Blood pressure; SpO_2: Pulse oxygen saturation; PCA: Postoperative continuous analgesia; NRS: Numerical rating scale; $EtCO_2$: End-tidal carbon dioxide concentration; PaO_2: Partial pressure of arterial oxygen; $PaCO_2$: Partial pressure of arterial carbon dioxide; ETI: Endotracheal intubation; VILI: Ventilator-induced lung injury; BMI: Body mass index; IAP: Inferior Articular Process; TPVS: Thoracic paravertebral space; PONV: Postoperative nausea and vomiting; Vt: Tidal volume; RR: Respiratory rate; MAC: Minimum alveolar concentration; SAPB: Serratus anterior plane block; INB: Intercostal nerve block; IC: Intercostal; PL: Paralaminar; ED_{95}: 95% effective dose; PPCs: Postoperative pulmonary complications

Acknowledgments
Not applicable.

Authors' contributions
This study was designed by JC and JFZ, and was conducted by JC, XYG, XLZ. XYG and JL collected the data. JC analyzed the data and drafted the manuscript. All authors read and approved the final manuscript.

References
1. Pieracci FM, et al. Consensus statement: surgical stabilization of rib fractures rib fracture colloquium clinical practice guidelines. Injury. 2017;48:307–21.
2. Dos Santos CC, Slutsky AS. Invited review: mechanisms of ventilator-induced lung injury: a perspective. J Appl Physiol (1985). 2000;89:1645–55.
3. Murphy GS, Szokol JW, Marymont JH, Greenberg SB, Avram MJ, Vender JS. Residual neuromuscular blockade and critical respiratory events in the postanesthesia care unit. Anesth Analg. 2008;107:130–7.
4. Gonzalez-Rivas D, Bonome C, Fieira E, et al. Non-intubated video-assisted thoracoscopic lung resections: the future of thoracic surgery? Eur J Cardiothorac Surg. 2016;49:721–31.
5. Luftig J, Mantuani D, Herring AA, et al. Successful emergency pain control for posterior rib fractures with ultrasound-guided erector spinae plane block. Am J Emerg Med. 2018;36:1391–6.
6. Rosero EB, Joshi GP. Nationwide incidence of serious complications of epidural analgesia in the United States. Acta Anaesthesiol Scand. 2016; 60:810–20.
7. Ban CH, Tsui AF, Munshey F, et al. The erector spinae plane (ESP) block: a pooled review of 242 cases. J Clin Anesth. 2019;53:29–34.
8. Taketa Y, Irisawa Y, Fujitani T. Comparison of analgesic efficacy between two approaches of paravertebral block for thoracotomy: a randomised trial. Acta Anaesthesiol Scand. 2018;62:1274–9.
9. Thomas Collin, Julie Cox. Innervation of the chest wall. Chapter 53. Gray's Anatomy: the anatomical basis of clinical practice, 41st edn. In: Jonathan D Spratt, Standring S, eds. Amsterdam, The Netherlands: Elsevier; 2015. p. 944–5.
10. Krediet AC, Moayeri N, van Geffen GJ, et al. Different approaches to ultrasound-guided thoracic paravertebral block: an illustrated review. Anesthesiology. 2015;123:459–74.
11. Sebastian G, Russo SC, Galli T, et al. Randomized comparison of the i-gel™, the LMA Supreme™, and the Laryngeal Tube Suction-D using clinical and fibreoptic assessments in elective patients. BMC Anesthesiol. 2012;12:18.
12. Noda M, Okada Y, Maeda S, et al. Is there a benefit of awake thoracoscopic surgery in patients with secondary spontaneous pneumothorax? J Thorac Cardiovasc Surg. 2012;143:613–6.
13. Tokics L, Hedenstierna G, Svensson L, et al. V/Q distribution and correlation to atelectasis in anesthetized paralyzed humans. J Appl Physiol (1985). 1996; 81(4):1822–33.
14. O'Toole D, Hassett P, Contreras M, et al. Hypercapnic acidosis attenuates pulmonary epithelial wound repair by an NF- kB dependent mechanism. Thorax. 2009;64:976–82.
15. Sinclair SE, Kregenow DA, Lamm WJ, et al. Hypercapnic acidosis is protective in an in vivo model of ventilator-induced lung injury. Am J Respir Crit Care Med. 2002;166:403–8.

16. Broccard AF, Hotchkiss JR, Vannay C, et al. Protective effects of hypercapnic acidosis on ventilator-induced lung injury. Am J Respir Crit Care Med. 2001; 164:802–6.

17. Jonathan M, Eddy F. Carbon Dioxide in the Critically Ill: Too Much or Too Little of a Good Thing? Respir Care. 2014;59:1597–605.

18. Bataille B, Nucci B, De Selle J, et al. Paravertebral block restore diaphragmatic motility measured by ultrasonography in patients with multiple rib fractures. J Clin Anesth. 2017;42:55–6.

19. Koo CH, Park EY, Lee SY, Ryu JH. The Effects of Intraoperative Inspired Oxygen Fraction on Postoperative Pulmonary Parameters in Patients with General Anesthesia: A Systemic Review and Meta-Analysis. J Clin Med. 2019; 28(8):583.

20. Althausen PL, Shannon S, Watts C, et al. Early surgical stabilization of flail chest with locked plate fixation. J Orthop Trauma. 2011;25:641–7.

21. Das S, Bhattacharya P, Mandal MC, et al. Multiple-injection thoracic paravertebral block as an alternative to general anaesthesia for elective breast surgeries: a randomized controlled trial. Indian J Anaesth. 2012;56:27–33.

22. Yeying G, Liyong Y, Yuebo C, et al. Thoracic paravertebral block versus intravenous patient-controlled analgesia for pain treatment in patients with multiple rib fractures. J Int Med Res. 2017;45:2085–91.

17

GlideScope® versus C-MAC®(D) videolaryngoscope versus Macintosh laryngoscope for double-lumen endotracheal intubation in patients with predicted normal airways

Ping Huang[†], Renlong Zhou[†], Zhixing Lu, Yannan Hang, Shanjuan Wang[*] and Zhenling Huang[*]

Abstract

Background: The double lumen endotracheal tube (DLT) is the most widely-used device for single lung ventilation in current thoracic anesthesia practice. In recent years, the routine application of the videolaryngoscope for single lumen endotracheal intubation has increased; nevertheless there are few studies of the use of the videolaryngoscope for DLT. We wondered whether there were benefits to using the videolaryngoscope for DLT placement in patients with predicted normal airways. Therefore, this study was designed to compare the performances of the GlideScope®, the C-MAC®(D) videolaryngoscope and the Macintosh laryngoscope in DLT intubation.

Methods: This was a randomized, controlled, prospective study. We randomly allocated 90 adult patients with predicted normal airways into three groups. All patients underwent routine anesthesia using different laryngoscopes according to group allocation. We compared DLT insertion times, first-pass success rates, numerical rating scales (NRS) of DLT delivery and DLT insertion, Cormack-Lehane degrees (C/L), hemodynamic changes and incidences of intubation complications. All outcomes were analyzed using SPSS13.0.

Results: Compared with the GlideScope, the Macintosh gave shorter times for DLT insertion (median: 96 (IQR: 51 [min–max: 62–376] s vs 73 (26 [48–419] s, $p = 0.003$); however, there was no difference between the Macintosh and C-MAC(D) ($p = 0.610$). The Macintosh had a significantly higher successful first attempt rate than did the GlideScope or C-MAC(D) ($p = 0.001$, $p = 0.028$, respectively). NRS of DLT delivery and insertion were significantly lower in the Macintosh than in the others ($p < 0.001$). However, the C/L degree in the Macintosh was significantly higher than in the others ($p < 0.001$). The incidences of oral bleeding, hoarseness, sore throat and dental trauma were low in all groups ($p > 0.05$). There were no significant differences in DLT misplacement, fiberoptic time or hemodynamic changes among the groups.

(Continued on next page)

* Correspondence: Shanjuanwang@shsmu.edu.cn;
Zhenlinghuang@shsmu.edu.cn
†Ping Huang and Renlong Zhou contributed equally to this work.
Department of Anesthesiology, Renji Hospital, School of Medicine, Shanghai
Jiaotong University, Shanghai 200001, China

(Continued from previous page)

Conclusions: Compared with the Macintosh laryngoscope, the GlideScope® and C-MAC®(D) videolaryngoscopes may not be recommended as the first choice for routine DLT intubation in patients with predicted normal airways.

Keywords: GlideScope® videolaryngoscope, C-MAC®(D) videolaryngoscope, Macintosh laryngoscope, Double lumen tracheal tube, Endotracheal intubation

Background

The double lumen endotracheal (DLT) tube is the most widely-used device for single lung ventilation in current thoracic anesthesia practice [1]. Nevertheless, on account of its relatively large diameter, larger volume of oral cavity occupation, and rotating insertion technique, the DLT is generally more difficult to insert and advance than is the single lumen endotracheal tube.

In recent years, videolaryngoscopes have become the new standard of care for intubation because they provide clear views of the glottis using a video-camera or video-chip that is positioned close to the tip of the laryngoscope blade. Each available videolaryngoscope is unique in terms of design [2, 3]. They can be divided into three types according to blade type: the standard Macintosh-shaped blade, the angulated blade, and a channel for tube passage [4].

The GlideScope® is a videolaryngoscope with a highly-angulated blade form that offers an obligatory indirect view of the epiglottis [5]. Several authors described use of the GlideScope® in patients with difficult airways during anesthesia [6–9]. Most authors found that the GlideScope® gave better laryngoscopic views than did either conventional direct laryngoscopy or Macintosh videolaryngoscopy in patients with predicted difficult airways [5]. Serocki et al. concluded that the GlideScope® and the C-MAC® may be useful in the management of predicted difficult airways [6]. Stroumpoulis et al. suggested that it could be a logical alternative in the management of difficult airways for single-lumen endotracheal intubation [7]. Sun et al. found that the GlideScope® provided laryngoscopic views equal to or better than those of direct laryngoscopy in 200 patients; however, the device required additional 16 s to achieve tracheal intubation [8]. In a systematic review and meta-analysis, Donald et al. found that, compared to direct laryngoscopy, Glidescope® videolaryngoscopy was associated with improved glottic visualization, particularly in patients with potential or simulated difficult airways [9].

The C-MAC® videolaryngoscope was introduced with conventional Macintosh blades, and has been used appropriately for routine airway intubation [10]. To manage difficult airways, the C-MAC® system recently introduced the highly angulated D-Blade [11]. The GlideScope® and C-MAC®(D) videolaryngoscope are generally of the same type, possessing angulated blades. They are the only videolaryngoscopes available in anesthesiology departments in China.

There are a few studies investigating angulated videolaryngoscopes for DLT intubation. The potential advantages of the GlideScope® for DLT insertion include a better view of the vocal cords, a clear view of the DLT when it passes the vocal cords, and an external video screen for teaching purposes and for the assistant providing external laryngeal pressure [12]. Nevertheless, at present, it remains controversial as to whether the GlideScope® videolaryngoscope possesses advantages for double lumen endotracheal intubation [12, 13]; to our knowledges, there has been only one article reporting the performance of the C-MAC®(D) for double lumen endotracheal intubation [14]. Therefore, in the present study, we compared the performances of the GlideScope®, C-MAC®(D) videolaryngoscope and the Macintosh laryngoscope in DLT intubation in normal airways.

Methods

Approval for the study was granted by the Shanghai Renji Hospital Ethics Committee (Ethical number: 2016[036]). Written informed consent was obtained from patients undergoing elective intra-thoracic surgeries requiring double lumen intubation. The present trial was registered at http://www.chictr.org.cn (registration number ChiCTR1 900025718; principal investigator: Z.L.H.; date of registration: September 6, 2019).

Inclusion criteria were as follows: age 18–75 years old; ASA I–II, BMI < 35 kg/m^2, with Mallampati score of 1 or 2. All Mallampati scores were assigned by the same observer. Exclusion criteria were as follows: presence of any predictors of difficult intubation; Mallampati score > =3; inter-incisor distance < 3 cm; thyromental distance < 6 cm; neck extension < 80°from neck flexion; cervical spine instability; history of difficult endotracheal intubation or difficult mask ventilation; and severe pulmonary ventilation dysfunction or risk of pulmonary aspiration.

Eligible patients were enrolled on the basis of the CONSORT Statement Extension for Randomized Controlled Trials of Nonpharmacological Trials, as displayed in the flowchart in Fig. 1. We randomly assigned 90 patients to GlideScope (Verathon Medical, Bothwell, UT, USA), C-MAC(D) (Karl Storz GmbHand Co.KG, Tuttlingen, Germany), or Macintosh groups. This was done using a

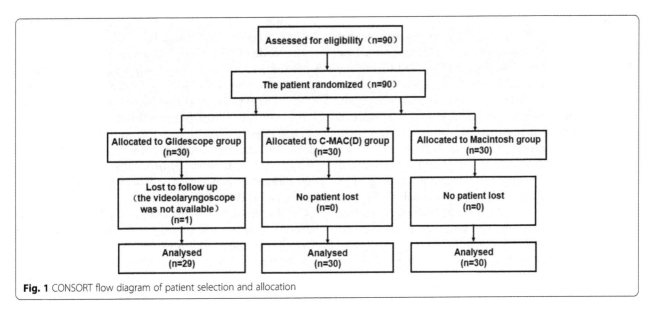

Fig. 1 CONSORT flow diagram of patient selection and allocation

closed envelope technique using a computer-generated block randomization method in blocks of 15. Before the study, the computerized randomization was performed and the allocation results were placed in individual numbered and sealed envelopes. The researcher responsible for recruitment blinded to the allocation result. After a patient was consented for the study, allocation was revealed. All endotracheal intubations were performed by five anesthesiologists with 10 years' working experience skilled in videolaryngoscopy.

Left-side or right-side 32Fr/35Fr Mallinckrodt™ DLTs (Mallinckrodt Medical, Athlone, Ireland) were selected for female patients and 35Fr/37Fr DLTs for male patients depending on whether their heights were below or above 155 cm for females and 165 cm for males. If the operation side was the left, right-side DLT was used; otherwise, the left-side DLT was used. To facilitate intubation, the distal 10–12 cm concavity of the DLT (with the stylet in situ) was molded along the blade convexity in each group. The tracheal and the bronchial cuffs of the DLT tubes were lubricated with sterile Surgilube.

No premedication was given before induction. Standard monitoring prior to induction included ECG, invasive arterial blood pressure, SpO_2, and end-tidal carbon dioxide. After pre-oxygenation with 100% oxygen, anesthesia was induced with intravenous midazolam 0.05 $mg\cdot kg^{-1}$, propofol 1.5 $mg\cdot kg^{-1}$, fentanyl 5 $\mu g\cdot kg^{-1}$, and rocuronium 0.6 $mg\cdot kg^{-1}$. Ninety seconds after rocuronium administration, DLT intubation was performed using the allocated laryngoscope. The DLT was inserted with the distal concavity facing anteriorly until the bronchial lumen cuff passed the vocal cords. The stylet was then removed, and rotation was performed while tube was advanced. The left DLT rotated 90° counter-clockwise, and the right DLT was rotated 90° clockwise to enter the respective mainstem

bronchus. Hemodynamic changes were monitored during induction. If systolic blood pressure fell below 80 mmHg, ephedrine 5 mg was administrated intravenously. Atropine 0.5 mg was given for heart rate below 50 beats per minute. After the tip of the DLT was located in the targeted bronchus, the tracheal cuff was inflated and ventilation of the lungs started. Fiberoptic bronchoscopic assessment of adequate bronchial cuff placement was followed by DLT placement.

DLT insertion time was defined as from the time the laryngoscope passed the patient's lips until three complete end-tidal carbon dioxide cycles were displayed on the monitor. Intubation success rate at the first attempt was recorded by the same observer. The difficulty of DLT insertion and delivery were assessed by the operator, using NRS ranging from 0 to 10. The NRS results were grouped as 0 = none, 1–3 = mild, 4–6 = moderate, and 7–10 = severe. C/L degrees were classified as four degrees (I, II_A, II_B, and III) and were assessed by the same operator. If the degree was not class I, external laryngeal pressure was provided by an assistant. The time taken for fiberoptic bronchoscopy was defined as the time from endobronchial intubation to placement confirmation using fiberoptic bronchoscopy. The operators examined blade surfaces for blood after removal. Hemodynamic parameters (mean arterial blood pressure and heart rate) were recorded 10 min before induction and 1, 3, and 5 min after intubation. After the assessment by fiberoptic bronchoscopy, the oral cavity, pharynx, larynx and teeth were examined for signs of laceration or bleeding by an independent investigator who was unaware of the type of laryngoscope used. One day after surgery, an independent investigator interviewed patients to assess the presence of sore throat and hoarseness of voice.

Statistical analysis

Based on previous studies [13, 14], we determined that the mean intubation time for the GlideScope would be 45.6 s with a standard deviation of 10.7 s, and that of the C-MAC(D) would be 32.27 s with a standard deviation of 11.13 s [12]. Factoring possible drop-outs, we recruited 30 patients in each group, with an alpha value of 0.05 and a beta value of 0.2.

Data were expressed as median (interquartile range (IQR) [min–max]), mean ± SD, or absolute numbers, as required. Statistical analysis was performed using SPSS 13.0 (SPSS Inc., Chicago, IL). The Kruskal–Wallis test was used to analyze independent samples (the success rate at the first attempt, the times of intubation attempts, the DLT insertion time, the number of external laryngeal pressure applications, C/L degree, and NRS of DLT delivery and insertion). The Chi-square and Student–Newman–Keuls tests were used to analyze demographic data and the incidence of complications. For the analysis of hemodynamic response to intubation, a repeated-measures analysis of variance was used. Statistical significance was considered at $P < 0.05$.

Results

The CONSORT flow diagram of the study is shown in Fig. 1. Of the 90 patients recruited, 89 completed the study. One patient in the GlideScope group was excluded because the videolaryngoscope was not available. Characteristics of patients and intubation conditions were similar in all three groups (Table 1).

The median DLT insertion time was 96 s (51 [62–376] s) with the GlideScope, 73 s (26 [48–419] s) with the Macintosh ($p = 0.003$) and 72.5 s (46 [47–467] s) with the C-MAC(D) ($p = 0.022$). There was no difference between the Macintosh and C-MAC(D) ($p = 0.610$) (Fig. 2).

The number of successes at the first attempt was 24 (80%) with the Macintosh, 11 (38%) with the GlideScope ($p = 0.001$), and 16 (53%) with the C-MAC(D) ($p = 0.028$).

There was no difference between the GlideScope and the C-MAC(D) ($p = 0.235$) (Table 2).

The median NRS of DLT delivery was 2 (1.75 [0–3]) with the Macintosh, 5 (3 [1–9]) with the GlideScope ($p = 0.000$), and 3 (2 [0–6]) with the C-MAC(D) (p = 0.001). The P-value for the difference between the GlideScope and the C-MAC(D) was 0.000. The median NRS of DLT insertion was 1 (2 [0–10]) with the Macintosh, 3 (3 [0–9]) with the GlideScope (p = 0.001), and 3 (1.75 [0–6]) with the C-MAC(D) ($p = 0.026$). The P-value for the difference between the GlideScope and the C-MAC(D) was 0.039 (Fig. 3).

C/L degrees ($I/II_A/II_B/III$) were 14/14/1/0 with the GlideScope, 26/4/0/0 with the C-MAC (D) ($p = 0.006$), and 9/9/5/7 with the Macintosh ($p = 0.008$). The P-value for the difference between the C-MAC(D) and the Macintosh was 0.000. The data indicate that external laryngeal pressure was used most often in the Macintosh group (Table 2).

There were no differences in the number of DLT misplacements or fiberoptic times. Blood was observed on the laryngoscopes in only one patient in each of the GlideScope and the C-MAC(D) groups. We found a low incidence of oral bleeding, sore throat, and dental trauma in all three groups, with no significant differences. One patient each required ephedrine in the GlideScope and C-MAC(D) groups; however, no patient in any group required atropine (Table 2).

Heart rate increased 1 min after intubation in all three groups and increased 3 min after intubation in the C-MAC(D) group (Fig. 4). Mean arterial pressure decreased 3 min after intubation in all three groups (Fig. 5). There was no difference between groups with respect to hemodynamic responses to intubation.

Discussion

In our study comparing the GlideScope® and C-MAC®(D) videolaryngoscopes with the Macintosh laryngoscope to assist DLT intubation, we found that the

Table 1 Characteristics and intubation conditions of patients assigned to GlideScope, C-MAC(D) or Macintosh group

	GlideScope group (n = 29)	C-MAC(D) group (n = 30)	Macintosh group (n = 30)
Age (yr)	58.45 ± 8.80	57.20 ± 9.60	54.57 ± 11.78
BMI (kg/m^2)	23.33 ± 3.29	22.82 ± 2.67	24.32 ± 3.78
Male/Female (n)	11/18	18/12	20/10
ASA I/II (n)	17/12	18/12	20/10
DLT left/right (n)	17/12	21/9	21/9
Malampati I/II (n)	17/11	17/13	19/11
Inter–incisor distance (cm)	4.29 ± 0.60	4.43 ± 0.77	4.53 ± 0.88
Thyromental distance (cm)	7.77 ± 0.78	7.97 ± 0.79	7.72 ± 0.75
Neck extension> 90^0 (n)	29	30	30

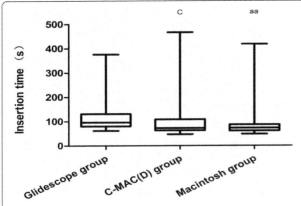

Fig. 2 The time taken for bronchial insertion with GlideScope was significantly longer compared with those taken for Macintosh and C-MAC(D). GlideScope vs C-MAC(D) vs Macintosh: 96 s (51 [62–376] s) vs 72.5 s (46 [47–467] s) vs 73 s (26 [48–419] s); ^{aa} $P < 0.01$, between the GlideScope and Macintosh groups. ^{c} $P < 0.05$, between the GlideScope and C-MAC(D) groups

Macintosh was associated with shorter insertion time, higher success rate at the first attempt, less difficulty score of DLT delivery and insertion, higher C/L degree and more use of external laryngeal pressure. To the best of our knowledge, no study has compared the Glide-Scope® and C-MAC®(D) videolaryngoscopes with the Macintosh laryngoscope for DLT intubation, highlighting the novelty of the present trial.

The GlideScope® videolaryngoscope was the first obligatory indirect videolaryngoscope with a pronounced anterior angulation of 60° of its blade [5]. The C-MAC®(D) videolaryngoscope has a pronounced angulation of 40°. In contrast to the GlideScope®, the D-Blade's camera and light socket are located closer (40 mm) to the blade's tip, which is bent another 20° [15].

With the attached cables and the angulated blade form, the GlideScope® and C-MAC®(D) videolaryngoscopes often require more delicate manipulation than the conventional Macintosh laryngoscope when they are introduced into the mouth and advanced further. Nevertheless, manipulation inside the oropharyngeal space is restricted because of the high degree of blade angulation. When proceeding in a relatively steep angle through the glottic opening, the DLT may get caught at the arytenoids or the ventral tracheal wall. The use of both videolaryngoscopes requires hand-eye coordination on the part of the operator. The operator should identify the glottis and vocal cords on the screen, then manipulate the DLT to enter into the mouth and past the vocal cords into trachea; doing so may prolong insertion time. Videolaryngoscopes with large bending blades often require larger angles of the distal stylet to enable the tracheal tube to reach the glottis through the "corner field" of the blade [16]. This increases the difficulty of tube delivery and insertion time. Nevertheless, in the present study, the insertion time of the C-MAC(D) was similar to that of the Macintosh. The reason may be that both blades are relatively thin. This increased room in the oral cavity for intubation and made the double lumen canal rotation relatively convenient. Second, because the images obtained by C-MAC®(D) videolaryngoscope include the tip of the blade, the device can be placed in the epiglottic valley under monitor vision. This also shortens insertion time. Because of the large outer

Table 2 Details of intubation with a double-lumen tube using the GlideScope, C-MAC(D) or Macintosh group

	GlideScope group($n = 29$)	C-MAC(D) group($n = 30$)	Macintosh group($i = 30$)	P value
Number of intubation attempts (1/2/3)	11/12/6	16/11/3	24/3/3 ^{aab}	0.010
The success at the first attempt (n)	11 (37.93%)	16 (53.33%)	24 (80.00%) ^{aab}	0.004
Cormack-Lehane degree(I/II$_A$/II$_B$/III)	14/14/1/0 ^{cc}	26/4/0/0	9/9/5/7 ^{aabb}	0.000
Number of external laryngeal pressure (n)	4 (13.79%) ^{c}	0 (0)	14 (46.67%) ^{aabb}	0.000
Number of DLT misplacement (n)	4 (13.79%)	9 (30.00%)	5 (16.67%)	0.252
Fibreoptic time (s)	54.07 ± 25.46	63.13 ± 23.77	57.43 ± 21.8	0.309
Oral bleeding (n)	1 (3.45%)	1 (3.33%)	0 (0)	0.594
Hoarseness (n)	0 (0)	0 (0)	1 (3.33%)	0.370
Sore throat (n)	1 (3.45%)	3 (10%)	1 (3.33%)	0.441
Dental trauma (n)	0 (0)	0 (0)	0 (0)	
Atropine (n)	0 (0)	0 (0)	0 (0)	
Ephedrine (n)	1 (3.45%)	1 (3.33%)	0 (0)	0.594

^{aa}p < 0.01 between Glidescope and Macintosh
^{bb}p < 0.01 between C-MAC(D) and Macintosh
^{b}p < 0.05 between C-MAC(D) and Macintosh
^{cc}p < 0.01 between Glidescope and C-MAC(D)
^{c}p < 0.05 between Glidescope and C-MAC(D)

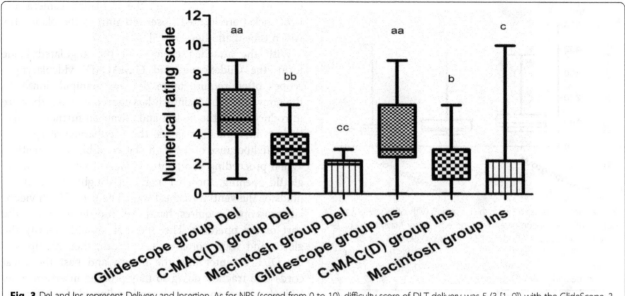

Fig. 3 Del and Ins represent Delivery and Insertion. As for NRS (scored from 0 to 10), difficulty score of DLT delivery was 5 (3 [1–9]) with the GlideScope, 3 (2 [0–6]) with the C-MAC(D) (p = 0.000), 2 (1.75 [0–3]) with the Macintosh (p = 0.000). C-MAC(D) vs the Macintosh (p = 0.001). Difficulty score of DLT insertion was 3 (3 [0–9]) with the GlideScope, 3 (1.75 [0–6]) with C-MAC(D) (p = 0.039) and 1 (2 [0–10]) with Macintosh (p = 0.001). C-MAC(D) vs Macintosh p = 0.026. aaP < 0.01, between the GlideScope and Macintosh groups; bbP < 0.01, between the C-MAC(D) and Macintosh groups; bP < 0.05, between the GlideScope and C-MAC(D) groups; ccP < 0.01, between the C-MAC(D) and Macintosh groups; cP < 0.05, between the C-MAC(D) and Macintosh groups

diameter and more rigid design of DLTs, they are relatively harder to insert alongside the angulated and thick blade of the GlideScope®, which necessitates angulation of the tip of the DLT to follow the curve of its angulated blade, together with sequential rotation of the DLT. This potentially could prolong the time required for DLT insertion [17].

The advantages of the GlideScope® and C-MAC®(D) videolaryngoscope for DLT insertion include the following: improved views of vocal cords and of the DLT when the devices pass the vocal cords; external video monitors for assisting staff who apply external pressure to the larynx; and finally, these devices are ideal for teaching purposes. Their disadvantages include increased blade angulation and

thickness that may cause difficulty in manipulating the DLT to enter into the mouth and pass the vocal cords into the trachea [12]. This decreases the success rate of the first attempt. At the same time, forward movement of the videolaryngoscope lens and requirement for hand-eye coordination on the part of the operator decrease the success rate at the first attempt. Although the Macintosh laryngoscope showed a higher C/L degree, that is unfavorable to endotracheal intubation, glottic views were improved by application of external laryngeal pressure. These data suggest that the Macintosh laryngoscope had a higher success rate at the first attempt.

Due to the thicker blade of GlideScope® and the larger DLT diameter, difficulty with DLT manipulation and

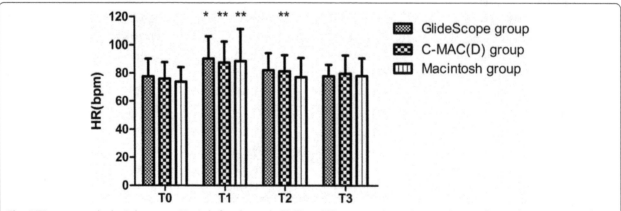

Fig. 4 T0 represents the basic heart rate 10 min before the study. T1, T2 and T3 represent 1 min, 3 min and 5 min after intubation, respectively. Heart rate increased 1 min after intubation in all three groups and increased 3 min after intubation in the C-MAC(D) group. Compared with T0, GlideScope *P < 0.05, C-MAC(D) **P < 0.01, Macintosh **P < 0.01 in T1, C-MAC(D) P < 0.01 in T2

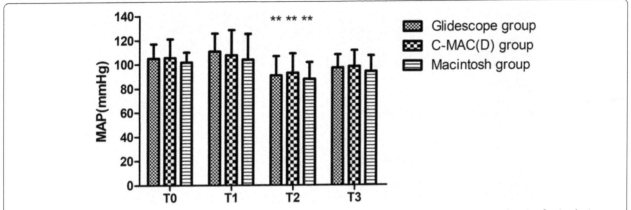

Fig. 5 T0 represents the basic mean arterial pressure 10 min before the study. T1, T2 and T3 represent 1 min, 3 min and 5 min after intubation, respectively. Mean arterial pressure decreased 3 min after intubation in all three groups. Compared with T0, three groups **$P < 0.01$ in T2

difficulty in fitting the device and entering into patient's mouth were the most common reasons for GlideScope intubation failures, as previously reported [12]. Blades with large cambers and forward movement of the C-MAC®(D) lens increased difficulty of DLT delivery and insertion. DLT delivery and insertion scores were lower with the Macintosh than with the GlideScope or C-MAC(D). Our findings support the common view that tube delivery and advancement into the trachea are the most difficult steps when using non-channeled hyper-angulated videolaryngoscopes [16].

There was no difference between left or right DLT with respect to the incidence of the DLT entering the wrong bronchus among the groups, suggesting that misplacement had no obvious association with any laryngoscope. The original preformed shape of the anterior concavity of the DLT was slightly altered to conform to the greater angulation of the D-blade and the GlideScope before intubation, possibly increasing DLT misplacement. Nevertheless, this could be easily rectified using the fiberoptic bronchoscopy.

Postoperative sore throat and hoarseness are common complications after using DLT [18]; nevertheless, we found a low incidence of oral bleeding, hoarseness, sore throat and dental trauma in all three groups. This may be the case for two reasons. First, the DLT tubes were adequately lubricated and operated by experienced anesthesiologists. Second, 90° rotation aligned the axis of the tracheal lumen with the patient's tracheal axis. This facilitated the passage of the tracheal cuff through the vocal cords and reduced the incidence of vocal cord injury. Hsu et al. described the method to rotate the DLT counterclockwise 180° to facilitate passage of the bronchial cuff. After the tracheal cuff passed through vocal cords, an additional 90° clockwise rotation was performed to align the tube with the left main bronchus [13]. The number of rotations was less in our study than in Hsu's; this may explain the lower incidence of hoarseness and sore throat.

There were no differences in hemodynamic changes among the groups, suggesting that videolaryngoscopy did not reduce the stress response caused by DLT intubation.

Limitations

There are a few limitations in our study. First, the intubating anesthesiologist or independent observer was unblinded to the randomization of the videolaryngoscope. This could lead to bias. Nevertheless, the primary outcome and most of the other outcomes were objective and well-defined. Second, the operators were five anesthesiologists who had substantial experience of using the GlideScope® and the C-MAC®(D) videolaryngoscopes as well as practical techniques of DLT for administration of thoracic anesthesia. This study excluded young anesthesiologists who were inexperienced; this may have been another source of bias. Third, recruited patients had normal airways. It is not possible to comment as to whether these findings would be consistent with DLT intubation of difficult airways. Such a study should be performed in the future. Finally, we did not include videolaryngoscopes with standard Macintosh shaped blades.

Conclusion

Compared with the Macintosh laryngoscope, the GlideScope® and C-MAC®(D) videolaryngoscopes may not be recommended as the first choice for routine DLT intubation in patients with predicted normal airways.

Abbreviations
DLT: Double lumen endotracheal tube; NRS: Numerical rating scale; C/L degree: Cormack-Lehane degree; ASA: American Society of Anesthesiologists; BMI: Body mass index; ECG: Electrocardiogram; SpO2: Pulse oximetry saturation

Acknowledgements
We wishes to acknowledge Yanyan Song (Department of statistics, School of Medicine, Shanghai Jiaotong University, Shanghai 200125, China), and Anqi Lv (Division of Anesthesiology and Perioperative Medicine, Singapore General Hospital, Singapore 169608) for their assistance in preparing and instructing this manuscript.

Authors' contributions
ZLH and SJW were responsible for the conception and design of the study. PH and RLZ were responsible for analysis of data and manuscript. PH and ZXL were responsible for performing the experiement and the collection of data. Furthermore, YNH made substantial contribution in writing and revising the manuscript. All authors have read and approved the final manuscript.

References
1. Campos JH. Lung isolation techniques for patients with difficult airway. Curr Opin Anaesthesiol. 2010;23:12–7.
2. Ng I, Hill AL, Williams DL, Lee K, Segal R. Randomized controlled trial comparing the McGrath videolaryngoscope with the C-MAC videolaryngoscope in intubating adult patients with potential difficult airways. Br J Anaesth. 2012;109:439–43.
3. Ahmed-Nusrath A. Focus on: ophthalmic anesthesia videolaryngoscopy. Curr Anaesth Crit Care. 2010;21:199–205.
4. Niforopoulou P, Pantazopoulos I, Demestiha T, Koudouna E, Xanthos T. Video-laryngoscopes in the adult airway management: a topical review of the literature. Acta Anaesthesiol Scand. 2010;54:1050–61.
5. Serocki G, Neumann T, Scharf E, Dörges V, Cavus E. Indirect videolaryngoscopy with C-MAC D-blade and GlideScope: a randomized, controlled comparison in patients with suspected difficult airways. Minerva Anestesiol. 2013;79:121–9.
6. Serocki G, Bein B, Scholz J, Dorges V. Management of the predicted difficult airway: a comparison of conventional blade laryngoscopy with video-assisted blade laryngoscopy and the GlideScope. Eur J Anaesthesiol. 2010; 27:24–30.
7. Stroumpoulis K, Pagoulatou A, Violari M, Ikonomou I, Kalantzi N, Kastrinaki K, et al. Videolaryngoscopy in the management of the difficult airway: a comparison with the Macintosh blade. Eur J Anaesthesiol. 2009;26:218–22.
8. Sun DA, Warriner CB, Parsons DG, Klein R, Umedaly HS, Moult M. The GlideScope video laryngoscope: randomized clinical trial in 200 patients. Br J Anaesth. 2005;94:381–4.
9. Griesdale DEG, Liu D, McKinney J, Choi PT. Glidescope® video-laryngoscoppy versus direct laryngoscopy for endotracheal intubation: a systematic review and meta-analysis. Can J Anesth. 2012;59:41–52.
10. Cavus E, Thee C, Moeller T, Kieckhaefer J, Doerges V, Wagner K. A randomised, controlled crossover comparison of the C-MAC videolaryngoscope with direct laryngoscopy in 150 patients during routine induction of anesthesia. BMC Anesthesiol. 2011;11:6–13.
11. Williams K, Carli F, Cormack RS. Unexpected, difficult laryngoscopy: a prospective survey in routine general surgery. Br J Anaesth. 1991;66:38–44.
12. Russell T, Slinger P, Roscoe A, McRae K, Rensburg AV. A randomised controlled trial comparing the GlideScope and the Macintosh laryngoscope for double lumen endobronchial intubation. Anaesthesia. 2013;68:1253–8.
13. Hsu HT, Chou SH, Wu PJ, Tseng KY, Kuo YW, Chou CY, Cheng KI. Comparison of the GlideScope videolaryngoscope and the Macintosh laryngoscope for double lumen tube intubation. Anaesthesia. 2012;67:411–5.
14. Shah SB, Bhargava AK, Hariharan U, Mittal AK, Goel N, Choudhary M. A randomized clinical trial comparing the standard McIntosh laryngoscope and the C-mac D blade video laryngoscope™ for double lumen tube insertion for one lung ventilation in Onco surgical patients. Indian J Anaesth. 2016;60:312–8.
15. Batuwitage B, McDonald A, Nishikawa K, Lythgoe D, Mercer S, Peter CP. Comparison between bougies and stylets for simulated tracheal intubation with the C-MAC D-blade videolaryngoscope. Eur J Anaesthesiol. 2015;32:400–5.
16. Levitan RM, Heitz JW, Sweeney M, Cooper RM. The complexities of tracheal intubation with direct laryngoscopy and alternative intubation devices. Ann Emerg Med. 2011;57:240–7.
17. El-Tahan MR, Khidr AM, Gaarour IS, Alshadwi SA, Alghamdi TM, Al'ghamdi A. Comparison of 3 Videolaryngoscopes for double lumen tube intubation in humans by users with mixed experience: a randomized controlled study. J Cardiothorac Vasc Anesth. 2018;32:277–86.
18. Park SH, Han SH, Do SH, Kim JW, Rhee KY, Kim JH. Prophylactic dexamethasone decreases the incidence of sore throat and hoarseness after tracheal extubation with a double lumen endobronchial tube. Anesth Analg. 2008;107:1814–8.

18

Nasotracheal intubation-extubation-intubation and asleep-awake-asleep anesthesia technique for deep brain stimulation

Wenxi Tang[1], Penghui Wei[1], Jiapeng Huang[2], Na Zhang[1], Haipeng Zhou[1], Jinfeng Zhou[1], Qiang Zheng[1], Jianjun Li[1*] and Zhigang Wang[3*]

Abstract

Background: The asleep-awake-asleep (AAA) technique and laryngeal mask airway (LMA) is a common general anesthesia technique for deep brain stimulation (DBS) surgery. However, the LMA is not always the ideal artificial airway. In this report, we presented our experiences with nasotracheal intubation-extubation-intubation (IEI) and AAA techniques in DBS surgery for Parkinson's disease (PD) patients to meet the needs of surgery and ensure patients' safety and comfort.

Case presentation: Three PD patients scheduled for DBS surgery had to receive general anesthesia for various reasons. For the first asleep stage, general anesthesia and nasotracheal intubation was completed with routine methods. During the awake stage, we pulled the nasotracheal tube back right above the epiglottis under fiberoptic bronchoscope (FOB) guidance for microelectrode recording (MER), macrostimulation testing and verbal communication. Once monitoring is completed, we induced anesthesia with rapid sequence induction and utilized the FOB to advance the nasotracheal tube into the trachea again. To minimize airway irritations during the process, we sprayed the airway with lidocaine before any manipulation. The neurophysiologists completed neuromoinitroing successfully and all three patients were satisfied with the anesthesia provided at follow-up.

Conclusion: Nasotracheal IEI and AAA anesthetic techniques should be considered as a viable option during DBS surgery.

Keywords: Asleep-awake-asleep, Deep brain stimulation, Nasotracheal intubation, Parkinson's disease

Background

Monitored Anesthesia Care (MAC) is the most popular anesthesia technique in DBS surgery for PD patients. However, general anesthesia might be the only option for some patients. The major challenge with DBS under general anesthesia is the requirement of a fully awake and communicative patient for microelectrode recording and macrostimulation testing. The Asleep-Awake-Asleep (AAA) technique may be suitable in this situation. There have been multiple reports of this technique with laryngeal mask airway (LMA) for other neurosurgical surgeries [1]. However, LMA does not always guarantee a secure airway [2]. In this report, we presented our experiences with nasotracheal IEI and AAA techniques in PD patients to meet the needs of surgery and ensure patient safety and comfort.

Case presentation

The first patient was a 63-yr-old female with Body Mass Index (BMI) 19.8 kg/m^2. She presented to our hospital for DBS implantation. Unfortunately, she suffered severe kyphosis and could not tolerate supine position. The second patient was a 56-yr-old male with BMI 24.4 kg/m^2 suffering from severe back pain and anxiety. Both patients refused MAC for surgery. The third patient was a 64-yr-old male and the BMI was 28.7 kg/m^2. This patient had

* Correspondence: ljj9573@163.com; wangzhigang367@163.com
[1]Department of Anesthesiology, Qilu Hospital of Shandong University (Qingdao), No.758 Hefei Road, Qingdao, People's Republic of China
[3]Department of Neurosurgery, Qilu Hospital of Shandong University (Qingdao), Qingdao, People's Republic of China

severely uncontrollable motor symptoms and Obstructive Sleep Apnea syndrome (OSA) (Apnea Hypopnea Index is 33). His OSAS was triggered and the head movements associated with snoring also hampered the preoperative MRI scan when we gave dexmedetomidine to reduce the body movement. Only after the OSAS was eliminated by placing a nasopharyngeal airway to overcome the upper airway obstruction, the MRI scan was finished successfully. This made MAC is a poor choice for his DBS surgery. All three patients agreed with our proposed IEI and AAA technique. Written consent from patients and Institutional Review Board approval were obtained. During preoperative interview, we described the protocol of arousing, extubation, macrostimulation testing and reintubation in great details. On the day of surgery, The Leksell stereotactic head frame was placed under local anesthesia before entering the operation room.

The first asleep stage
After entering the operation room, dexmedetomidine 0.4μg/kg was given within 15 min. We kept the first patient in the supine position with multiple cushions (Fig. 1, Part A). The other two patients were placed in routine supine position (Fig. 1, Part B). The oxygen saturation, expired carbon dioxide, ECG and invasive blood pressure were monitored. One nostril was sprayed with 1% ephedrine, then the nasal and oral mucosa were anesthetized with 1% dyclonine gel. After glycopyrrolate 0.2 mg and palonosetron 0.25 mg i.v., general anesthesia was induced with dexamethasone 5 mg, fentanyl 2μg/kg, propofol 1-2 mg/kg and atracurium 1 mg/kg. After 3 min of mask ventilation, the laryngeal and tracheal mucosa was anesthetized with 2% lidocaine (5 ml) through a disposable endolaryngeal anesthetic tube sprayer (Henan Tuoren Medical Device Co., Ltd., China) under video laryngoscope guidance (Aircraft Medical Ltd., Ediburgh, United Kindom). A nasotracheal tube (ID 6.5 for male and ID 6.0 for female) was advanced past the vocal cords and the distance between the nare and the epiglottis was recorded. General anesthesia was maintained with 4 mg/kg/h propofol, remifentanil 0.1μg/kg/min and dexmedetomidine 0.2μg/kg/h. Local anesthesia to operative sites was provided with 0.325% ropivacaine by surgeons.

The awake stage
Ten minutes before the anticipated microelectrode recording (MER), dexmedetomidine, propofol and remifentanil were discontinued. After patient's spontaneous respiration was restored, we deflated the cuff of endotracheal tube and injected atomized 2% lidocaine 3 ml via a catheter mount and a simple atomizer (Jiangsu Sona Care Medical Science-Technology Co., LTD, Nantong, China) (Fig. 1, Part G). The endotracheal tube was retracted to the top of epiglottis (at level of the tongue base) under the guidance of FB-10 V FOB (HOYA Corporation, PENTAX Lifecare Division, Tokyo, Japan) and kept there as a nasopharyngeal airway. When the patient woke up fully, MER, macrostimulation testing and language communication were performed. All

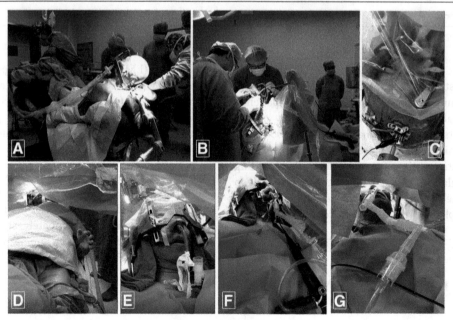

Fig. 1 a The severe hunchback of the first patient and methods to keep the patient in the supine position, **b** The other two patients were in routine supine position. **c-e** During macrostimulation testing, patients were calm and cooperative, able to move fingers, limbs, and to communicate verbally with the operator. **f** The reintubations guided by FOB. **g** Inhaling atomized 2% lidocaine via nasotracheal tube with catheter mount and a simple atomizer

three patients opened their eyes upon commands (7 ± 0.66 min) and their spontaneous respiration restored within 5–10 min after stopping sedation. They all tolerated nasal endotracheal tube well (Fig. 1, Part C). Both blood pressure and heart rate were significantly higher than asleep stage. Compared with baseline blood pressure, the fluctuation of mean arterial pressure (MAP) of the first patient and third patient were within 30% and we did nto give any treatment. The MAP of the second patient was higher than 30% baseline blood pressure, we gave nicardipine (0.1 mg) and esmolol (0.5µg/Kg) intermittently to maintain hemodynamic stability (the total dose of nicardipine was 0.3 mg, esmolol was 100µg).

The neurophysiologists finished MER successfully and were satisfied with the quality of signals. During the macrostimulation testing, all the patients were calm and cooperative, able to move fingers, limbs, to count numbers upon instructions and to communicate orally with the operator easily (Fig. 1, Part C, D, E).

The second asleep stage
Once the electrophysiological test was complete, atomized 2% lidocaine 3 ml via nasotracheal tube was injected again. Midazolam 0.04 mg/kg, fentanyl 2µg/kg, propofol 1 mg/kg were utilized to sedate patients and maintained spontaneous respirations. The glottis was identified with FOB and oxygen was supplemented through the catheter mount. Once the FOB entered the trachea, the nasotracheal tube was passed over the FOB into the trachea (Fig. 1, Part F). Rocuronium 1 mg/kg, remifentanil 0.5µg/kg and propofol 1 mg/kg were injected intravenously to induce general anesthesia. The rest of the procedure, such as implantation of electrodes and pacemakers, was continued under general anesthesia. The reintubation guided by FOB were successful on the first attempt in all three patients (Fig. 1, Part F).

Total AAA time were 235–280 min, including first asleep stage 80–100 min, wake-up test time of 58–70 min, and the second asleep stage 97–110 min. No patient had coughing or body movement. One patient suffered mild nose bleeding but had no significant impact on nasotracheal reintubation guided by FOB. No patient suffered hypoxia during the whole process. All patients were extubated within 10mins after operation without complication. Anesthesia follow up on postoperative day 2 demonstrated that all patients were satisfied with their anesthesia experiences.

Discussion and conclusions
We did not find reports on nasotracheal IEI and AAA technique after Huncke K, et al. published their technique for intractable seizure resection in 1998 [3]. Our technique has several noticeable improvements compared to Huncke's method. First, we did not remove nasotracheal tube during awake stage. Instead, we kept the nasotracheal tube above the epiglottis in the nose, which could keep airway unobstructed. This could prevent additional trauma and bleeding from placing another nasopharyngeal airway in patients with airway obstructions. In addition, this technique will not impair the necessary oral communication testing and could make reintubation easier by reducing the difficulty to find the glottis with FOB. Second, both intubation and reintubation by Huncke K were performed while patients were awake. For the first asleep stage, intubation by us was performed after induction of general anesthesia. For the second stage, we identified the glottis and intubated trachea using FOB when the patient was heavily sedated. Patient safety and comfort during the intubation are improved and the difficulty of anesthesia management is reduced. High-flow nasal oxygen therapy or high frequency ventilation during the apnea period might be useful to prevent hypoxia [4]. Third, Huncke K, et al. used a spirally attached catheter around the endotracheal tube to provide airway anesthesia, we used a disposable endolaryngeal anesthetic tube spray before the first intubation, a simple atomizer before the first extubation and second intubation. Endotracheal surface anesthesia before intubation is the most important factor to make patient tolerable to intubation or extubation. Fourth, Huncke K used propofol, sulfentanyl or inhaled agents and they needed to be discontinued at least 1 h before the wake-up. We maintained general anesthesia with short acting propofol, remifentanil and low-dose dexmedetomidine. Only 10mins was required before the wake-up. All of our patients were able to wake up quickly and cooperated with neurological tests. Dexmedetomidine could reduce anxiety, airway sensitivity and increase analgesic effects but had no significant impact on MER monitoring [5, 6]. Finally, DBS was performed in the supine position and the airway was easily accessible to the anesthesiologist. In other neurosurgical cases, it may require extra personnel or devices to tent the surgical drape to facilitate airway management as reported by Huncke K.

Possible advantages of our IEI technique in comparison with LMA techniques are: First, the supra-epiglottis position of the endotracheal tube could serve as a nasopharyngeal airway and reduce the risk of hypoxemia. Second, the depth of anesthesia required is lower in IEI and can be performed when patients are conscious. Third, the successful rate for a secure airway with video laryngoscopy may be higher than that of LMA when the head position is fixed. Finally, this technique can potentially prevent aspiration with a secured airway. Potential disadvantages include: First, the possibility of significant nasal bleeding causing laryngeal irritation. Second, airway swelling from repeated instrumentations. Third, advanced skills to manipulate the FOB are required.

Our experiences suggest that nasotracheal IEI and AAA techniques should be considered as a viable option for some certain patients undergoing DBS surgery. Compared with local anesthesia alone, this technique could shorten the awake time and improved patient's satisfaction. In addition, the secured airway with an endotracheal tube may be safer than LMA. The advantages and disadvantages of this technique should be verified by more rigorous research.

Abbreviations
AAA: Asleep-awake-asleep; DBS: Deep brain stimulation; FOB: Fiberoptic bronchoscope; IEI: Intubation-extubation-intubation; LMA: Laryngeal mask airway; MAC: Monitored Care Anesthesia; MER: Microelectrode recording; PD: Parkinson's disease

Acknowledgements
Not applicable

Authors' contributions
JJL and ZGW conceived and designed the case report; and agreed to be accountable for all aspects of the work in ensuring that questions related to the accuracy or integrity of any part of the work were appropriately investigated and resolved. WXT contributed to writing the manuscript. PHW and JPH contributed to revising it critically for important intellectual content. NZ contributed to collection of data. HPZ and JFZ and QZ performed the anesthesia. All authors read and approved the final manuscript.

Author details
[1]Department of Anesthesiology, Qilu Hospital of Shandong University (Qingdao), No.758 Hefei Road, Qingdao, People's Republic of China. [2]Department of Anesthesia, Jewish Hospital and Department of Anesthesiology & Perioperative Medicine, University of Louisville, Louisville, KY, USA. [3]Department of Neurosurgery, Qilu Hospital of Shandong University (Qingdao), Qingdao, People's Republic of China.

References
1. Gadhinglajkar S, Sreedhar R, Abraham M. Anesthesia management of awake craniotomy performed under asleep-awake-asleep technique using laryngeal mask airway: report of two cases. Neurol India. 2008;56:65–7.
2. Meng L, McDonagh DL, Berger MS, Gelb AW. Anesthesia for awake craniotomy: a how-to guide for the occasional practitioner. Can J Anaesth. 2017;64:517–29.
3. Huncke K, Van de Wiele B, Fried I, Rubinstein EH. The asleep-awake-asleep anesthetic technique for intraoperative language mapping. Neurosurgery. 1998;42:1312–6 discussion 1316-1317.
4. Renda T, Corrado A, Iskandar G, Pelaia G, Abdalla K, Navalesi P. High-flow nasal oxygen therapy in intensive care and anaesthesia. Br J Anaesth. 2018;120:18–27.
5. Kwon WK, Kim JH, Lee JH, Lim BG, Lee IO, Koh SB, Kwon TH. Microelectrode recording (MER) findings during sleep-awake anesthesia using dexmedetomidine in deep brain stimulation surgery for Parkinson's disease. Clin Neurol Neurosurg. 2016;143:27–33.
6. Martinez-Simon A, Alegre M, Honorato-Cia C, Nunez-Cordoba JM, Cacho-Asenjo E, Troconiz IF, Carmona-Abellan M, Valencia M, Guridi J. Effect of Dexmedetomidine and Propofol on basal ganglia activity in Parkinson disease: a controlled clinical trial. Anesthesiology. 2017;126:1033–42.

19

Awake intubation and extraluminal use of Uniblocker for one-lung ventilation in a patient with a large mediastinal mass

Zhuo Liu*👤, Qianqian Jia and Xiaochun Yang

Abstract

Background: The anesthesia of patients with large mediastinal mass is at high-risk. Avoidance of general anesthesia in these patients is the safest option, if this is unavoidable, maintenance of spontaneous ventilation is the next safest technique. In these types of patients, it is not applicable to use double-lumen tube (DLT) to achieve one-lung ventilation (OLV) because the DLT has a larger diameter and is more rigid than single-lumen tube (SLT), so the mass may rupture and bleed during intubation. Even using a bronchial blocker, a small size of SLT is required for once the trachea collapses the SLT can pass through the narrowest part of trachea. However, it is difficult to control the fiberoptic bronchoscopy (FOB) and the bronchial blocker simultaneously within the lumen of a small size SLT with traditional intubation methods.

Case presentation: The current study presented a 66 years old female patient with a large mediastinal mass that presented with difficulty breathing when lying flat. In this case, we combined use of dexmedetomidine and remifentanil to preserve the patient's spontaneous ventilation during intubation and achieved one-lung ventilation with extraluminal use of Uniblocker.

Conclusions: Extraluminal use of Uniblocker and maintenance of spontaneous ventilation during intubation may be an alternative to traditional methods of lung isolation in such patients with a large mediastinal mass.

Keywords: One-lung ventilation, Awake intubation, Extraluminal use of Uniblocker, Mediastinal mass

Background

Large mediastinal masses can cause airway collapse and hemodynamic collapse and these feared complications occur particularly during positional changes and with induction of anesthesia or muscle relaxation, which is why the anesthesia of these patients with large mediastinal mass is at high-risk [1]. We presented a single case report of a patient whose airway management was especially challenging.

---

* Correspondence: liuzhuo2011@yeah.net
Department of Anesthesiology, The First Hospital of Qinhuangdao, N.O. 258, Wenhua Road, Qinhuangdao, Hebei, China

Case presentation

A 66 years old female patient, weight 52 kg, height 150 cm was scheduled for mediastinal mass resection surgery. Because the mediastinal mass had been compressed the weakened trachea and interfered with the patient's breathing, so the surgery needed to be performed as soon as possible. The patient had a general anaesthetic 14 years ago for laparoscopic cholecystectomy without complications. Pre-operative blood pressure (BP) was 101/72 mmHg, heart rate (HR) was 85 min^{-1}, respiratory rate (RR) was 20 per minute and SpO_2 was 94%. Pre-operative chest computed tomographic (CT) scans showed that a large mediastinal mass (10.1 cm × 7.4 cm × 4.9 cm) compressed the trachea and carina. The narrowest part of the trachea was located at 4.9 cm above the carina, where the cross section of the trachea was a fissure (0.45 cm × 1.41 cm) (Fig. 1a,b,c).

The patient without premedication and received standard monitoring in the operating room. After preoxygenation the patient was intravenously injected with midazolam 0.03 mg·kg^{-1} and then an arterial catheter and an internal jugular vein catheter were placed under local anesthesia. A transtracheal injection of 1% lidocaine (3-4 ml) was administered and the patient was suggested to open mouth then the oral cavity and hypopharynx mucosa were sprayed with 1% lidocaine.

After intratracheal surface anesthesia, the patient was received dexmedetomidine at a loading dose of 1 µg·kg^{-1} (the infusion was completed in 10 min) then remifentanil at a loading dose of 0.5 µg·kg^{-1}, followed by a continuous infusion at a speed of 0.1 µg·kg^{-1}·min^{-1}. During this process, the patient was received continuous oxygen by mask. After deep sedation (patient breathing spontaneously but cannot be awakened by calling her name), the intubation was performed and the steps were as follows: First, inserted a Uniblocker (9-French) into the trachea via a visual laryngoscope and advanced the Uniblocker toward the right main-stem bronchus after the tip passed the glottis; Second, inserted a single lumen tube (SLT, inner-diameter 6.0 mm) into the trachea until the cuff of SLT passed the glottis (Fig. 1d,e); Third, fixed the Uniblocker and SLT to the patient's mouth separately with a cloth tape; Finally, inserted the fiberoptic bronchoscopy (FOB, external diameter 3.8 mm, MDHAO Medical Technology, Zhuhai, China) into the lumen of SLT to adjust the Uniblocker to optimal position.

After 4 attempts of adjustment, the Uniblocker to optimum position (Fig. 1f). Anesthesia maintenance with 1–2% sevoflurane and continuous infusion of remifentanil and propofol at a speed of 0.1–0.2 µg·kg^{-1}·min^{-1} and 30-80 µg·kg^{-1}·min^{-1}. The narrowest part of the trachea was monitored: if there was a sudden increase of peak airway pressure, the FOB would be inserted into the tube to detect the stenosis of trachea; if the airway collapsed and the SLT could pass through the narrowest part of the trachea via FOB then the SLT would be advanced through the stenosis as soon as posible; If the airway collapsed after anesthesia and the SLT could not be advanced through the narrowest part of the trachea, our plan is to change the patient's position and use high frequency jet ventilation via the Uniblocker to maintain the patient's oxygen supply then the emergent extracorporeal circulation would be established and the operation would be performed under extracorporeal circulation; If the airway collapsed intraoperative we would recommend the surgeon to lift up the mass or drain the cyst fluid as soon as possible then advance the SLT through the narrowest part of trachea.

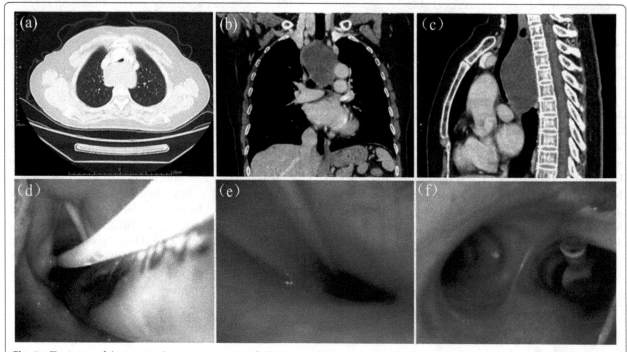

Fig. 1 a The image of the mass in the transverse position; **b** The image of the mass in the coronary position; **c** The image of the mass in the sagittal position; **d** The Uniblocker and single lumen tube passed the glottis; **e** The Uniblocker passed through the narrowest part of the trachea; **f** the cuff of the Uniblocker located below the carina

During the operation, the airway was not collapsed. After 1.5 h, the mass was successfully removed without any complications and the SLT was also successfully removed in the post anesthesia care unit.

Discussion and conclusions

The most feared complications of mediastinal mass resection surgery are airway collapse and hemodynamic collapse. Avoidance of general anesthesia is a prevailing recommendations in such patients [2–5]. If general anesthesia is required, avoidance of paralytic agents and maintenance of spontaneous ventilation are emphasized [2–5]. In this case, we combined use of dexmedetomidine and remifentanil to preserve the patient's spontaneous ventilation during intubation.

Large mediastinal masses increase the complexity of one lung ventilation. In this patient, the chest CT revealed that the trachea was severely compressed and the narrowest part of the trachea was only 0.45 cm, so the DLT may not pass through the narrowest part of the trachea (Fig. 1e) and bronchial blockers (BBs) may be more suitable for this patient [6]. However, even using BBs, a small size of SLT should be chosen for this patient, for once the airway was obstructed, the SLT could be advanced through the narrowest part of trachea via FOB. With the conventional intubation method, both the BBs and FOB are inserted into the lumen of the SLT then the BBs are guided to the optimal position, so it is difficult to contral the FOB and rotate BBs simultaneously in the lumen of a small size SLT. Compared with conventional intubation method, extraluminal use of BBs has more advantageous, especially in this case: First, with this method, we were able to choose a small size of SLT (ID 6.0 mm), so the SLT might be easy to pass through the narrowest part of trachea via FOB once the airway collapsed. Second, the Uniblocker could be easily positioned without the interference of FOB and the limitations of narrow spaces of SLT when adjusted the Uniblocker to the optimal position, especially in this case the trachea was compressed and displaced. Third, the lumen of SLT was unobstructed, so a suction catheter could be easily inserted into the SLT to clear the hemorrhage once the mass ruptures and bleeds.

In conclusion, this case highlights that in the patient with large mediastinal masses, extraluminal use of Uniblocker and the combination use of dexmedetomidine and remifentanil to preserve the patient's spontaneous ventilation during intubation increase the patient's safety and this novel method may be an alternative to traditional methods of lung isolation in the patients with airway stenosis.

Abbreviations
OLV: One-lung ventilation; DLT: Double-lumen tube; SLT: Single-lumen tube; CT: Computed tomography; FOB: Fiberoptic bronchoscopy

Acknowledgements
None.

Authors' contributions
ZL collected all the patient initial data and drafted the manuscript, QQJ and XCY completed the anesthesia management. All authors gave their comments on the article and approved the final version.

References
1. Hartigan PM, Ng J-M, Gill RR. Anesthesia in a patient with a largemediastinal mass. N Engl J Med. 2018;379:587–8.
2. Hack HA, Wright NB, Wynn RF. The anaesthetic management of children with anterior mediastinal masses. Anaesthesia. 2008;63:837–46.
3. Slinger P, Karsli C. Management of the patient with a large anterior mediastinal mass: recurring myths. Curr Opin Anaesthesiol. 2007;20:1–3.
4. Slinger P. Management of the patient with a central airway obstruction. Saudi J Anaesth. 2011;5(3):241–3.
5. Blank RS, de Souza DG. Anesthetic management of patients with an anterior mediastinal mass: continuing professional development. Can J Anaesth. 2011;58:853–9.
6. Campos JH. Lung isolation techniques for patients with difficult airway. Curr Opin Anaesthesiol. 2010;23:12–7.

20

Suitability and realism of the novel Fix for Life cadaver model for videolaryngoscopy and fiberoptic tracheoscopy in airway management training

Michael W. van Emden[1]*[iD], Jeroen J. G. Geurts[1], Patrick Schober[2] and Lothar A. Schwarte[2]

Abstract

Background: Videolaryngoscopy is increasingly advocated as the standard intubation technique, while fibreoptic intubation is broadly regarded as the 'gold standard' for difficult airways. Traditionally, the training of these techniques is on patients, though manikins, simulators and cadavers are also used, with their respective limitations. In this study, we investigated whether the novel 'Fix for Life' (F4L) cadaver model is a suitable and realistic model for the teaching of these two intubation techniques to novices in airway management.

Methods: Forty consultant anaesthetists and senior trainees were instructed to perform tracheal intubation with videolaryngoscopy and fibreoptic tracheoscopy in four F4L cadaver models. The primary outcome measure was the verbal rating scores (scale 1–10, higher scores indicate a better rating) for suitability and for realism of the F4L cadavers as training model for these techniques. Secondary outcomes included success rates of the procedures and the time to successful completion of the procedures.

Results: The mean verbal rating scores for suitability and realism for videolaryngoscopy was 8.3 (95% CI, 7.9–8.6) and 7.2 (95% CI, 6.7–7.6), respectively. For fibreoptic tracheoscopy, suitability was 8.2 (95% CI, 7.9–8.5) and realism 7.5 (95% CI, 7.1–7.8). In videolaryngoscopy, 100% of the procedures were successful. The mean (SD) time until successful tracheal intubation was 34.8 (30.9) s. For fibreoptic tracheoscopy, the success rate was 96.3%, with a mean time of 89.4 (80.1) s.

Conclusions: We conclude that the F4L cadaver model is a suitable and realistic model to train and teach tracheal intubation with videolaryngoscopy and fibreoptic tracheoscopy to novices in airway management training.

Keywords: Videolaryngoscopy, Fibreoptic intubation, Airway management training, Cadaver model

* Correspondence: m.vanemden@amsterdamumc.nl
[1]Department of Anatomy and Neurosciences, Amsterdam UMC, Vrije Universiteit, PO Box 7057, 1007 MB, De Boelelaan 1117, 1081, HV, Amsterdam, The Netherlands

Background

Videolaryngoscopy (VLS) is an established standard airway technique, while the use of flexible fibreoptic or video tracheoscopy (FOT) is broadly regarded as the 'gold standard' when confronted with a difficult airway [1–3]. Traditionally, novice airway practitioners learn these techniques on patients in the operating room, though synthetic manikins or simulators are also being used, with their respective limitations [4]. The advantage of training outside the operating room is an environment free of risks to patients, and the option of constructing clinical scenarios not regularly encountered in practice [5]. However, mimicking the characteristics of human anatomy in synthetic manikins and simulators is difficult [6]. Human cadavers of persons who donated their body to science after death are potentially of added value in the training of VLS and FOT [7–9]. Such cadaver models reflect the variance in anatomy also encountered in real patients. However, the method of conservation of these cadaver models is crucial, because the traditional embalmment with large amounts of formaldehyde causes the tissues to be rigid and makes airway management training rather unrealistic. Recently, a new cadaver model has been described, embalmed with 'Fix for Life' (F4L), which trainee and specialist airway practitioners have found to be realistic and suited for teaching basic airway management techniques, e.g., mask ventilation [10]. In the present study, we investigated the suitability and realism of the F4L cadaver model for the training of two advanced video airway techniques, i.e., VLS and FOT for tracheal intubation.

Methods

The study was approved by the biobank and ethics committee of the Amsterdam UMC, Vrije Universiteit, Amsterdam, the Netherlands. All data were collected in the anatomy laboratory of the department of Anatomy and Neurosciences.

Participants

Forty consultant anaesthetists and senior trainees (4th and 5th year of the 5-year training program) were recruited to participate in the study. Inclusion criteria were familiarity with VLS and FOT for tracheal intubation, i.e., the participants are familiar with and have received training in these techniques. Due to formaldehyde being used at the anatomical facility, exclusion criteria were pregnancy and lactation. Before participating, all consultants and trainees gave written informed consent. Age, sex, number of years of professional experience and an estimation of the number of tracheal intubations with VLS and FOT (including anaesthetised and awake procedures) of the participants were recorded.

F4L cadaver models

The four F4L cadavers used in this study were from body donors who donated their body to science after death through written consent, in accordance with Dutch legislation. Embalmment was performed within 24–72 h after demise. The cadavers were embalmed with the F4L embalmment fluids, according to the embalmment protocol for F4L fixation [11]. Basic characteristics of the cadavers (age at demise, sex, length, weight, body mass index) and morphometric predictors of difficult intubation (dental status, neck circumference, thyromental and sternomental distance) were recorded. The Cormack-Lehane grade of each F4L cadaver model was assessed in agreement by 2 senior consultant anaesthetists via direct laryngoscopy (Macintosh blade size 3) before the start of the study.

Study protocol

Each participant performed the VLS and FOT procedures individually, with no other participants present in the room at the same time. The participants were instructed to first intubate the tracheas of the F4L cadaver models with the VLS (GlideScope®, Verathon Medical, Burnaby, Canada) with a size 3 blade. After completion of the VLS procedures on all cadaver models, the participants performed tracheal intubation via FOT (Ambu® aScope™ 4, Ambu A/S, Ballerup, Denmark, regular size, outer diameter 5.5 mm) on all four F4L cadaver models. Tracheal tubes were available in different sizes from 6.0 mm to 8.0 mm (Covidien™, Mansfield, MA). The procedures using VLS and FOT were performed in the same order for all participants on all four F4L cadavers. The participants were allowed to optimize the position of the head of the cadaver according to their own preferences (e.g., sniffing position or ramping). Any fluids present in the oropharyngeal cavity of the cadavers were suctioned before starting the procedures. One of the researchers present served as a 'non-obstructive' assistant to the participant to provide instruments (e.g., tracheal tube), or to apply jaw thrust or backward, upward, or rightward pressure (BURP) of the larynx, or other optimizing manoeuvres, if requested. For the FOT procedure, the participants were instructed to perform a nasotracheal intubation. The tracheal tube was allowed to be pre-fixed ('loaded') on the tracheoscope or pre-inserted through the nose of the cadaver model prior to the start of the FOT procedure, according to the preference of the participant. Lubricant was applied to the FOT device and tracheal tube, as required. Also, the participants were allowed to take their preferred position relative to the cadaver model (e.g., standing behind the 'patient' or next to the 'patient').

The time of the procedure (in seconds, [s]) was recorded for each intubation attempt. For the VLS intubation procedure, recording of time started when the tip of the VLS entered the mouth of the cadaver model and stopped when the tracheal tube was cuffed. Time of the FOT procedure was measured when the tip of the tracheoscope entered the cadaver's nose (or the pre-inserted tracheal tube) and also stopped when the tracheal tube was cuffed. Active assistance upon request of the participant (e.g., jaw thrust) was recorded. Success of the VLS or FOT procedure was defined as a correct intubation of the trachea. In the VLS, correct placement of the tracheal tube was ascertained by direct view of the passing of the tube through the vocal cords on the GlideScope videoscreen by 2 of the present researchers. For the FOT procedures, correct placement of the tracheal tube was ascertained by confirming view of the carina on the aScope videoscreen. Failure of the procedures were additionally recorded if the participant resigned the task or if the time of the VLS procedure exceeded 5 min, or 10 min for the FOT procedure.

After completion of the intubation procedures on all cadaver models with VLS, and subsequently with FOT, the participants were asked to give an overall verbal rating score (VRS) for each technique [7, 10, 12]. The participants were asked to rate the F4L cadaver model for suitability as a training model to learn VLS or FOT ("Considering real-life patients as a reference, how suitable is the F4L cadaver model as a teaching model to teach novices the use of VLS or FOT with regard to the technical aspects?"). Thereafter, they were asked to score the model on realism ("Considering real-life patients as a reference, how realistic is the F4L cadaver model as a teaching model to teach novices the use of VLS or FOT with regard to look, feel and flexibility?"). The VRSs were given on a scale of 1 to 10 (1 = worst score, 10 = best score). Any relevant narrative feedback was also recorded.

Outcome measures and statistical analysis

The primary outcome measures were the VRSs for suitability and for realism of the F4L cadaver as training model for VLS and FOT respectively. Secondary outcomes were success rates of the procedures, the time to successful intubation of the trachea and whether assistance was needed.

For this study we used a convenience sample of 40 consultant anaesthetists and senior trainees, and four F4L cadavers per participant. Statistical analysis was performed using SPSS, version 26 (IBM Corp, Armonk, NY). The mean VRSs are presented with calculated 95% confidence intervals (95% CI). Success rates of the VLS and FOT procedures are presented as proportions. Time, given in seconds, until successful intubation of the trachea is presented in mean with standard deviation (SD). The Mann-Whitney U-test was used to compare the VRSs given by consultant anaesthetists and the senior trainees. A P value < 0.05 was considered significant.

Results

The participants included 26 consultant anaesthetists and 14 senior trainees with a mean (SD) professional experience of 11.7 (8.0) years. The male/female ratio was 20/20. Mean (SD) age was 40.2 (9.4) years. Self-estimated previous experience with VLS assisted tracheal intubations was < 20 in 5% of participants, and ≥ 20 in 95% of participants. Experience with FOT on patients was < 20 in 47.5% of participants, and ≥ 20 in 52.5% of participants. The characteristics of the 4 F4L cadaver models are presented in Table 1. All 40 participants completed all of the procedures on the 4 F4L cadaver models for a total of 160 VLS and 160 FOT assisted tracheal intubation attempts.

For suitability of training VLS, the mean VRS was 8.3 (95% CI, 7.9–8.6). For realism, the mean VRS was 7.2 (95% CI, 6.7–7.6). The suitability of the F4L cadaver model for FOT was rated with a mean VRS of 8.2 (95% CI, 7.9–8.5) and for realism, the mean VRS was 7.5 (95% CI, 7.1–7.8).

The results in proportion of successful procedures, time until successful completion and proportion of assistance needed are presented in Table 2.

No significant differences were observed in the mean (SD) VRSs given by consultant anaesthetists versus trainees respectively for suitability for VLS (8.5 [1.1] versus 7.9 [1.1], $P = 0.190$), realism for VLS (7.2 [1.4] versus 7.1 [1.5], $P = 0.604$), suitability for FOT (8.2 [1.0] versus 8.2 [0.8], $P = 0.747$), and realism for FOT (7.3 [1.1] versus 7.6 [1.0], $P = 0.332$). Additional comparative analyses of mean (SD) VRSs given by participants with < 20 and ≥ 20 FOT performed in patients respectively, revealed no significant differences in suitability for FOT (8.2 [1.1] versus 8.3 [0.8], $P = 0.979$) or for realism for FOT (7.7 [1.1] versus 7.2 [1.0], $P = 0.161$). For the mean (SD) VRSs given by participants with < 20 and ≥ 20 VLS performed in patients respectively, also no significant differences were observed in suitability for VLS (8.5 [0.7] versus 8.3 [1.2], $P = 0.785$), and realism for VLS (6.5 [0.7] versus 7.2 [1.4], $P = 0.369$).

The additional, narrative feedback provided by the participants was that the F4L cadaver model was 'more rigid', had a 'paler or different colour', and was 'dryer' in regard to real patients. Other remarks were the 'setting differences' (e.g., no beeping sounds of monitors), and the 'not awake patient'.

Table 1 Characteristics of the 4 Fix for Life (F4L) cadaver models

	Cadaver 1	Cadaver 2	Cadaver 3	Cadaver 4
Age at demise (y)	89	70	68	90
Sex	Male	Male	Female	Female
Weight (kg)	75	54	52	66
Length (m)	1.75	1.73	1.70	1.67
Body mass index (kg.m^{-2})	24.5	18	18	23.7
Neck circumference (cm)	47	38	42	52
Thyromental distance (cm)	6.5	7.5	6	5.5
Sternomental distance (cm)	13.5	15	14	13.5
Dental status	Toothless	Toothless	Incomplete	Toothless
Cormack-Lehane grade	4	2	2	3

A typical example of the laryngeal view with VLS is presented in Fig. 1.

Discussion

This is the first study to investigate the suitability and the realism of the novel F4L cadaver model as airway management training model for both VLS and FOT. Our results suggest that experienced airway practitioners regard the F4L cadaver as a suitable and realistic training model for both VLS and FOT procedures.

Different models for VLS and FOT training have been described, ranging from manikins, simulators [13–15], animals [16] and cadaver models [7, 9, 17]. Learning these airway techniques on different types of models outside the operating room could be effective, and time efficient [4, 5, 18]. In our study, the participants rated the F4L cadaver model high with regard to suitability and realism, considering real patients as a reference. This finding is comparable to an earlier study in which the F4L cadaver model was found to be a realistic and suitable model for more basic airway manoeuvres [10]. For example, suitability and realism as a teaching model for mask ventilation were scored as 7.2 and 7.0 respectively, which is consistent with our current findings. These scores are promising, and support the use of the

F4L cadaver model for airway management training programmes. The results of the present study suggest extending the application spectrum of F4L cadavers from these more basic airway manoeuvres to the advanced airway manoeuvres, i.e., VLS and FOT. The F4L cadaver could be a useful asset to reduce the learning period of VLS and FOT procedures outside the operating theatre.

Simulation training has found a place in anaesthesia training programmes, although there is discussion about the degree of reality a simulation model should have [6, 19, 20]. Using the F4L cadaver in addition to simulators and manikins in airway management training could provide for optimal preparation of novice airway practitioners before executing these techniques on actual patients. In addition, experienced airway practitioners can refresh or optimize their technical skills outside the operating room. In the ever faster evolving market of novel airway devices, the F4L cadaver model may provide a safe 'test field' to test and train new devices before their first application in a real patient.

Table 2 Results in Verbal Rating Scores (VRS) for suitability and for realism, success rates, time until successful completion, and requested assistance of the videolaryngoscopy (VLS) and flexible tracheoscopy (FOT) in the F4L cadaver model

	VLS	FOT
VRS suitability	8.3 (7.9–8.6)	8.2 (7.9–8.5)
VRS realism	7.2 (6.7–7.6)	7.5 (7.1–7.8)
Success rate	160 (100%)	154 (96.3%)
Time until completion; s	34.8 (30.9)	89.4 (80.1)
Assistance needed	22 (13.8%)	126 (78.8%)

Values are mean (95% confidence interval or standard deviation) or number (proportion).

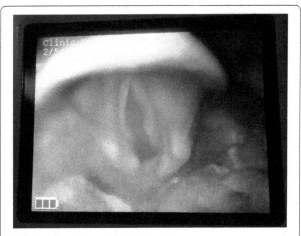

Fig. 1 Laryngeal view with the videolaryngoscope

The success rate of intubation with VLS was 100%, which is within the range of reported success rates of 73–100% in a recent meta-analysis of Glidescope VLS [21]. Also, the mean time to successfully complete the VLS procedure did not exceed those previously reported [21, 22]. For the FOT procedures, the success rate was 96.3%, which is comparable with reported success rates from an analysis of 1612 fibreoptic intubation cases [23]. In this study, 93.9% of FOT procedures were successfully completed within 3 min. In our study on the F4L cadaver models, this was 90.9% within the same timeframe. In a recent manikin study, the success rate for nasotracheal intubation of the trachea with the Ambu aScope 3 was 95% [24]. In this report, the mean (SD) time for proper tracheal tube placement was 70 (33) seconds, which is on average 20 s faster compared to our measured mean time of approximately 90 s. However, only a single manikin was used in that study. In our study, occasionally oropharyngeal fluid collections were encountered during the procedure and were suctioned with the Ambu aScope, which adds time to the duration of the procedure. However, the F4L cadaver model probably resembles the clinical setting more closely, where blood or secretions may be encountered in the airway of patients.

There are some limitations to our study. The F4L cadaver model was not compared with other cadaveric preparations or manikins with regard to the performance of VLS and FOT, thus no conclusions can be drawn on its performance in comparison to these other models. We used only one type of VLS (Glidescope) and FOT (Ambu aScope 3) device, while there are multiple types available in practice. Our results are therefore not necessarily generalizable to other device types, but we did use broadly distributed devices, also mostly used in our hospital. We are aware that not every hospital has the availability of a cadaver lab, but a university hospital as ours serves also as a regional training centre, and airway courses are given to an (inter-)national public where the cadaver lab can be integrated in the curriculum. However, currently used standard formaldehyde-based fixation techniques result in very rigid cadavers, which are not useful for airway management training [10, 25]. While fresh frozen cadavers have the advantage that they are realistic after thawing, and are used in airway management training [26], continuing decomposition remains a major limitation. Ideally, a preservation technique would avert decomposition while at the same time preserve the natural characteristics of human tissue. The F4L preservation method appears to come quite close to this ideal as it provides for a flexible human cadaver model with comparable tissue quality as fresh frozen cadavers, yet without the disadvantage of ongoing decomposition. In contrast to the use of

formaldehyde preserved cadaveric preparations, the necessary amount of formaldehyde in F4L cadaver models is much smaller, which reduces toxicity. A main advantage of formaldehyde preserved cadaveric preparation is the long duration these specimens can be used, usually for multiple years. In our experience, a well preserved F4L cadaver model can generally be used for a minimum of 2 years before the tissue quality diminishes. Due to these properties, the F4L cadaver is utilised at our facilities for the training and teaching of surgical procedures, and also for ultrasonography airway management courses in identifying anatomical structures in patients (e.g. the cricothyroid membrane for front-of-neck access) [27]. Regarding our field of interest, the F4L cadaver model can also be used to learn to handle different airway devices, while providing a rather realistic anatomical view. For this first study of VLS and FOT in F4L cadaver models, we selected cadavers with rather normal habitus and morphology. For follow-up studies and our airway training courses, cadavers with more challenging characteristics (e.g., obesity) can also be selected and preserved.

Conclusions
In conclusion, our results suggest that the F4L cadaver model is a realistic and suitable model for the training and teaching of VLS and FOT airway manoeuvres to novices in airway management. We see potential for the F4L cadaver model to be incorporated in airway training curricula.

Abbreviations
CI: Confidence Interval; F4L: Fix for Life; FOT: Fibreoptic tracheoscopy; SD: Standard Deviation; VLS: Videolaryngoscopy; VRS: Verbal Rating Scale

Acknowledgements
Not applicable.

Authors' contributions
Study design: ME, JG, PS, LS. Recruitment: PS, LS. Data collection: ME, PS, LS. Statistical analysis: ME, PS, LS. Drafting of manuscript: ME, JG, PS, LS. All authors read and approved the final manuscript.

Author details
[1]Department of Anatomy and Neurosciences, Amsterdam UMC, Vrije Universiteit, PO Box 7057, 1007 MB, De Boelelaan 1117, 1081, HV, Amsterdam, The Netherlands. [2]Department of Anaesthesiology, Amsterdam UMC, Vrije Universiteit, De Boelelaan 1117, 1081, HV, Amsterdam, The Netherlands.

References
1. Frerk C, Mitchell VS, McNarry AF, Mendonca C, Bhagrath R, Patel A, O'Sullivan EP, Woodall NM, Ahmad I. Difficult airway society intubation guidelines working g: difficult airway society 2015 guidelines for management of unanticipated difficult intubation in adults. Br J Anaesth. 2015;115(6):827–48.
2. Lewis SR, Butler AR, Parker J, Cook TM, Smith AF. Videolaryngoscopy versus direct laryngoscopy for adult patients requiring tracheal intubation. Cochrane Db Syst Rev. 2016;(11):CD011136.

3. Pieters BMA, Maas EHA, Knape JTA, van Zundert AAJ. Videolaryngoscopy vs. direct laryngoscopy use by experienced anaesthetists in patients with known difficult airways: a systematic review and meta-analysis. Anaesthesia. 2017;72(12):1532–41.

4. Goldmann K, Z Ferson D. Education and training in airway management. Best Pract Res Clin Anaesthesiol. 2005;19(4):717–32.

5. Baker PA, Weller JM, Greenland KB, Riley RH, Merry AF. Education in airway management. Anaesthesia. 2011;66(Suppl 2):101–11.

6. Schebesta K, Hupfl M, Rossler B, Ringl H, Muller MP, Kimberger O. Degrees of reality: airway anatomy of high-fidelity human patient simulators and airway trainers. Anesthesiology. 2012;116(6):1204–9.

7. Laszlo CJ, Szucs Z, Nemeskeri A, Baksa G, Szuak A, Varga M, Tassonyi E. Human cadavers preserved using Thiel's method for the teaching of fibreoptically-guided intubation of the trachea: a laboratory investigation. Anaesthesia. 2018;73(1):65–70.

8. Olesnicky BL, Rehak A, Bestic WB, Brock JT, Watterson L. A cadaver study comparing three fibreoptic-assisted techniques for converting a supraglottic airway to a cuffed tracheal tube. Anaesthesia. 2017;72(2):223–9.

9. Boedeker BH, Nicholsal TA, Carpenter J, Singh L, Bernhagen MA, Murray WB, Wadman MC. A comparison of direct versus indirect laryngoscopic visualization during endotracheal intubation of lightly embalmed cadavers utilizing the GlideScope(R), Storz Medi pack Mobile imaging system and the new Storz CMAC videolaryngoscope. J Spec Oper Med. 2011;11(2):21–9.

10. van Emden MW, Geurts JJ, Schober P, Schwarte LA. Comparison of a novel cadaver model (fix for life) with the formalin-fixed cadaver and manikin model for suitability and realism in airway management training. Anesth Analg. 2018;127(4):914–9.

11. Dam AJv, Munsteren JCv, DeRuiter MC. Fix for Life. The development of a new embalming method to preserve life-like morphology. FASEB J. 2015; 29(1 Supplement):547–10.

12. Szucs Z, Laszlo CJ, Baksa G, Laszlo I, Varga M, Szuak A, Nemeskeri A, Tassonyi E. Suitability of a preserved human cadaver model for the simulation of facemask ventilation, direct laryngoscopy and tracheal intubation: a laboratory investigation. Br J Anaesth. 2016;116(3):417–22.

13. Baker PA, Weller JM, Baker MJ, Hounsell GL, Scott J, Gardiner PJ, Thompson JM. Evaluating the ORSIM(R) simulator for assessment of anaesthetists' skills in flexible bronchoscopy: aspects of validity and reliability. Br J Anaesth. 2016;117(Suppl 1):i87–91.

14. Giglioli S, Boet S, De Gaudio AR, Linden M, Schaeffer R, Bould MD, Diemunsch P. Self-directed deliberate practice with virtual fiberoptic intubation improves initial skills for anesthesia residents. Minerva Anestesiol. 2012;78(4):456–61.

15. Chandra DB, Savoldelli GL, Joo HS, Weiss ID, Naik VN. Fiberoptic oral intubation: the effect of model fidelity on training for transfer to patient care. Anesthesiology. 2008;109(6):1007–13.

16. Forbes RB, Murray DJ, Albanese MA. Evaluation of an animal model for teaching fibreoptic tracheal intubation. Can J Anaesth. 1989;36(2):141–4.

17. Dodd KW, Kornas RL, Prekker ME, Klein LR, Reardon RF, Driver BE. Endotracheal intubation with the king laryngeal tube in situ using video laryngoscopy and a Bougie: a retrospective case series and cadaveric crossover study. J Emerg Med. 2017;52(4):403–8.

18. Naik VN, Matsumoto ED, Houston PL, Hamstra SJ, Yeung RY, Mallon JS, Martire TM. Fiberoptic orotracheal intubation on anesthetized patients: do manipulation skills learned on a simple model transfer into the operating room? Anesthesiology. 2001;95(2):343–8.

19. Krage R, Erwteman M. State-of-the-art usage of simulation in anesthesia: skills and teamwork. Curr Opin Anaesthesiol. 2015;28(6):727–34.

20. Lorello GR, Cook DA, Johnson RL, Brydges R. Simulation-based training in anaesthesiology: a systematic review and meta-analysis. Br J Anaesth. 2014; 112(2):231–45.

21. Griesdale DE, Liu D, McKinney J, Choi PT. Glidescope(R) video-laryngoscopy versus direct laryngoscopy for endotracheal intubation: a systematic review and meta-analysis. Can J Anaesth. 2012;59(1):41–52.

22. Niforopoulou P, Pantazopoulos I, Demestiha T, Koudouna E, Xanthos T. Video-laryngoscopes in the adult airway management: a topical review of the literature. Acta Anaesthesiol Scand. 2010;54(9):1050–61.

23. Heidegger T, Gerig HJ, Ulrich B, Schnider TW. Structure and process quality illustrated by fibreoptic intubation: analysis of 1612 cases. Anaesthesia. 2003; 58(8):734–9.

24. Fukada T, Tsuchiya Y, Iwakiri H, Ozaki M. Is the Ambu aScope 3 slim single-use fiberscope equally efficient compared with a conventional bronchoscope for management of the difficult airway? J Clin Anesth. 2016; 30:68–73.

25. Balta JY, Cronin M, Cryan JF, O'Mahony SM. Human preservation techniques in anatomy: a 21st century medical education perspective. Clin Anat. 2015; 28(6):725–34.

26. Yang JH, Kim YM, Chung HS, Cho J, Lee HM, Kang GH, Kim EC, Lim T, Cho YS. Comparison of four manikins and fresh frozen cadaver models for direct laryngoscopic orotracheal intubation training. Emerg Med J. 2010;27(1):13–6.

27. van Emden MW, Geurts JJG, Craenen AMC, Schwarte LA, Schober P. Cricothyroid membrane identification with ultrasonography and palpation in cadavers with a novel fixation technique (fix for life): a laboratory investigation. Eur J Anaesthesiol. 2020;37(6):510–2.

21

Supraglottic airway versus endotracheal tube during interventional pulmonary procedures

Kyle M. Behrens[1]*◉ and Richard E. Galgon[2]

Abstract

Background: As the field of interventional pulmonology (IP) expands, anesthesia services are increasingly being utilized when complex procedures of longer duration are performed on sicker patients with high risk co-morbidities and lung pathology. Yet, evidence on the optimal anesthetic management for these patients remains lacking. Our aim was to characterize the airway management and, secondarily anesthetic maintenance patterns used for IP procedures at our institution.

Methods: From 2894 identified encounters, charts of 783 patients undergoing an IP procedure with general anesthesia over a 5-year period, employing an endotracheal tube (ETT) or a supraglottic airway (SGA) for airway maintenance, were identified and reviewed after exclusions. Patients posted for a concurrent thoracic surgical procedure and those already intubated at presentation were excluded. Baseline patient demographics, procedure, proceduralist type, anesthesia maintenance modality, neuromuscular blocking drug (NMBD) use, and airway management characteristics were extracted and analyzed.

Results: Inhaled general anesthesia with an ETT for airway maintenance was most commonly employed; however, SGAs were used in one-third of patients with a very low conversion rate (0.4%), and their use was associated with a significant reduction in NMBD use.

Conclusions: In this large series of patients receiving general anesthesia for IP procedures, inhaled anesthetic agents and ETTs were favored. However, in appropriately selected patients, SGA use was effective for airway maintenance and allowed for a reduction in NMBD use, which may have implications in this patient population who may have an increased risk for pulmonary complications and warrants further investigation.

Keywords: Supraglottic airway, Endotracheal tube, Airway maintenance, Interventional pulmonology, Neuromuscular blocking

Background

The field of interventional pulmonology (IP) is rapidly expanding as new technologies and techniques are invented with nearly 500,000 bronchoscopies being performed in the United States each year [1, 2]. Sicker patients with high risk co-morbidities and lung pathology are now able to undergo less invasive procedures resulting in shorter hospital stays. It is common for patients with less co-morbidities to be managed effectively using conscious sedation during these procedures, which can even be administered/directed by the interventionalist. However, many US and European medical centers have made it standard practice to have an anesthesiologist provide either sedation or general anesthesia to selected high risk patients undergoing IP procedures to safely manage them [3, 4].

It has been nearly 35 years since supraglottic airways (SGAs) have been released for anesthetic practice; however, SGAs have not been the standard of care to facilitate IP procedures due to the increased potential for dislodgement and less airway control compared to endotracheal tube (ETT). Over time, anesthesia providers and interventionalist with experience using SGAs have allowed their

* Correspondence: kyle.behrens@my.rfums.org
[1]Chicago Medical School, Rosalind Franklin University of Medicine and Science, 3333 Green Bay Road, North Chicago, IL 60064, USA

scope to be advanced. Advantages of using SGAs (compared to ETT) include (1) quicker and easier placement, (2) reduction in neuromuscular blocking drug (NMBD) usage, residual paralysis, hemodynamic variability, anesthetic requirement for device placement, emergence coughing, and laryngeal and subglottic trauma, and (3) preservation of laryngeal competence and mucociliary function [5]. In a report in 2016, Arevalo-Ludena et al reported observing no difference in leakage between SGAs and ETT during bronchoscopic lung volume reduction procedures [6]. However, data on the use of SGAs for other procedures remains lacking.

Over the course of the last five to ten years, the scope of SGA usage at our institution for IP procedures has grown, particularly because the use of an SGA for IP procedures affords versatility over use of an ETT in selected patients by providing the ability to (1) perform a complete airway exam, including visualization of glottic structures, (2) biopsy more proximal lymph nodes, and (3) manipulate endobronchial devices more easily through the airway conduit. The purpose of our study was to characterize the use of SGA versus ETT, and secondarily anesthetic maintenance patterns, during IP procedures at our institution.

Methods

For this study, after Institutional Review Board review and exemption from informed consent, we performed a retrospective chart review. Consecutive patients who underwent an IP procedure at our institution and were cared for by an anesthesia provider during the period of April 15, 2008 through April 14, 2013 (5 years) were identified and included using anesthesia departmental billing records. A priori exclusion criteria included patients who underwent airway management by facemask, rigid bronchoscopy, or jet ventilation, those who underwent a concurrent surgical procedure and those already intubated at presentation. The primary analysis was focused on comparing the use of an SGA versus ETT for airway maintenance, and the need to convert use of an SGA to an ETT during the procedure (i.e., SGA failure). SGA failure was defined as a need to place an ETT during the procedure secondary to poor airway seal performance. SGA failure did not include incidence of airway placement failure at the initial start of the procedure. The determination to use an SGA or ETT was made by the attending anesthesiologist at the time of the procedure. Data including (1) patient characteristics (e.g., age, gender, weight, height, co-morbid diseases, such as diabetes mellitus, gastroesophageal reflux disease, hiatal hernia, or a history of neck radiation, known airway management difficulties, and airway exam findings), (2) procedure type (e.g., flexible bronchoscopy, endobronchial ultrasound, endobronchial tumor debulking, super dimensional bronchoscopy, etc.), and (3) anesthetic management characteristics (e.g., intravenous versus inhalational agent

use, ventilation mode, and NMBD), were defined a priori and extracted for secondary exploratory analyses. NMBD use was recorded if an intermediate acting NMBD was administered or re-dosed during the procedure. If a short acting NMBD (succinylcholine) was given to facilitate airway management device placement and no other NMBDs were administered, NMBD use was not counted. Descriptive statistics (mean (SD) and percent) were used to characterize group data. Intergroup comparisons (SGA versus ETT) were performed using t-tests for continuous data and chi square or Fisher's exact tests for categorical data, using GraphPad Prism (Version 5.0, GraphPad Software Inc., La Jolla, CA). Statistical significance was considered at a p-level < 0.05.

Results

During the study period, 2081 encounters meeting the study inclusion criteria were identified. From these, 783 records were analyzed after exclusions (see Fig. 1 for study flow diagram). Overall, 39.3, 57.3, and 3.4% of the patients underwent flexible diagnostic bronchoscopy with or without transtracheal fine needle aspiration biopsy, endobronchial ultrasound (EBUS) guided transtracheal fine needle aspiration biopsy, and tracheal and/or bronchial laser debulking and/or placement procedures, respectively. Interventional pulmonologists performed these procedures 72.2% of the time, while a thoracic surgeon performed 27.8% of the procedures. General anesthesia was maintained using inhalational agents in the majority of cases (85.7% versus 14.3% for intravenous agents). Five hundred seventeen patients were managed using an ETT, while 266 patients were managed using an SGA, providing study groups for intergroup comparisons.

For the intergroup comparisons, baseline patient demographics and device performance characteristics are shown in Table 1. There were no significant differences noted between the comparison groups amongst the baseline characteristics, including characteristics that might suggest an increase risk for pulmonary aspiration, poor SGA fit, or difficult airway management. Endotracheal tube was preferred for flexible bronchoscopy procedures, while SGA was preferred for endobronchial ultrasound guided diagnostic procedures. Tracheal and/or bronchial laser debulking and/or stent procedures showed no preference between airway device usage. With respect to device performance, SGA conversion rate (to ETT) was 0.4% [95% CI: 0.0, 2.3%]. SGA versus ETT use was also associated with a significant reduction in NMBD administration (9.0% [6.1, 13.1%] versus 78.3% [74.6, 81.7%]).

Discussion

The main finding of this study is that usage of SGAs for IP procedures can be highly successful with a low conversion rate to ETT when used in appropriately selected

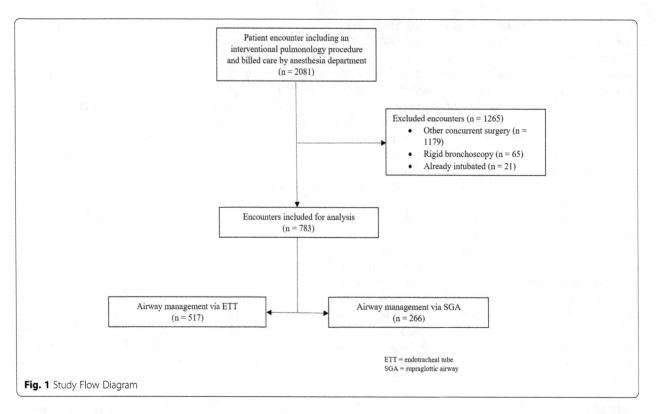

Fig. 1 Study Flow Diagram

patients. Secondarily, when SGAs are used for IP procedures in our institution, the avoidance of NMBDs and the potential for consequent residual paralysis in a patient population that may have significant underlying pulmonary co-morbidities is achieved.

With the advancement of therapeutic and interventional procedures in the field of IP in recent years, there has been limited literature showing the usage and successfulness of SGAs compared to ETTs in anesthetized patients. Previously, Du Plessis et al found that during 140 adult patients undergoing fiberoptic bronchoscopy with general anesthesia using an SGA, only one patient required tracheal intubation due to laryngospasms, a conversion rate of 0.7% [7]. In a different retrospective study of 200 patients having underwent awake diagnostic bronchoscopies, use of an SGA facilitated successful bronchoscopies in every patient except one, where device placement was not tolerated [8]. Finally, in a recent publication by Schmutz et al, an SGA failure rate was found to be 3.1% in 132 patients that underwent transbronchial lung cryobiopsy, which the authors attributed to impossible placement of SGA ($n = 1$), high oropharyngeal leakage ($n = 1$), massive endobronchial bleeding ($n = 1$), and acute right heart failure requiring resuscitation ($n = 1$) [9]. In our study, which includes a broader range of IP procedures, we found similar success in the use of SGAs for airway maintenance during general anesthesia.

Previous authors have discussed some advantages of SGA use during fiberoptic bronchoscopy under general anesthesia [10]. Beyond the use of decreased NMBDs use, advantages of using an SGA over an ETT for IP procedures based on clinical experience includes easier placement, examination of glottis and upper trachea, easier device placement including bronchoscope, lighter depth of anesthesia requirement, and smoother emergence. Additionally, based on our experience, we suggest several ideal features of SGAs for IP procedures. First, an SGA with a good oropharyngeal seal and stable fit enables positive pressure ventilation when needed at a higher airway pressure and may be less prone to dislodgement. Second, an SGA with a relatively short, straight, and large internal diameter air tube reduces resistance to bronchoscopic device movements, facilitating the IP procedure. Third, an SGA with a built-in bite block protects the bronchoscopic equipment from damage due to potential patient biting during the procedure. Finally, an SGA with a gastric channel enables decompression of a patient's stomach if desired, and also provides a means to reseat a dislodged SGA over an orogastric tube if left in situ.

Although our study provides evidence to support the use of SGAs for IP procedures, it is not without limitations. First, several different types of SGAs (Ambu® AuraStratight™, Ambu® AuraFlex™, LMA® Supreme™, LMA® ProSeal™, i-gel®, and air-Q®) were in use in our institution during the study period, and the specific SGA used for each case was not routinely recorded in the chart. Therefore, we cannot ascribe any success to a particular device. During the last two years of the study period, however, it

Table 1 Baseline Characteristics and Device Performance Comparisons

	ETT (n = 517)	SGA (n = 266)	p-value[‡]
Age, yrs	61 (13)	62 (13)	0.43
Gender, n (%)			
Male	294 (56.9%)	143 (53.8%)	0.45
Female	223 (43.1%)	123 (46.2%)	
ASA, n (%)			
1	2 (0.4%)	2 (0.8%)	0.77
2	187 (36.2%)	91 (34.2%)	
3	300 (58.0%)	161 (60.5%)	
4	28 (5.4%)	12 (4.5%)	
Co-morbidities, n (%)			
DM	81 (15.7%)	39 (14.7%)	0.75
GERD	155 (30.0%)	88 (33.1%)	0.37
OSA	39 (7.5%)	27 (10.2%)	0.22
Known difficult intubation	10 (1.9%)	6 (2.3%)	0.42
BMI, kg·m⁻²	28 (6)	28 (7)	0.55
Mallampati score, n (%)			
I	115 (32.1%)	62 (28.6%)	0.55
II	199 (55.6%)	123 (56.7%)	
III	44 (12.3%)	27 (12.4%)	
IV	0 (0%)	5 (2.3%)	
Mouth opening, n (%)			
< 4 cm	27 (6.5%)	20 (9.2%)	0.59
> 4 cm	388 (93.5%)	211 (90.8%)	
Upper lip bite test, n (%)			
Achieved	184 (94.4%)	103 (96.3%)	0.34
Not Achieved	11 (5.6%)	4 (3.7%)	
Thyromental distance, n (%)			
< 6 cm	42 (10.6%)	25 (11.5%)	0.79
> 6 cm	355 (89.4%)	193 (88.5%)	
Neck range of motion, n (%)			
Full	271 (79.2%)	149 (76.8%)	0.51
Limited	70 (20.8%)	45 (23.2%)	< 0.0001

Table 1 Baseline Characteristics and Device Performance Comparisons (Continued)

	ETT (n = 517)	SGA (n = 266)	p-value[‡]
Procedure type, n (%)			
Flexible bronchoscopy y	233 (45%)	74 (28%)	< 0.0001
Endobronchial ultrasound	263 (51%)	185 (70%)	0.42
Tracheal/bronchial laser/stent	20 (4%)	7 (3%)	
Anesthetic type, n (%)			
Inhalational	438 (84.7%)	233 (87.6%)	0.33
TIVA	79 (15.3%)	33 (12.4%)	
[†]Neuromuscular blocking drug use, n (%)	405 (78.3%)	24 (9.0%)	< 0.0001
Failed primary airway, n (%)	1 (0.4%)		

Data are mean (SD) unless otherwise noted. ASA American Society of Anesthesiologists, DM diabetes mellitus, GERD gastroesophageal reflux disease, OSA obstructive sleep apnea, BMI body mass index, TIVA total intravenous anesthesia, ETT endotracheal tube, SGA supraglottic airway. [†]Includes intermediate or long-acting neuromuscular blocking drugs; excludes succinylcholine used for airway placement. [‡] Intergroup comparisons were performed using t-tests and chi square or Fisher's exact tests for continuous and categorical data, respectively. A p-value < 0.05 was considered statistically significant

is known that the i-gel® (over the Ambu® AuraStraight™) started to be used routinely for IP procedures, and continues to enjoy predominant use today, as it incorporates many of the ideal features noted above. Second, our study is a retrospective study, which can suffer from selection biases, variations in intra-operative management techniques, and missing data specifics, amongst others. It can be noted that at the time of these procedures patient characteristics, previous anesthesia and surgical experience, and local culture may have led to the anesthesiologist preferentially using one airway device over the others. The results of our study also do not show a correlation between airway device selection and general anesthesia maintenance (i.e. inhalational versus total intravenous anesthesia). Although prior reports indicate some advantages to total intravenous anesthesia, the majority of IP procedures at our institution continue to be performed using inhalation anesthesia due to attending anesthesiologist preferences [11]. Finally, two main modes of ventilation were used during the study period. For patients in the ETT group, the most common mode of ventilation was mandatory volume control ventilation (VCV) (56%), followed by mandatory pressure control ventilation (PCV) (39%). In the SGA group, the most common primary mode of ventilation was mandatory PCV (50%), followed by mandatory VCV (22%). Less commonly in both groups, patients were intermittently managed with other modes of ventilation. Specific ventilator parameters were not recorded in the database. Generally during the procedure, a standard bronchoscope with a sideport connection was placed on the proximal end of airway device facilitating passage of the bronchoscope into the patient's trachea and pulmonary tree. Patient ventilation and oxygenation was monitored using end-tidal carbon dioxide and pulse oximetry. If inadequate ventilation or oxygenation was a concern, the anesthesiologist communicated to the interventionalist to halt the procedure and withdrawal the bronchoscope to allow for collection of adequate monitor data. Adjustments in oxygen delivery and/or ventilation parameters were then made. Operating room pollution from inhalation agents was controlled using a standard gas scavenger system. Anesthesia providers who were uncomfortable with the performance of the SGA during the procedure due to air leak, exchanged the device for an ETT. This occurred in 0.4% of patients whose airways were managed with an SGA. We would like to acknowledge that high frequency jet ventilation has been commonly used during interventional pulmonology procedures at other institutions, however, this was not a mode of ventilation available at our institution and was not used during the study period. Nonetheless, despite the limitations of our study, our study is the largest study on the topic, and we believe the results provide support for the use of SGAs for airway maintenance during IP procedures, particularly given the limited availability of other data.

Conclusions

In summary, our study has shown ETT are more commonly used in practice for IP procedures, but evidence of successful SGA usage and the potential reduction in NMBD administration can be achieved in appropriate patient populations.

Abbreviations
ETT: Endotracheal tube; IP: Interventional pulmonology;
NMBD: Neuromuscular blocking drugs; PCV: Pressure control ventilation;
SGA: Supraglottic airway; VCV: Volume control ventilation

Acknowledgements
We would like to thank Michael Sookochoff for his help collecting study data.

Author' contributions
KMB analyzed and interpreted the patient data, and was a major contributor in writing the manuscript. REG was responsible for the study conception and design, and acquisition, analysis, and interpretation of the study data. All authors read and approved the final manuscript, and agreed to be accountable for all aspects of their work.

Author details
[1]Chicago Medical School, Rosalind Franklin University of Medicine and Science, 3333 Green Bay Road, North Chicago, IL 60064, USA. [2]Department of Anesthesiology, University of Wisconsin School of Medicine and Public Health, 600 Highland Ave., B6/319, Madison, WI 53792, USA.

References
1. Ross A, Ferguson J. Advances in interventional pulmonology. Curr Opin Anaesthesiol. 2009;22(1):11–7.
2. Ernst A, Silvestri G, Johnstone D. Interventional Pulmonary Procedures. Chest. 2003;123(5):1693–4.
3. Sarkiss M. Anesthesia for bronchoscopy and interventional pulmonology: from moderate sedation to jet ventilation. Curr Opin Pulm Med. 2011;4:274–8.
4. Abdelmalak B, Gildea T, Doyle D. Anesthesia for bronchoscopy. Curr Pharm Des. 2012;18(38):6314–24.
5. Brimacombe J. The advantages of the LMA over the tracheal tube or facemask: a meta-analysis. Can J Anaesth. 1995;42(11):1017–23.
6. Arevalo-Ludena J, Arcas-Bellas J, Alvarez-Rementeria R, et al. A comparison of the I-gel supraglottic device with endotracheal intubation for bronchoscopic lung volume reduction coil treatment. J Clin Anesth. 2016;31:137–41.
7. Du Plessis M, Barr A, Verghese C, Lyall J. Fibreoptic bronchoscopy under general anaesthesia using the laryngeal mask airway. Eur J Anaesthesiol. 1993;10(5):363–5.
8. Brimacombe J, Tucker P, Simons S. The laryngeal mask airway for awake diagnostic bronchoscopy. A retrospective study of 200 consecutive patients. Eur J Anaesthesiol. 1995;12(4):357–61.
9. Schmutz A, Durk T, Idzko M, Koehler T, Kalbhenn J, Loop T. Feasibility of a Supraglottic airway device for Transbronchial lung Cryobiopsy – a retrospective analysis. J Cardiothorc Vasc Anesth. 2017;31:1342–7.
10. Tuck M, Phillips R, Corbett J. LMA for fibreoptic bronchoscopy. Anaesth Intensive Care. 1991;19(3):472–3.
11. Yamaguchi S, Koguchi T, Midorikawa Y, Okuda Y, Kitajima T. Comparative evaluation of TIVA with propofol-fentanyl and thiopental-sevoflurane anesthesia using laryngeal mask airway for diagnostic bronchoscopy. J Anesth. 1998;12:53–6.

22

The median effective dose (ED50) of *cis*-Atracurium for laryngeal mask airway insertion during general Anaesthesia for patients undergoing urinary surgery

Xiaohua Wang[1,2,3]*, Ke Huang[1,2,3], Hao Yan[4], Fei Lan[1,2,3], Dongxu Yao[1,2,3], Yanhong Li[1,2,3], Jixiu Xue[1,2,3] and Tianlong Wang[1,2,3]*

Abstract

Background: In clinical practice, the laryngeal mask airway is an easy-to-use supraglottic airway device. However, the *cis*-atracurium dosage for laryngeal mask insertion has not been standardised. We aimed to determine the optimal dose of *cis*-atracurium using a sequential method for successful laryngeal mask insertion.

Methods: The cohort study protocol is registered at clinicaltrial.gov (NCT-03668262). Twenty-three patients undergoing elective urinary surgery were sequentially administered *cis*-atracurium doses as follows: 150, 100, 70, 50, 30, and 20 $\mu g \cdot kg^{-1}$. The main outcome involved the determination of the response to laryngeal mask airway insertion: ≥16 points and < 16 points indicated "satisfactory" and "unsatisfactory" responses, respectively. The median effective dose was estimated using the mean of the seven crossovers from "satisfactory" and "unsatisfactory" responses. The primary outcome involved the determination of the median effective dose (ED50) of *cis*-atracurium for laryngeal mask airway insertion.

Results: The median effective dose of *cis*-atracurium was 26.5 $\mu g \cdot kg^{-1}$ (95% CI 23.6–29.8) using the sequential method. Heart rate was decreased in the 50 $\mu g \cdot kg^{-1}$ group compared to that in the 30 $\mu g \cdot kg^{-1}$ group at timepoints T7, T8, and T10 ($P = 0.0482$, $P = 0.0460$, and $P = 0.0236$, respectively), but no difference was observed in the 20 $\mu g \cdot kg^{-1}$ group. Systolic blood pressure was decreased in the 50 $\mu g \cdot kg^{-1}$ group compared to that in the 20 $\mu g \cdot kg^{-1}$ group at timepoints T2, T3, and T4 ($P = 0.0159$, $P = 0.0233$, and $P = 0.0428$, respectively). The train-of-four value was significantly lower in the 50 $\mu g \cdot kg^{-1}$ group than in the 30 $\mu g \cdot kg^{-1}$ group at timepoint T3 ($P = 0.0326$).

Conclusions: The ED50 of *cis*-atracurium was 26.5 $\mu g \cdot kg^{-1}$ for laryngeal mask airway insertion.

Keywords: Sequential method, ED50, *cis*-Atracurium, Urinary surgery, Laryngeal mask

* Correspondence: 15910851623@163.com; w_tl5595@yahoo.com
[1]Department of Anesthesiology, Xuanwu Hospital, Capital Medical University, Beijing 100053, China

Background

The laryngeal mask airway (LMA) is a supraglottic ventilation device that is more effective than mask airway for difficult airway management and includes the characteristics of mask and endotracheal intubation [1]. LMA insertion has more advantages than endotracheal intubation: it has little influence on the patient's circulation during insertion, reduces the dosage of analgesics required to maintain anaesthesia during surgery, and is well-tolerated [2]. Therefore, the laryngeal mask is widely used in elective minor surgery, particularly in minor urinary surgery [3]. The use of muscle relaxants is necessary to improve the conditions of laryngeal mask insertion [4]. Without muscle relaxants, the pharyngeal tissues are not relaxed, and appropriate laryngeal mask placement is difficult owing to resistance to mouth opening and biting [5]. Moreover, muscle relaxation is needed to avoid excessive airway reactivity of laryngeal mask insertion (e.g., laryngeal spasm, hypersalivation, coughing), to reduce laryngeal mask insertion-related complications (e.g., postoperative throat pain), and to reduce the incidence of airway complications such as hypoxia, ineffective ventilation, and sternal muscle stiffness that are induced by opioid analgesics [6–8]. Analgesic and narcotic agents are required in high dosages without the use of muscle relaxants, and an overdose of analgesic agents can inhibit the patient's haemodynamics [9]. Small doses of neuromuscular blocking agents (NMBAs) may improve mandibular relaxation and shorten the time required for laryngeal mask placement, thereby improving the laryngeal mask placement conditions [10].

Cis-atracurium is a non-depolarizing NMBA and has been widely used adjunctively during anaesthesia to facilitate endotracheal intubation and provide a longer duration of muscle relaxation [11]. It is spontaneously degraded at physiological pH via Hofmann elimination, which is an organ-independent degradative mechanism that yields laudanosine and plasma esterase-mediated hydrolysis [12]. Little or no risk is associated with the use of *cis*-atracurium in patients with renal diseases; therefore, it is frequently used in general anaesthesia during urinary surgery. Furthermore, *cis*-atracurium has unique advantages and is approximately three times more potent than atracurium as a muscle relaxant [13]. It has less propensity to induce histamine release, which causes subsequent cutaneous flushing, hypotension, and tachycardia complications [14], and it significantly reduces the use of proinflammatory markers during surgery [15]. However, an overdose of *cis*-atracurium may increase the risk of aspiration, airway obstruction, and delayed recovery. The dosages of muscle relaxants used in trachea intubation vary greatly and range from 10 to 200 µg·kg^{-1} [16–19]. However, a reasonable dosage of *cis*-atracurium under LMA has not been reported.

This study aimed to determine the median effective dose (ED50) of *cis*-atracurium for laryngeal mask insertion in anesthetised adults using Dixon's up-and-down method [20] and to determine the dose-response curves for laryngeal mask insertion in urinary surgery.

Methods
Patient characteristics

This prospective observational study was approved by the university's institutional review board (IRB no.: CINI-AD-20180808). All individuals participating in the trial provided written informed consent. The trial is also registered at http://ClinicalTrials.gov (registry no.: NCT-03668262; date of registration: September 11, 2018). The methodology in this study followed the international guidelines for observational studies according to the Strengthening the Reporting of Observational Studies in Epidemiology (STROBE) 2010 statement (Supplementary-STROBE checklist). We recruited 23 prospective consecutive patients who were scheduled for elective minor urological surgery under general anaesthesia between 15 September, 2018, and 30 January, 2019, at Xuanwu Hospital (Beijing, China). All patients met the criteria for the American Society of Anesthesiologists (ASA) Physical Status I–III; Body Mass Index (BMI), 18.5–30 kg/m^2; age, 20–60 years; predicted operation duration < 180 min; and estimated blood loss < 5 ml·kg^{-1}. The exclusion criteria were as follows: neuromuscular diseases; metabolic diseases; preoperative condition complicated with electrolyte disorders, serious hepatic insufficiency (i.e., liver transaminase level > 40 U·L^{-1}), or renal insufficiency (i.e., serum creatinine level > 1.2 mg·dL^{-1}); serious heart and lung disease; predicted difficult airway; use of preoperative medications that interact with non-depolarising NMBAs (e.g., aminoglycosides, polymyxin, steroids, phenytoin sodium, neuroleptics, carbamazepine); history of allergy to NMBAs; and history of alcoholism or drug abuse.

Anaesthesia protocol

After the patient entered the operating room, lactate Ringer's solution was infused at a rate of 5 ml·kg^{-1}·h^{-1}. After 3 min of oxygen supplied via the mask, intravenous sufentanil (dose, 0.25 µg·kg^{-1}; injection time, 30 s) and etomidate (dose, 0.2 mg·kg^{-1}; injection time, 30 s) were administered. The bispectral index (BIS) reaching a value below 60 and loss of the eyelash reflex indicated that the patient had lost consciousness, and the train-of-four (TOF) value was calibrated. The calibration of TOF as the baseline was 100. After calibration, *cis*-atracurium was administered (injection time, 5 s). Three minutes after the *cis*-atracurium injection, and once the BIS reached a value of 40–60, an experienced anaesthesiologist placed a flexible LMA (Teleflex Medical, Wayne,

PA, USA; Athlone Co., Westmeath, Ireland) of the appropriate type (LMA® Flexible criteria: 30–50 kg for No. 3; 50–70 kg for No. 4; and 70–100 kg for No. 5). The patients' responses were jointly evaluated by another anaesthesiologist who was blinded to the *cis*-atracurium concentrations when the LMA was inserted. The tidal volume setting was 7 ml·kg^{-1}, and the respiration rate setting was 12 RR·min^{-1}. If laryngeal mask insertion was unsuccessful, anaesthesia was deepened with further increments of *cis*-atracurium, or an inhalation agent, or both, until the laryngeal mask was tolerated; however, the patient was placed in the "unsatisfactory" group in these cases. Propofol combined with remifentanil was used to maintain the BIS at 40–60 throughout the operation. The range of blood pressure and heart rate (HR) fluctuation did not exceed the 20% baseline value. Body temperature was maintained at > 36 °C using a warm air blanket.

Cis-Atracurium administration and evaluation of the LMA placement conditions

Administration of cis-Atracurium and subdivision of groups

The first patient enrolled in the study was exposed to an initial *cis*-atracurium concentration of 0.15 mg·kg^{-1}. The step size of the concentration was calculated by a common ratio 1.5; thus, the administered doses were $0.1 = [0.15/(1.5)]$, $0.06667 = [0.15/(1.5)^2]$, $0.04444 = [0.15/(1.5)^3]$, 20 µg·kg^{-1} 962 $= [0.15/(1.5)^4]$, and $0.01975 = [0.15/(1.5)^5]$ mg. In the clinical setting, the

actual administered doses were 0.15, 0.1, 0.07, 0.05, 0.03, and 0.02 mg kg^{-1}, which are equal to 150, 100, 70, 50, 30, and 20 µg·kg^{-1} in this study. We categorized the patients into six groups as follows: 150 µg·kg^{-1} group, 100 µg·kg^{-1} group, 70 µg·kg^{-1} group, 50 µg·kg^{-1} group, 30 µg·kg^{-1} group, and 20 µg·kg^{-1} group. Depending on the previous patient's response to the laryngeal mask, using a modified Dixon's up-and-down method, we adjusted the subsequent dose in the remaining patients [20]. Beginning with the first case of unsatisfactory response, the number of observation units was counted. A "satisfactory-satisfactory" response was noted at seven exchange points. This marked the completion of the test (Fig. 1). When self-contained respiration occurred during the operation, additional doses of *cis*-atracurium were re-administered to the patient.

Laryngeal mask placement conditions

The insertion condition was evaluated only when the laryngeal mask was inserted the first time. Using the recognised six-point-three scale proposed by Sivalingam [21], which has been used successfully in previous research, the following were graded: resistance to mouth opening, resistance to insertion, coughing, swallowing, laryngospasm/airway obstruction (including Paw pressure more than 40 mmHg after insertion immediately), and head and body movement. Each item was scored 3 points, 2 points, and 1 point, based on the severity. A full score was 18 points. A score of ≥16 points was

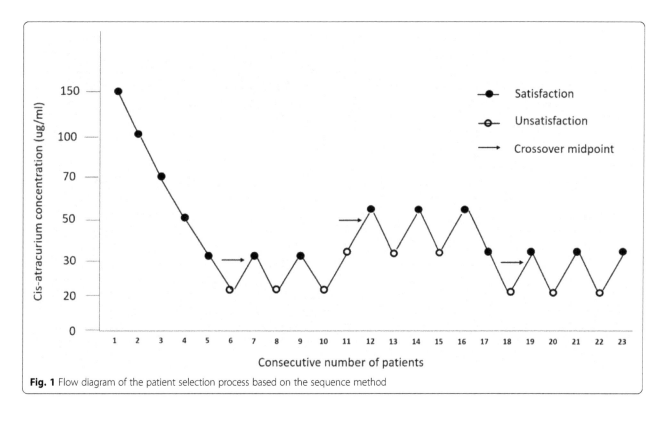

Fig. 1 Flow diagram of the patient selection process based on the sequence method

considered to be a "satisfactory" response, and a score of < 16 points was considered to be an "unsatisfactory" response (Supplementary) (Table_S1). If the response was "unsatisfactory", the *cis*-atracurium dosagr was increased in the next patient. After approximately 60 s of successful laryngeal mask insertion, the position and ventilation condition of the laryngeal mask and whether the patient had a "satisfactory" or "unsatisfactory" response were recorded.

Muscle relaxation (TOF) monitoring, general parameter monitoring, and blood sample analysis

The patient's upper limb was extended and fixed. After degreasing the skin with alcohol, surface electrodes were placed on the side of the ulnar nerve of the wrist for TOF stimulation monitoring (TOF-Watch; Organon Ireland, Ltd., Swords, Dublin, Ireland). The sensor probe of the TOF monitor was placed between the thumb and forefinger with no resistance between them. When the patient lost consciousness, the calibration scale of T1 was 100, the stimulation current was 45–75 mA, the interval was 5 s, and the frequency was 2 Hz. The nasopharyngeal temperatures, electrocardiography, blood pressure, HR, pulse oxygen saturation (SpO_2), and BIS of patients were routinely monitored. We set 10 timepoints to record variations during the operation as follows: upon administration of *cis*-atracurium (T1), and 3 min (i.e., at LMA insertion) (T2), 10 min (at the beginning of the operation) (T3), 20 min (T4), 30 min (T5), 40 min (T6), 50 min (T7), 60 min (T8), 70 min (T9), and 80 min after the administration of cis-atracurium (T10). Systolic blood pressure (SBP), diastolic blood pressure (DBP), HR, SpO_2, BIS, TOF and airway peak pressure (Paw peak pressure) were recorded at each timepoint. Intraoperative haemodynamic changes and adverse reactions such as cough, respiratory depression, dizziness, nausea, and vomiting were also recorded.

Statistical analysis

The ED50 of *cis*-atracurium was determined by calculating the midpoint concentration of the crossover point from the "satisfactory" or "unsatisfactory" responses. To facilitate the dose-response analysis, the laryngeal mask insertion conditions were recorded as dichotomous outcomes. A probit analysis linear regression plot of the log dose versus the percentage response was generated, and interpolation (with 95% CIs) was used to determine the laryngeal mask condition. The average of the midpoints of all pairs was used to calculate the ED50 using Dixon's up-and-down method. The number of responders at each dose was used to plot a sigmoid dose-response curve and a log-dose probit response relation. The other parameters were analysed using repeated measures ANOVA. The patient characteristics are presented as

the mean (± SD) or the number (proportion). A *P*-value of < 0.05 was considered to represent significant difference among outcomes. These data were analysed using SPSS version 17.0 (SPSS Inc., Chicago, IL, USA). The sample size of 23 patients was based on α = 0.05 for the two-sided chi-square test to analyse trends in proportions and a logistic model of β = 0.1 to detect the insertion success rates. The sample size of this study also was based on the fact that a minimum of seven independent pairs of participants exhibited a crossover point from a "satisfactory" response to an "unsatisfactory" response. In similar studies in the field of airway device insertion, the number of crossover points varied from six to eight, with six crossover points being the most common. For this study, seven crossovers were sufficient to determine the ED50 of *cis*-atracurium required to insert a laryngeal mask. A minimum of seven pairs of failure-success was required for the statistical analysis. The total score for the insertion conditions was calculated by addition. A score of ≥16 represented the optimal condition for LMA insertion.

Results
Patient profile, Haemodynamics, TOF value, and ventilation condition for each dosage

Age, sex, weight, height, BMI, and the ASA Physical Status were similar among the three groups (Table 1). No significant differences were noted in the pH values and nasopharyngeal temperatures in all patients. Haemoglobin values, globulin fraction of plasma protein, and albumin fraction of plasma protein were similar among the groups (Table 1). The preoperative Mallampati variable did not differ among the groups. The operation duration, anaesthesia duration, and blood loss were nonsignificantly different among groups (Table 1). There was no statistical difference in the DBP among groups. The SBP was significantly decreased in the 20 µg·kg^{-1} group compared with the 50 µg·kg^{-1} group at T2, T3, and T4 (*P* = 0.0159, *P* = 0.0233, and *P* = 0.0428, respectively; Fig. 2a and b). For each group, the HR did not significantly differ at most timepoints; however, the HR was significantly decreased at T7, T8, and T10 in the 50 µg·kg^{-1} group compared to the 30 µg·kg^{-1} group (*P* = 0.0482, *P* = 0.0460, and *P* = 0.0236, respectively). This finding indirectly reflected the lower stress at these timepoints (Fig. 2c).

The BIS value did not significantly differ among the three groups and was maintained at 40–60 during surgery (Fig. 2d). TOF and airway peak pressure (Paw peak pressure) were recorded at T1-T8, because after T8, muscle relaxation subsided in most cases in the 20 µg·kg^{-1} group, and participants were unable to tolerate the laryngeal mask. Additional doses of *cis*-atracurium were re-administered to patients after the T8

Table 1 Population Demographics and Intraoperative and Preoperative Data

Variable	50 μg·kg^{-1}	30 μg·kg^{-1}	20 μg·kg^{-1}
Female sex	1 (25)	1 (10)	2 (33.3)
Age (years)	54.50 (14.08)	50.60 (12.65)	48.83 (13.23)
Weight (kg)	77.00 (12.36)	76.90 (5.28)	75.67 (14.90)
Height (cm)	168.75 (7.14)	171.40 (4.97)	169.00 (6.20)
BMI	26.90 (2.37)	26.21 (2.02)	26.32 (3.93)
Haemoglobin (g·L^{-1})	137.5 (19.16)	140.30 (9.59)	138.67 (25.45)
Globin fraction of plasma protein (g·L^{-1})	30.98 (4.89)	24.21 (3.45)	23.87 (5.61)
Albumin fraction of plasma protein (g·L^{-1})	40.19 (4.24)	39.82 (3.67)	41.22 (6.23)
pH value	7.37 (0.04)	7.38 (0.03)	7.39 (0.03)
Nasopharyngeal temperature (°C)	36.33 (0.25)	36.34 (0.28)	36.38 (0.10)
Operation duration (min)	93 (42.42)	67.20 (41.58)	56.17 (90.27)
Anaesthesia duration (min)	122.25 (41.16)	104.20 (45.85)	99.33 (81.02)
Blood loss (ml)	141.03 (13.52)	139.01 (10.18)	138.89 (20.11)
Mallampati class			
I	0 (0)	1 (10)	1 (16.67)
II	0 (0)	2 (20)	1 (16.67)
III	4 (100)	7 (70)	3 (50)
IV	0 (0)	0 (0)	1 (16.67)
ASA class			
II	2 (50)	2 (20)	1 (16.67)
III	2 (50)	8 (80)	5 (83.33)

ASA American Society of Anesthesiologists, *BMI* Body Mass Index
The numerical values (e.g., Mallampati class, ASA score, sex) are expressed as the number (%) or number (proportion). All other values are expressed as the mean (SD)
*$P < 0.05$; **$P < 0.01$

timepoint. TOF and airway peak pressure (Paw peak pressure) were affected by re-administration of *cis*-atracurium; therefore, we did not include the TOF and airway peak pressure (Paw peak pressure) at T9 and T10 in the statistical analysis. The TOF value at T3 was significantly lower in the 50 μg·kg^{-1} group than that in the 30 μg·kg^{-1} group ($P = 0.0226$) (Fig. 2e). The TOF values in the 30 μg·kg^{-1} group and in the 20 μg·kg^{-1} group showed no difference at each timepoint, and the TOF values in the 50 μg·kg^{-1} group and in the 20 μg·kg^{-1} group also showed no difference at each timepoint (Fig. 2e). The Paw pressure is indicative of airway protection and the supraglottic airway device placement condition. In this study, the airway peak pressure (i.e., mean Paw pressure) did not significantly differ between the 50 μg·kg^{-1} group and the 30 μg·kg^{-1} group at any timepoint. However, it was significantly higher at T8 in the 20 μg·kg^{-1} group than that in the 30 μg·kg^{-1} group ($P = 0.0423$; Fig. 2f). There were no severe intraoperative haemodynamic changes or adverse reactions such as respiratory depression, nausea, or vomiting in any group.

The ED50 and ED95 of cis-Atracurium

In our patients, the ED50 (95% CI) of *cis*-atracurium for laryngeal mask insertion, which was obtained using the up-and-down method, was 26.5 μg·kg^{-1} (95% CI, 23.6–29.8). We found that the laryngeal mask, based on a probit regression analysis, can be successfully inserted in 50% (95% CI) of anaesthetised adults at a *cis*-atracurium concentration of 26.5 μg·kg^{-1} (95% CI, 23.6 μg·kg^{-1}-29.8 μg·kg^{-1}). The log dosage probit response curves for *cis*-atracurium for the insertion of the laryngeal mask (probability unit vs. concentration) are shown in Fig. 3. We generated the dose response curves and determined the effective doses of *cis*-atracurium required for the insertion of the laryngeal mask in adult patients (Fig. 3).

Discussion

In this study, we aimed to determine the optimal cis-atracurium dosage for LMA insertion in anaesthetised adults using Dixon's up-and-down method and to determine the dose-response curves for LMA insertion in patients undergoing urinary surgery. We found that the ED50 of *cis*-atracurium for LMA insertion in the patients in this study was 26.5 μg·kg^{-1}. Based on our findings, we concluded that laryngeal mask insertion requires the same *cis*-atracurium dosage as tracheal intubation and is an important adjuvant to general anaesthesia. A previous study reported that the calculated ED50 value was 0.0262 mg·kg^{-1} (95% CI: 0.0258–0.0265)

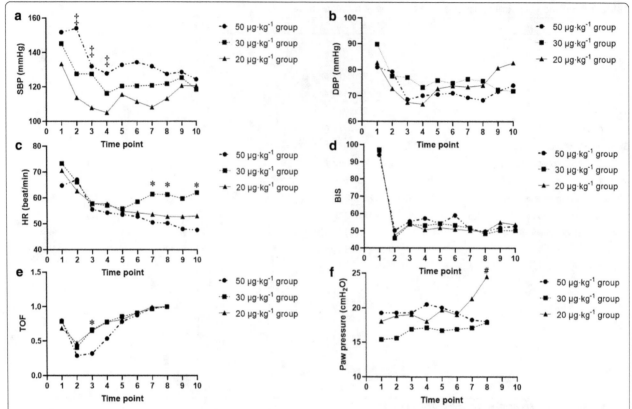

Fig. 2 Haemodynamic value fluctuation, train-of-four, Paw pressure and bispectral index value changes in three groups. Data are presented as mean ± SD. * statistical significance between the 50 μg·kg^{-1} group vs. 30 μg·kg^{-1} group, $P < 0.05$; ‡statistically significant difference between the 50 μg·kg^{-1} and 20 μg·kg^{-1} groups, $P < 0.05$; # statistically significant difference between the 30 μg·kg^{-1} and 20 μg·kg^{-1} groups, $P < 0.05$. There were ten timepoints: T1: administration of *cis*-atracurium, T2: 3 min after administration of *cis*-atracurium (LMA insertion), T3: 10 min after administration of *cis*-atracurium (i.e., beginning of the operation), T4: 20 min after administration of *cis*-atracurium, T5: 30 min after administration of *cis*-atracurium, T6: 40 min after administration of *cis*-atracurium, T7: 50 min after administration of *cis*-atracurium, T8: 60 min after administration of *cis*-atracurium, T9: 70 min after administration of *cis*-atracurium, and T10: 80 min after administration of *cis*-atracurium. Diastolic blood pressure (DBP) did not significantly differ among the groups. Systolic blood pressure (SBP) was significantly decreased in the 50 μg·kg^{-1} group compared to that in the 20 μg·kg^{-1} group at T2, T3, and T4 ($P = 0.0159$, $P = 0.0233$, and $P = 0.0428$, respectively). The heart rate (HR) significantly differed among the groups. The HR was significantly decreased in the 50 μg·kg^{-1} group compared to that in the 20 μg·kg^{-1} group at T7, T8, and T10 ($P = 0.0482$, $P = 0.0460$, and $P = 0.0236$, respectively). The train-of-four [TOF] onset, the time to TOF ratio = 0 TOF value). The TOF value at T3 was significantly lower in the 50 μg·kg^{-1} group than in the 30 μg·kg^{-1} group ($P = 0.0326$). The Paw pressure at each timepoint did not significantly differ between the 50 μg·kg^{-1} and 30 μg·kg^{-1} groups. However, the Paw pressure was significantly higher at T8 in the 30 μg·kg^{-1} group than in the 20 μg·kg^{-1} group ($P = 0.0423$)

[22]. In another study, the ED50 (SD) and ED95 (SD) values of *cis*-atracurium were 0.021 (0.04) and 0.051 (0.013) mg·kg^{-1}, respectively, for tracheal intubation under total intravenous anaesthesia [23]. Tracheal intubation is required when the neuromuscular response is abolished, which is also an indication for laryngeal mask insertion. No consensus exists regarding the appropriate dose of muscle relaxant required for placing a laryngeal mask; the dose ranges from 1/10 dose to the full dose for normal tracheal intubation [18]. One study [18] also demonstrated that the dose of muscle relaxants required for laryngeal mask placement was smaller than that of the muscle relaxants required for endotracheal intubation. This finding coincided with our results. The estimated ED50 for the total patient group was 35.11 μg·kg^{-1} [24]. The effective dose in our study differed from the

48 μg·kg^{-1} that was estimated as the ED95 of *cis*-atracurium by Belmont et al. [25] and differed from the ED50 and ED95 of 30 μg·kg^{-1} and 53 μg·kg^{-1}, respectively, reported by Lepage et al. [26].

In our study, the SBP was significantly lower in the 20 μg·kg^{-1} group at T2 (i.e., anaesthesia induction timepoint), T3, and T4, and was indistinguishable from the SBP in the 30 μg·kg^{-1} group and the 50 μg·kg^{-1} group. No significant difference in SBP was observed between the 50 μg·kg^{-1} group and the 30 μg·kg^{-1} group. However, the propensity to maintain the SBP at a relatively stable level at the preoperative stage was the same among the three groups.

Over 50% of the patients in the 20 μg·kg^{-1} group had an unsatisfactory first response to laryngeal mask insertion. Placement of a laryngeal mask requires adequate

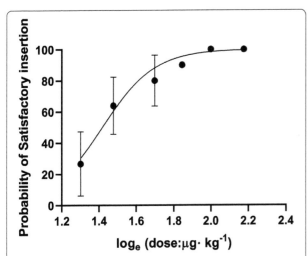

Fig. 3 Dose-response curve of *cis*-atracurium for the insertion of the laryngeal mask airway (probability unit vs. concentration). The median effective dose was 26.5 (95% CI: 33.6–29.8). Log dose/probit response curves of *cis*-atracurium for laryngeal mask airway insertion. The points along the lines represent the mean responses of subgroups of ten patients. Only four of six points are provided for the *cis*-atracurium group. In addition, 100% of the patients who received the higher dose (50 μg·kg^{-1}) had a satisfactory laryngeal mask airway insertion response

anaesthesia depth and mouth opening. Therefore, administration of additional doses of propofol and sufentanil was needed to achieve satisfactory insertion. The combination of an appropriate dose of muscle relaxants can improve laryngeal mask placement without increasing the incidence of associated adverse reactions, while reducing the amount of propofol or sufentanil anaesthetics and reducing their inhibitory effect on the circulation [27]. Without the use of muscle relaxants, it is necessary to increase the depth of anaesthesia, which prolongs the time of the patient's recovery of consciousness.

Our results indicated that the HR was significantly decreased in the 50 μg·kg^{-1} group compared to the 30 μg·kg^{-1} group at T7, T8, and T10. This finding indirectly reflected a lower stress in the 50 μg·kg^{-1} group compared to the 30 μg·kg^{-1} group and the 20 μg·kg^{-1} group. *Cis*-atracurium did not exert significant haemodynamic changes, even at different concentrations. However, the interaction among anaesthetic agents caused a statistically significant decline in some haemodynamic parameters at certain timepoints. However, this change was not a clinical effect and required no vasopressor agents. Using an appropriate NMBA did not affect the extubation time but reduced the stress reaction [28]. *Cis*-atracurium did not cause harmful autonomic nervous system effects and resulted in reduced secretion of histamine. Some investigators have demonstrated no cardiovascular system variations, even with histamine

secretion, when administering a double dose of ED95 to patients with coronary artery disease [29, 30]. The pharmacodynamics of NMBAs are affected by several factors such as temperature [31, 32], use of inhalation agents, magnesium, local anaesthetics [33], antiepileptic drugs, age [34], weight [35], and plasma clearance and volume of distribution [30, 36]. Our study revealed no difference among the three groups in terms of the ASA Physical Status, age, weight, height, and sex. The patients' body temperature in each group was maintained within the normal range. We restricted the use of inhalation anaesthesia throughout the operation.

Based on our findings, all three groups had recovered to the 100% TOF value by T6. The TOF value was significantly lower in the 50 μg·kg^{-1} group than in the 30 μg·kg^{-1} group. This finding indicates that the 50 μg·kg^{-1} group had more efficient muscle relaxation. At the earliest timepoint, the TOF value did not significantly differ between the 30 μg·kg^{-1} group and the 20 μg·kg^{-1} group. The use of a relatively high dose of muscle relaxants will also prolong the extraction of the laryngeal mask due to the prolonged TOF recovery time. The administration of 200% of the ED95 values of *cis*-atracurium, producing an onset duration of 5.2 min, and the time to 25% of T1 recovery at 45 min have been reported [25, 36]. Tulgar [37] demonstrated that the use of subclinical doses of muscle relaxants does not affect the anaesthetic recovery time. In this study, the airway peak pressure (mean Paw pressure) was insignificantly different between the 50 μg·kg^{-1} group and the 30 μg·kg^{-1} group at each timepoint. However, the airway peak pressure at T8 was significantly higher in the 20 μg·kg^{-1} group than in the 30 μg·kg^{-1} group ($P = 0.0423$). Hemmerling [38] reported that a certain degree of muscle relaxation could prevent reduced sealing of the laryngeal mask owing to recovery of strength in the throat muscles.

Our study was limited in that we did not analyse subgroups of these patients. We plan to determine the differences in the ED50 between younger and elderly patients in our future study because reactions and pharmacokinetics differ between young and elderly patients. We also plan to analyse the differences based on sex in the future. Our research provides information for anaesthesiologists, which could help them improve general anaesthesia induction and LMA insertion in patients undergoing minor surgeries.

Conclusion

In this study, the ED50 of *cis*-atracurium for effective muscle relaxation in urinary surgery for LMA insertion was 26.5 μg·kg^{-1}.

Appendix

The formula for ED50

The numbers of satisfactory (r) and unsatisfactory cases (s) of laryngeal mask insertion under different doses of *cis*-atracurium were determined. The logarithm (x) of each dose, total number of patients (n), satisfaction rate of laryngeal mask insertion (p), and difference (I) between the logarithms of two adjacent doses were calculated. The ED50 and its 95% CI were calculated using the following formula for half-dose sequential calculation:

$$P = r/(r+s)$$

Pair value lgED50 of ED50 = σ NX/σ n. Standard error of lgED 50 (SlgED50) = I √ σ [p (1–p)/(n–1)] with 95% CI of ED50 pairs of values (lED 50–1.96 SlgED50; lgED50 + 1.96 SlgED50.

Abbreviations

ASA: American Society of Anesthesiologists; BIS: Bispectral index; BMI: Body Mass Index; DBP: Diastolic blood pressure; ED50: The median effective dose; HR: Heart rate; IRB: Institutional review board; LMA: Laryngeal mask airway;; NMBAs: Neuromuscular blocking agents; SBP: The systolic blood pressure; SpO2: Pulse oxygen saturation; STROBE: Observational Studies in Epidemiology; TOF: Train-of-four

Acknowledgements

This research was supported by the National Natural Science Foundation of China and the department of Urinary surgery at Xuanwu Hospital. The authors thank Jiangtao Wu, Hao Yan, and Tongwen Ou for performing the operation and assisting in manuscript preparation.

Authors' contributions

XW; Contribution: contributed to data acquisition and analysis, and drafted manuscript. KH; Contribution: contributed to trial conduction, and helped prepare the *cis*-atracurium concentrations. HY; Contribution: contributed to performing the operation, writing manuscript and funding support. DY; Contribution: contributed to trial conduction, and helped place a flexible LMA of the appropriate type. JX; Contribution: contributed to trial conduction, and helped evaluate the patients' responses and was blinded to the *cis*-atracurium concentrations. FL; Contribution: contributed to substantially revised the manuscript. YL; Contribution: contributed to interpretation of data and helped to revise the manuscript. TW; Contribution: contributed to the design of the research and agreed to be accountable for all aspects of this work. All authors read and approved the final manuscript version.

Author details

[1]Department of Anesthesiology, Xuanwu Hospital, Capital Medical University, Beijing 100053, China. [2]Institute of Geriatrics, Beijing 100053, China. [3]National Clinical Research Center for Geriatric Disorders, Beijing 100053, China. [4]Department of Urinary surgery, Xuanwu Hospital, Capital Medical University, Beijing 100053, China.

References

1. Cattano D, Van Zundert TCRV, Wojtczak J. Laryngeal mask airway and the enigma of anatomical sizing. J Clin Monit Comput. 2019;33(5):757–8.
2. Hohlrieder M, Brimacombe J, von Goedecke A, et al. Postoperative nausea, vomiting, airway morbidity, and analgesic requirements are lower for the ProSeal laryngeal mask airway than the tracheal tube in females undergoing breast and gynaecological surgery. Br J Anaesth. 2007;99(4): 576–80.
3. Erhan E, Ugur G, Anadolu O, et al. General anaesthesia or spinal anaesthesia for outpatient urological surgery. Eur J Anaesthesiol. 2003;20(8):647–52.
4. Baker AR, Baker AB. Anaesthesia for endoscopic sinus surgery. Acta Anaesthesiol Scand. 2010;54(7):795–803.
5. Hu LQ, Leavitt OS, Malwitz C, et al. Comparison of laryngeal mask airway insertion methods, including the external larynx lift with pre-inflated cuff, on postoperative pharyngolaryngeal complications: a randomized clinical trial. Eur J Anaesthesiol. 2017;34(7):448–55.
6. Scanlon P, Carey M, Power M, et al. Patient response to laryngeal mask insertion after induction of anaesthesia with propofol or thiopentone. Can J Anaesth. 1993;40(9):816–8.
7. Chandra S, Pryambodho P, Melati AC, et al. Comparison Between Lidocaine Inhalation and Intravenous Dexamethasone in Reducing Postoperative Sore Throat Frequency After Laryngeal Mask Insertion. Anesth Pain Med. 2018; 8(5):e82131.
8. Eichelsbacher C, Ilper H, Noppens R, et al. Rapid sequence induction and intubation in patients with risk of aspiration: recommendations for action for practical management of anesthesia. Anaesthesist. 2018;67(8):568–83.
9. Michel J, Hofbeck M, Gerbig I, et al. Nurse-driven analgesia and sedation in pediatric patients with univentricular hearts requiring extracorporeal life support after first-stage palliation surgery: a pilot study. Paediatr Anaesth. 2017;27(12):1261–70.
10. Nasseri K. Effect of low-dose Atracurium on laryngeal mask airway insertion conditions: a randomized double-blind clinical trial. Adv Biomed Res. 2017; 6(1):119.
11. Ortiz JR, Percaz JA, Carrascosa F. Cisatracurium. Rev Esp Anestesiol Reanim. 1998;45(6):242–7.
12. Fuchs-Buder T. New muscle relaxants. Update on mivacurium, rocuronium and cis-atracurium. Anaesthesist. 1997;46(4):350–9.
13. Diefenbach C, Buzello W. New muscle relaxants. Anasthesiol Intensivmed Notfallmed Schmerzther. 1996;31(1):2–8.
14. Savarese JJ, Wastila WB. The future of the benzylisoquinolinium relaxants. Acta Anaesthesiol Scand Suppl. 1995;106:91–3.
15. Konrad FM, Unertl KE, Schroeder TH. Mastocytosis. A challenge in anaesthesiology. Anaesthesist. 2009;58(12):1239–43.
16. Kim KS, Chun YS, Chon SU, et al. Neuromuscular interaction between cisatracurium and mivacurium, atracurium, vecuronium or rocuronium administered in combination. Anaesthesia. 1998;53(9):872–8.
17. Bergeron L, Bevan DR, Berrill A, et al. Concentration–effect relationship of cisatracurium at three different dose levels in the anesthetized patient. Anesthesiology. 2001;95:314–23.
18. Naguib M, Samarkandi AH, Ammar A, et al. Comparative clinical pharmacology of rocuronium, cisatracurium, and their combination. Anesthesiology. 1998;89(5):1116–24.
19. Kim JH, Lee YC, Lee SI, et al. Effective doses of cisatracurium in the adult and the elderly. Korean J Anesthesiol. 2016;69(5):453–9.
20. Dixon WJ. Staircase bioassay: the up-and-down method. Neurosci Biobehav Rev. 1991;15(1):47–50.
21. Sivalingham P, Kandasamy R, Madhaven G, et al. Conditions for laryngeal mask insertion: a comparison of propofol versus sevoflurane with or without alfentanil. Anaesthesia. 1999;54:271–6.
22. Wulf H, Kahl M, Ledowski T. Augmentation of the neuromuscular blocking effects of cisatracurium during desflurane, sevoflurane, isoflurane or total i.v. anaesthesia. Br J Anaesth. 1998;80(3):308–12.
23. Park WY, Choi JC, Yun HJ, et al. Optimal dose of combined rocuronium and cisatracurium during minor surgery: a randomized trial. Medicine (Baltimore). 2018;97(10):e9779.
24. Belmont MR, Lien CA, Quessy S, et al. The clinical neuromuscular pharmacology of 51W89 in patients receiving nitrous oxide/opioid/ barbiturate anesthesia. Anesthesiology. 1995;82:1139–45.
25. Lepage JY, Malinovsky JM, Malinge M, et al. Pharmacodynamic dose-response and safety study of cisatracurium (51W89) in adult surgical patients during N2O-O2-opioid anesthesia. Anesth Analg. 1996;83:823–9.
26. George LR, Sahajanandan R, Ninan S. Low-dose succinylcholine to facilitate laryngeal mask airway insertion: a comparison of two doses. Anesth Essays Res. 2017;11(4):1051–6.
27. Smith SE, Hamblin SE, Dennis BM. Effect of neuromuscular blocking agents on sedation requirements in trauma patients with an open abdomen. Pharmacotherapy. 2019;39(3):271–9.
28. Naguib M, Lien CA, Meistelman C. Pharmacology of muscle relaxants and their antagonists. In: Miller RD, editor. Miller's Anesthesia. 8th ed. Philadelphia: Churchill Livingstone/Elsevier; 2015. p. 958–94.

29. Kisor DF, Schmith VD. Clinical pharmacokinetics of cisatracurium besilate. Clin Pharmacokinet. 1999;36:27–40.
30. Sorooshian SS, Stafford MA, Eastwood NB, et al. Pharmacokinetics and pharmacodynamics of cisatracurium in young and elderly adult patients. Anesthesiology. 1996;84:1083–91.
31. Amin AM, Mohammad MY, Ibrahim MF. Comparative study of neuromuscular blocking and hemodynamic effects of rocuronium and cisatracurium under sevoflurane or total intravenous anesthesia. Middle East J Anaesthesiol. 2009;20(1):39–51.
32. Kim YB, Sung TY, Yang HS. Factors that affect the onset of action ofnon-depolarizing neuromuscular blocking agents. Korean J Anesthesiol. 2017;70:500–10.
33. Ornstein E, Lien CA, Matteo RS, et al. Pharmacodynamics and pharmacokinetics of cisatracurium in geriatric surgical patients. Anesthesiology. 1996;84:520–5.
34. Leykin Y, Pellis T, Lucca M, et al. The pharmacodynamic effects of rocuronium when dosed according to real body weight or ideal body weight in morbidly obese patients. Anesth Analg. 2004;99:1086–9.
35. Arain SR, Kern S, Ficke DJ, et al. Variability of duration of action of neuromuscular-blocking drugs in elderly patients. Acta Anaesthesiol Scand. 2005;49:312–5.
36. Naguib M. Neuromuscular effects of rocuronium bromide and mivacurium chloride administered alone and in combination. Anesthesiology. 1994;81:388–95.
37. Tulgar S, Boga I, Cakiroglu B, et al. Short-lasting pediatric laparoscopic surgery: are muscle relaxants necessary? Endotracheal intubation vs. laryngeal mask airway. J Pediatr Surg. 2017;52(11):1705–10.
38. Hemmerling TM, Michaud G, Deschamps S, et al. Patients who sing need to be relaxed'–neuromuscular blockade as a solution for air-leaking during intermittent positive pressure ventilation using LMA. Can J Anaesth. 2005;52(5):549.

23

A randomized controlled comparison of non-channeled king vision, McGrath MAC video laryngoscope and Macintosh direct laryngoscope for nasotracheal intubation in patients with predicted difficult intubations

Haozhen Zhu, Jinxing Liu, Lulu Suo, Chi Zhou, Yu Sun[*] and Hong Jiang[*]

Abstract

Background: King Vision and McGrath MAC video laryngoscopes (VLs) are increasingly used. The purpose of this study was to evaluate the performance of nasotracheal intubation in patients with predicted difficult intubations using non-channeled King Vision VL, McGrath MAC VL or Macintosh laryngoscope by experienced intubators.

Methods: Ninety nine ASA I or II adult patients, scheduled for oral maxillofacial surgeries with El-Ganzouri risk index 1–7 were enrolled. Patients were randomly allocated to intubate with one of three laryngoscopes (non-channeled King Vision, McGrath MAC and Macintosh). The intubators were experienced with more than 100 successful nasotracheal intubations using each device. The primary outcome was intubation time. The secondary outcomes included first success rate, time required for viewing the glottis, Cormack-Lehane grade of glottis view, the number of assist maneuvers, hemodynamic responses, the subjective evaluating of sensations of performances and associated complications.

Results: The intubation time of King Vision and McGrath group was comparable (37.6 ± 7.3 s vs. 35.4 ± 8.8 s) and both were shorter than Macintosh group (46.8 ± 10.4 s, $p < 0.001$). Both King Vision and McGrath groups had a 100% first attempt success rate, significantly higher than Macintosh group (85%, $p < 0.05$). The laryngoscopy time was comparable between King Vision and McGrath group (16.7 ± 5.5 s vs. 15.6 ± 6.3 s) and was shorter than Macintosh group (22.8 ± 7.2 s, $p < 0.05$) also. Compared with Macintosh laryngoscope, Glottis view was obviously improved when exposed with either non-channeled King Vision or McGrath MAC VL ($p < 0.001$), and assist maneuvers required were reduced ($p < 0.001$). The maximum fluctuations of MAP were significantly attenuated in VL groups (47.7 ± 12.5 mmHg and 45.1 ± 10.3 mmHg vs. 54.9 ± 10.2 mmHg, $p < 0.05$ and $p < 0.01$). Most device insertions were graded as excellent in McGrath group, followed by Macintosh and King Vision group ($p = 0.0014$). The tube advancements were easier in VLs compared with the Macintosh laryngoscope ($p < 0.001$). Sore throat was found more frequent in Macintosh group compared with King Vision group ($p < 0.05$).

Conclusions: Non-channeled King Vision and McGrath MAC VLs were comparable and both devices facilitated nasotracheal intubation in managing predicted difficult intubations compared with Macintosh laryngoscope.

Keywords: Airway management - video laryngoscopes - Nasotracheal intubation

* Correspondence: dr_sunyu@163.com; dr_jianghong@163.com
Department of Anesthesiology, Shanghai Ninth People's Hospital Affiliated to
Shanghai Jiao Tong University School of Medicine, 639 Zhizaoju Road,
Shanghai 200011, China

Introduction

The video laryngoscope (VL) has been well established as an approach in airway management for patients with difficult direct laryngoscopy [1–5]. However, most of the literatures focused on their usage for oral intubation. Nasotracheal intubation (NTI), often required for oral and maxillofacial operation, may be complicated by causing injuries to the nasal passage and sinusitis [6]. In addition, a superior laryngoscopy does not guarantee a successful advancement of the tube into the trachea and external manipulation of the larynx, a Magill forceps, change in head position or partial inflation of cuff is required [6–9].

The success of a VL assisted intubation depends on multiple factors, such as blade design (acute angled or Macintosh like; channeled or non-channeled); quality of the image on the monitor, as well as the experience of the intubator [5, 10]. Recently, the McGrath MAC VL (Fig. 1a) (Aircraft Medical, Edinburgh, UK) has been widely used. It has a battery powered handle, on the top of which is an adjustable liquid crystal display monitor. It has an angulated single-use blade without a guiding channel. It was reported to facilitate routine NTIs in normal patients compared with Macintosh laryngoscope [11, 12]. The King Vision VL (Fig. 1b) (Ambu Inc., Denmark) is also a portable device with similar design with McGrath MAC VL. King Vision VL is relative newer and cheaper. Different from McGrath, its monitor is fixed to the handle. It has a channel integrated to the blade to facilitate tube guidance into the trachea though, channeled King Vision VL required longer time and provided lower success rates on first attempt for oral intubation in normal airway compared to McGrath MAC VL [13]. It is argued that channeled devices are often bulky and can be difficult to use in patients with limited mouth opening [2, 13, 14]. However, the King Vision VL is also available with standard non-channeled blade for NTI. Recent study also found time for tracheal intubation could be shortened by using a non-channeled blade [15]. In addition, the King Vision VL is reported that can provide a better vision condition which may be beneficial to NTI.

A recent systematic review comparing VL versus DL for NTI showed that VL is particularly beneficial for patients with difficult airways [16]. However, only two randomized controlled trials (Airtriq and C-MAC versus Macintosh) were enrolled [7, 17]. It remains unclear whether non-channeled King Vision or McGrath MAC VL, compared with conventional laryngoscope, provide shorter intubation time and a higher first success rate for NTI when used by experienced provider in management of predicted difficult intubation. It is also unclear whether non-channeled King Vision VL is superior to McGrath MAC VL when used for NTI. We therefore performed this randomized, controlled trial to fill the gap. Our hypothesis was that the non-channeled King Vision and McGrath MAC VL were comparable, and both video devices were superior to Macintosh laryngoscope in terms of shorter intubation time and higher first success rate.

Methods

Ethics approval and consent to participate

This trial was approved by IRB (2017–308-T228) from Shanghai Ninth People's Hospital Affiliated to Shanghai Jiao Tong University School of Medicine, and registered at clinicaltrials.gov (NCT03126344). Written consents to participate were obtained from all participants after enrollment. Our study was adhered to the applicable

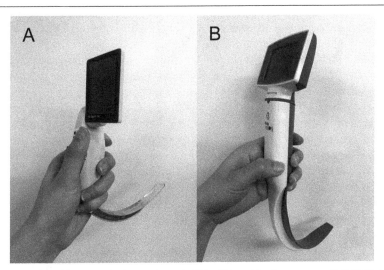

Fig. 1 The video laryngoscopes evaluated in our study. A: non-channeled King Vision video laryngoscope. B: McGrath MAC video laryngoscope

Consolidated Standards of Reporting Trials (CONSORT) guidelines.

Subjects

Consecutive patients, between 18 and 60 years old with American Society of Anesthesiologists (ASA) classification of I or II, and requiring NTI for elective oral and maxillofacial surgery, were screened in the Preoperative Evaluation Unit of our institute. Prediction of difficult intubation is graded by El-Ganzouri multivariate risk index (EGRI) based on seven parameters (body weight, modified Mallampati class, mouth opening, thyromental distance, neck movement, prognathism, and history of difficult airway) [17, 18] (Additional file 1). Patients were enrolled if EGRI score 1–7 [17]. In cases where an awake NTI was planned [i.e. EGRI score > 7, history of reflux or diagnosed oesophageal disease, severe obstructive sleep apnea (OSA) and morbid obesity (body mass index > 40 kg/m^2)] were excluded from the study.

Method of anesthesia

The study was designed as a single blind, three parallel arms, randomized controlled trial comparing NTIs using non-channeled King Vision VL, McGrath MAC VL and Macintosh DL in adults with predictors of difficult airways. The size 3 blades were used in both King Vision and McGrath group. The standard Macintosh blade (size 3 for female; size 4 for male) was used as control.

Patients were asked which nostril was clearer. If both sides were equal and the surgeon had no objection, the right nostril was chosen [19]. Patients were randomly assigned to King Vision group, McGrath group or Macintosh group via a computer generated randomization table. All NTIs were performed by attending anesthesiologists experienced with more than 100 successful NTIs with each device.

No premedication was administered. Lactated Ringer's solution infusion was started intravenously to deal with the fluid loss from the overnight fast after entering the operating theatre. A standard preparation was then performed, including heart rate (HR), lead II ECG, SpO$_2$ (pulse oximetry), and end expiratory carbon dioxide. A Bispectral (BIS) index sensor was attached to the patient's forehead in conjunction with the BIS Monitor. Cannulation of right radial artery was performed under local anesthesia for invasive blood pressure monitoring.

All patients were preoxygenated by a facemask in the position of neutral. Prior to anesthesia induction, the nasal mucosa was well prepared with 1% tetracaine hydrochloride jelly for 2 min and five drops of ephedrine hydrochloride nitrofurazone (containing approximately 2 mg ephedrine) in all patients. Baseline hemodynamic data were recorded by an investigator after a stabilization period of 10 min.

The nasotracheal tube used was reinforced endotracheal tube (ETT, Safety-Flex with Murphy Eye, oral/nasal, Athlone, Ireland; ID 6.5 mm in female and ID 7.0 mm in male patients) and was well lubricated with 1% tetracaine hydrochloride jelly. Dosing of induction medications was given at the discretion of the attending anesthesiologists. Induction agents included midazolam (0.02 mg/kg), propofol (1.5~2 mg/kg) and fentanyl (2 µg/kg). Upon loss of consciousness and jaw relaxation, manual ventilation was tested. If manual ventilation was available, cissatracurium besilate (0.15 mg/kg) was administrated and post induction values were recorded 3 min after induction. Unsuccessful manual ventilation led to study exclusion.

The anesthesiologist tried to intubate when the Train of Four (TOF) count reached zero and BIS value decreased to 50. NTI was performed in a standard manner. First, a preformed ETT was inserted into the nostril and advanced to the posterior nasopharyngeal wall. Second, a laryngoscope blade was introduced into the mouth to expose the glottis. If it's necessary, the BURP maneuver (backward, upward, right-sided pressure) on the thyroid cartilage was attempted to obtain good glottis visibility [20]. And ultimately, the ETT was inserted into the trachea with the aid of Magill's forceps, head flexion, or cuff inflation if necessary.

The primary outcome was the intubation time, defined as the interval between opening the mouth and the time when three consecutive end-tidal CO$_2$ waves were appeared on the monitor. Since the time required for SpO$_2$ to decrease during apnea was about 150 s [21], we defined a failure as the intubation time took longer than 150 s [22], SpO$_2$ less than 92% or oesophagus intubation. The patient was mask ventilated after a failed attempt. In VL groups, the intubator should try the other video device for the second attempt. In Macintosh group, the patient's airway was managed using either non-channeled King Vision or McGrath MAC VL at the discretion of the intubator. If the second attempt was still unsuccessful, the fiberoptic bronchoscope (FOB) was applied. If intubation is not possible with FOB, the patient was awakened.

Secondary outcome measures included time to expose the glottis (laryngoscopy time) and the view of glottis opening valued by Cormack-Lehane grade. A Cormack-Lehane grade IV was defined as laryngoscopy failure. A blinded investigator also recorded the hemodynamic changes (MAP, HR) during the procedure of NTI. The maximum values of invasive MAP were recorded. After successful intubation, the subjective sensation of the intubator (ease of device insertion, quality of view on display and ease of tube advancement) was graded as excellent, good, fair and poor. Other intubation parameters included incidences of bleeding or dental injury, number of assist maneuvers (use of BURP maneuver, Magill's forceps, or cuff inflation). Twenty four hours after the procedure, a nurse anesthetist blinded to group assignment recorded the severity of sore throat and hoarseness.

Statistical analysis

Our sample size estimation was based on previous studies [11, 23], in which the standard deviations (SD) of intubation time were estimated as 8 and 13.7 s. To detect a intergroup difference of 10 s in intubation time with α of 0.05 and β of 0.8, we estimated that 30 patients would be enough for each group. To compensate for patients dropping out during the study, additional patients (10%) were added. The final sample size of 33 patients was in each group.

Mean (SD) or Median (IQR [range]) was used to describe the parametric data. The number (percentage) was used to describe nonparametric data. Statistical analyses were performed with Prism 5.0 for Windows (GraphPad Software, Inc., La Jolla, California, USA). Binary data for three groups were analyzed using chi-square test and each two groups were compared with chi-square segmentation method or Fisher's exact test as appropriate. One-way analysis of variance (ANOVA) with post-hoc Bonferroni's Multiple Comparison test was used to analyze parameter data for changes within groups. The Kruskal-Wallis ANOVA with post-hoc Dunn's test was used to analyze ordinal data. A p value less than 0.05 was considered as significant.

Results

In total, 99 patients were enrolled in this study between June 2017 and January 2018(Fig. 2). The distribution of the patient characteristics and difficult intubation predictors were well balanced between three groups (Table 1). Five patients in Macintosh group were intubated successfully with VLs (two patients with King Vision and three patients with McGrath VL) after failed intubation attempt. All failures were due to poor glottis exposure and esophagus intubation. These patients were excluded from follow-up data analysis as these outcomes were not controlled.

Regarding the primary outcome measure intubation time, King Vision and McGrath groups were comparable (37.6 ± 7.3 s vs. 35.4 ± 8.8 s) and both were significantly shorter than Macintosh group (46.8 ± 10.4 s, $p < 0.001$, Table 2).

Regarding the secondary outcomes, both King Vision and McGrath groups had a 100% first attempt success rate, significantly higher than Macintosh group (85%, $p < 0.05$, Table 2). The laryngoscopy time was comparable

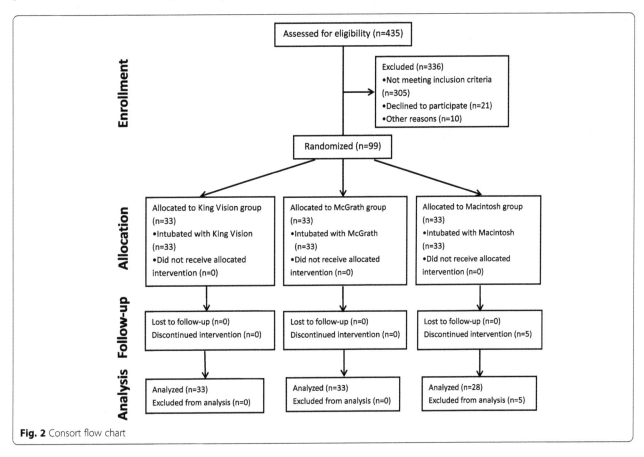

Fig. 2 Consort flow chart

Table 1 Patient characteristics and difficult intubation profiles

	King Vision n = 33	McGrath n = 33	Macintosh n = 33	p value
Men (%)	15 (45%)	19 (58%)	16 (48%)	NS
Age; years	38 (12)	36 (11)	40 (11)	NS
BMI; Kg·m^{-2}	22 (3)	22 (3)	22 (3)	NS
ASA class I/II (%)	11/22 (33/67%)	15/18 (45/55%)	13/20 (40/60%)	NS
Neck movement < 80° (%)	2 (6%)	1 (3%)	1 (3%)	NS
Mallampati III or IV (%)	30 (91%)	31 (94%)	30 (91%)	NS
Interincisor gap < 3 cm (%)	9 (27%)	10 (30%)	8 (27%)	NS
Thyromental distance < 6 cm (%)	8 (27%)	9 (27%)	11 (33%)	NS
Ability to prognath (%)	30 (91%)	28 (85%)	29 (88%)	NS
EGRI scores	3 (2,4.5)	3 (2.5,4)	3 (2,4)	NS

Data presented as mean (SD), median (IQR [range]) or number of patients (percentage). BMI: Body Mass Index. ASA class: American Society of Anesthesiologists classification. EGRI: El-Ganzouri risk index. NS: not significant

between King Vision and McGrath groups (16.7 ± 5.5 s vs. 15.6 ± 6.3 s) and were significantly shorter than Macintosh group (22.8 ± 7.2 s, $p < 0.05$, Table 2), also. Glottis view was obviously improved when exposed with either non-channeled King Vision or McGrath MAC VL: the percentage of Cormack-Lehane grade I or II was 100% in VLs groups and 48% in Macintosh group, respectively ($p = 0.0004$, Table 2). The number of assist maneuvers required was 5, 4 and 18 in King Vision, McGrath and Macintosh group, respectively ($p < 0.0001$, Table 2). The SpO_2 did not differ between groups.

Changes in hemodynamic responses during anesthesia induction and intubation were demonstrated in Fig. 3. Briefly, both MAP and HR decreased significantly in each group after anesthesia induction. Then glottis exposure with each laryngoscope and following ETT placement caused significantly increase in MAP and HR. Finally, MAP and HR descended slowly 1, 3, 5 min after successful intubation. Notably, the maximum fluctuations of MAP ($MAP_{max} - MAP_{post-induction}$) in King Vision and McGrath groups were comparable and both were significantly attenuated compared with Macintosh group (47.7 ± 12.5 mmHg and 45.1 ± 10.3 mmHg vs.

54.9 ± 10.2 mmHg, $p < 0.05$ and $p < 0.01$ respectively, Table 2).

Results of the subjective sensations between devices were listed in Table 3. Most device insertions were graded as excellent in McGrath group (91%), followed by Macintosh (82%) and King Vision group (54%) ($p = 0.0014$). Quality of view on display did not differ between King Vision and McGrath groups. The ease of tube advancement was comparable between King Vision and McGrath groups, and both were much better than Macintosh group ($p < 0.001$). There were no cases of desaturation and dental injury during NTIs. Sore throat was found more frequent in Macintosh group compared with King Vision group ($p < 0.01$). Occurrence of bleeding and hoarseness seemed more frequent in Macintosh group, but failed to show significance. These symptoms were minor and ceased spontaneously without intervention.

Discussion

Although many studies about indirect laryngoscopes were carried out, only two randomized controlled trial, to our knowledge, have compared the VLs (Airtraq and C MAC respectively) with Macintosh laryngoscope in

Table 2 Intubation profiles

	King Vision n = 33	McGrath n = 33	Macintosh n = 33	p value
Intubation time (sec) [1]	37.6 (7.3) ***	35.4 (8.8) ***	46.8 (10.4)	< 0.0001
First success of intubation (%)	33 (100%) *	33 (100%) *	28 (85%)	0.0017
Laryngoscopy time (sec) [1]	16.7 (5.5) *	15.6 (6.3) *	22.8 (7.2)	0.0002
C-L grade I/II/III/IV	29/4/0/0 ***	27/6/0/0 ***	6/10/12/5	< 0.0001
C-L grade I and II (%)	33 (100%) ***	33 (100%) ***	16 (48%)	0.0004
Assist maneuvers (%) [1]	5 (15%) ***	4 (12%) ***	18 (64%)	< 0.0001
Difference between $MAP_{maximum}$ and $MAP_{post-induction}$ (mmHg) [1]	47.7 (12.5)*	45.1 (10.3)**	54.9 (10.2)	0.0030

Data presented as mean (SD) or number (percentage). C-L: Cormack and Lehane. MAP: mean arterial pressure. NS: not significant. Assist maneuvers: use of the BURP maneuver, Magill's forceps or cuff inflation. [1]: n = 28 in Macintosh group. *$p < 0.05$; **$p < 0.01$; ***$p < 0.001$ compared with Macintosh group

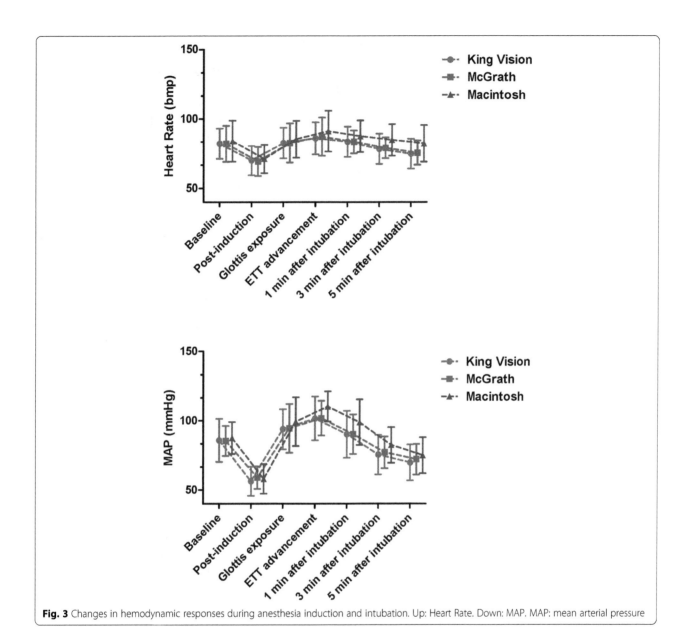

Fig. 3 Changes in hemodynamic responses during anesthesia induction and intubation. Up: Heart Rate. Down: MAP. MAP: mean arterial pressure

Table 3 Sensations of performances and any complications

	King Vision n = 33	McGrath n = 33	Macintosh n = 28	p value
Ease of device insertion (excellent/good/fair/poor)	18/13/2/0 # (54/40/6/0%)	30/3/0/0 (91/9/0/0%)	23/5/0/0 (82/18/0/0%)	0.0014
Quality of view on display (excellent/good/fair/poor)	33/0/0/0 (100/0/0/0%)	32/1/0/0 (97/3/0/0%)	/	NS
Ease of tube advancement (excellent/good/fair/poor)	28/5/0/0 *** (85/15/0/0%)	29/4/0/0 *** (88/12/0/0%)	13/10/4/1 (46/36/14/4%)	0.0001
Desaturation (%)	0 (0)	0 (0)	0 (0)	NS
Bleeding (%)	1 (3%)	0 (0)	4 (14%)	0.0357
Dental injury (%)	0 (0)	0 (0)	0 (0)	NS
Sore throat (%)	3 (11%) **	8 (24%)	12 (43%)	0.0093
Hoarseness (%)	2 (6%)	1 (3%)	5 (18%)	0.969

Data presented as number (percentage). NS: not significant. #$p < 0.05$ compared with McGrath group. *$p < 0.05$; **$p < 0.01$; ***$p < 0.001$ compared with Macintosh group

patients showing predictors of difficult nasal intubation [7, 17]. King Vison and McGrath MAC VLs are relative newer and are also well worth studying. We provided the first study about the non-channeled King Vision and McGrath MAC VLs for NTIs in predicted difficult patients.

Our main result was that the time to successful NTI with both VLs was significantly faster than with Macintosh DL. The intubation time mainly comprises two parts: time to view the vocal cords and time required for tube passage through glottis. Firstly, we confirmed both non-channeled King Vision and McGrath MAC VL significantly shortened the laryngoscopy time in predicted difficult patients, which was certainly a reason for a shortened intubation time. The result showed less association between predictors of difficult intubations and glottis exposure using non-channeled King Vision or McGrath MAC VL than using Macintosh DL. Secondly, laryngoscopy with non-channeled King Vision or McGrath MAC caused less anterior elevation of the larynx than invasive direct laryngoscopy because airway axes alignment was not needed. This might provide a more direct route from nasopharynx to glottis and therefore ease advancing the tube into the trachea. In current study, we confirmed it was easier to advance the ETT through the glottis, accordingly less frequency of assist maneuvers was required in VL groups. Thirdly, when doing oral intubation with VLs, we often bend the styletted tracheal tube to a greater degree ('hockey stick' like) to follow the curvature of the video blade, which always hinder stylet removal and increase intubation time [24, 25]. However, stylet was not required for NTI in our study. So use of VLs also saved time required for tube advancement by decreasing the frequency of additional assist maneuvers and stylet removal [7, 11, 24]. We noticed the laryngoscopy time was longer in King Vision group compared with McGrath group. Alvis et al., in a recent comparison with McGrath, suggested that it was difficult when inserting the channeled blade of King Vision VL into the mouth [13]. Here we found it also more difficult when introducing the non-channeled King Vision blade compared with McGrath blade. The blade of King Vision is longer and more acute angled. We agree with the author who claimed a specific angle to the patient's chest was required when insertion King Vision 'L' shaped blade [13]. On the contrary, the blade design of the McGrath VL is similar to the classic Macintosh DL. This provides the intubator with a familiar laryngoscopy experience. The channeled blade of King Vision may decrease the oral cavity for tube adjustment and advancement during oral intubation [2, 13]. During NTI, however, no such difficulty was observed when advancing the trachea tube with non-channeled King Vision VL. This was in contrast to oral intubation [13].

Although the intubation time was a little bit longer in King Vision group, the clinical relevant is debatable because SpO2 was not different between King Vision and McGrath VL.

The predictors of difficult airways used in our study are reliable [26]. To compare difficult intubation levels, EGRI was used in our study [17, 18]. It is reported that EGRI > 7 were more suitable for awake fiberoptic intubation [27]. Therefore, only patients with EGRI score 1–7 were included in our study. Although the variation of enrollment was big, the EGRI scores were similar between groups. In addition, the distributions of risk factor were also comparable. The proportion of Cormark-Lehane grade III and IV in Macintosh group suggested patients enrolled were predicted difficult intubations. The 15% failure rate of Macintosh DL seem quite high though, the success rate of Macintosh DL (85%) was similar to what has been described previously [3, 17].

Both non-channeled King Vision and McGrath MAC VLs improved the Cormack-Lehane grade significantly which was the main superiority of VLs. St Mont et al. demonstrated first attempt success rate of NTI by Airtraq was 94% in predicted difficult airway [7]. Hazarika H et al. reported a 98% first attempt success rate of NTI by C-MAC D-Blade VL for difficult nasal intubation [17]. Here, we demonstrated the success rate of first attempt of NTI was 100% in non-channeled King Vision and McGrath groups. The 'you see that you fail' situations of King Vision reported previously [2, 14] did not occur in present study. This could be explained by the fact that its 'L' shape blade conformed to the upper airway well though; it always hindered oral ETT advancement. While during NTI, the shape and size of the non-channeled King Vision blade has little influence on the tube advancement and oral cavity allowed for nasotracheal tube adjustment is big enough. Therefore, these results clearly demonstrate that both non-channeled King Vision and McGrath MAC VLs are good choices for NTIs. All failed Macintosh assisted NTIs were because of the poor glottis view, even with the help of assist maneuvers. These patients were eventually easily intubated on the first attempt with either non-channeled King Vision or McGrath MAC VLs. We believe that both of them can serve as a promising backup alternative for failed NTI using Macintosh DL. However, VLs are not the Holy Grail [28]. Actually, VLs will fail under certain conditions; the total success range was 37–98% in literature [2]. Although our results seem to suggest a 100% success rate of VLs intubation, our result should be interpreted with caution due to small sample size. Also, the results of this study may not be applicable to other types of patients, such as severe OSA or morbid obesity. The

NTIs in our study were done by experienced attending anesthesiologists. Hence, there may generalize bias in experience.

To avoid missing any hemodynamic response, invasive blood pressure was used in current study. In addition, the maximum fluctuation of MAP was chosen to reflect the hemodynamic change. This could partially explain why our data were different from previous study [17]. During NTI, stimulations of the nasopharyngeal structures, oropharyngeal structures and trachea induced by laryngoscopy or ETT advancement are three main stages of hemodynamic changes [29]. To optimizing glottis exposure in difficult laryngoscopy patients, enhanced upward lifting force of Macintosh blade was required [30]. The laryngeal prominence was excessively compressed and the oropharynx structure was therefore distorted. In such circumstance, assist maneuvers were often used to help the ETT through the glottis in the Macintosh group. However, the VLs allow to view glottis from the monitor, intubate tube using less maneuvers and potentially less force which minimized stimuli applied to the oropharyngeal structures during intubation [31]. Our data strongly demonstrated that the non-channeled King Vision and McGrath MAC VLs might provide clinical advantages in attenuating the hemodynamic changes to potential difficult NTI patients.

Most participants felt McGrath blade insertions were easiest. That was because of its slim design as we discussed before. McGrath MAC was lightest and more portable than the others. The monitor could be adjusted to an optimized angle for intubation. Although it was claimed that the King Vision VL could provide a better vision condition, we did not see the difference. Quality of view on display did not differ between King Vision and McGrath VLs. Reducing the usage of assist maneuvers, fewer demanding of the physical workload and lower anterior pressure exerted on the soft structures could be linked to reduced sore throat and hoarseness occurrences in both VL groups. The King Vision group had the fewest cases of sore throat. We guessed the length and angle of the King Vision non-channeled blade might be more beneficial to exposure of glottis compared with Macintosh like blade, and accordingly less workload was required. However, oral surgical procedures might confound these results since they tend to cause similar symptoms, and further study is required.

Some limitations of our study should be considered carefully. First, neither the intubator nor the independent observer could be blinded from the groups. However, we have minimized adverse effects by defining robust outcome measures. Second, if we compared both Cormark-Lehane and POGO scores, our results should be more convincing. Third, our results might be biased by the variable experience of the intubator with different

laryngoscope. It is believed that intubation with VL require a complex hand-eye-coordination competencies which grow with a learning curve [32]. On the other hand, it was suggested that novices could translate direct laryngoscopy technique to video laryngoscopy if it is similar to classic Macintosh laryngoscope [33]. Therefore, the results might not necessarily be obtained by novice users. Finally, the participants included did not represent genuine difficult airways. We believe it ethically questionable to test a new intubation device on genuine difficult airway patients. Therefore, further studies may be carried out to clarify these issues.

Conclusion

In summary, we observed that NTIs with non-channeled King Vision and McGrath VLs in the setting of predicted difficult intubations resulted in shorter intubation time, higher first success rate, better qualities of glottis view, attenuated hemodynamic responses, and fewer incidences of side effect compared with Macintosh DL. These data provided evidence that NTI using King Vision and McGrath were comparable, and both devices were superior to Macintosh DL in managing the difficult intubations.

Abbreviations

ASA: America Society of Anesthesiologists; BMI: Body Mass Index; DL: Direct laryngoscope;; EGRI: El-Ganzouri risk index; HR: Heart rate; MAP: Mean arterial pressure; NTI: Nasotracheal intubation; VL: Video larynogoscope

Acknowledgements

We would like to thank all the participants in this study for their willing cooperation.

Authors' contributions

YS and HJ contributed to the study design, study coordination, and writing of the manuscript. HZ, LS, JL and CZ contributed to the data collection. HZ and YS contributed to the data analysis. All authors approved the final version of the manuscript.

References

1. Lewis SR, Butler AR, Parker J, et al. Videolaryngoscopy versus direct laryngoscopy for adult patients requiring tracheal intubation. Cochrane Database Syst Rev. 2016;11:CD011136.
2. Kleine-Brueggeney M, Greif R, Schoettker P, et al. Evaluation of six videolaryngoscopes in 720 patients with a simulated difficult airway: a multicentre randomized controlled trial. Br J Anaesth. 2016;116:670–9.
3. Aziz MF, Dillman D, Fu R, Brambrink AM. Comparative effectiveness of the C-MAC video laryngoscope versus direct laryngoscopy in the setting of the predicted difficult airway. Anesthesiology. 2012;116:629–36.
4. Malik MA, Subramaniam R, Maharaj CH, et al. Randomized controlled trial of the Pentax AWS, Glidescope, and Macintosh laryngoscopes in predicted difficult intubation. Br J Anaesth. 2009;103:761–8.
5. Pieters BMA, Maas EHA, Knape JTA, van Zundert AAJ. Videolaryngoscopy vs. direct laryngoscopy use by experienced anaesthetists in patients with known difficult airways: a systematic review and meta-analysis. Anaesthesia. 2017;72:1532–41.

6. Hall CE, Shutt LE. Nasotracheal intubation for head and neck surgery. Anaesthesia. 2003;58:249–56.

7. St Mont G, Biesler I, Pfortner R, et al. Easy and difficult nasal intubation--a randomised comparison of Macintosh vs Airtraq(R) laryngoscopes. Anaesthesia. 2012;67:132–8.

8. Staar S, Biesler I, Muller D, et al. Nasotracheal intubation with three indirect laryngoscopes assisted by standard or modified Magill forceps. Anaesthesia. 2013;68:467–71.

9. Kumar R, Gupta E, Kumar S, et al. Cuff inflation-supplemented laryngoscope-guided nasal intubation: a comparison of three endotracheal tubes. Anesth Analg. 2013;116:619–24.

10. Huitink JM, Bouwman RA. The myth of the difficult airway: airway management revisited. Anaesthesia. 2015;70:244–9.

11. Kwak HJ, Lee SY, Lee SY, et al. McGrath video laryngoscopy facilitates routine Nasotracheal intubation in patients undergoing Oral and maxillofacial surgery: a comparison with Macintosh laryngoscopy. J Oral Maxillofac Surg. 2016;74:256–61.

12. Sato Boku A, Sobue K, Kako E, et al. The usefulness of the McGrath MAC laryngoscope in comparison with Airwayscope and Macintosh laryngoscope during routine nasotracheal intubation: a randomaized controlled trial. BMC Anesthesiol. 2017;17:160.

13. Alvis BD, Hester D, Watson D, et al. Randomized controlled trial comparing the McGrath MAC video laryngoscope with the king vision video laryngoscope in adult patients. Minerva Anestesiol. 2016;82:30–5.

14. Kleine-Brueggeney M, Buttenberg M, Greif R, et al. Evaluation of three unchannelled videolaryngoscopes and the Macintosh laryngoscope in patients with a simulated difficult airway: a randomised, controlled trial. Anaesthesia. 2016;72:370–8.

15. Kriege M, Alflen C, Noppens RR. Using king vision video laryngoscope with a channeled blade prolongs time for tracheal intubation in different training levels, compared to non-channeled blade. PLoS One. 2017;12:e0183382.

16. Jiang J, Ma DX, Li B, et al. Videolaryngoscopy versus direct laryngoscopy for nasotracheal intubation: a systematic review and meta-analysis of randomised controlled trials. J Clin Anesth. 2019;52:6–16.

17. Hazarika H, Saxena A, Meshram P, Kumar Bhargava A. A randomized controlled trial comparing C mac D blade and Macintosh laryngoscope for nasotracheal intubation in patients undergoing surgeries for head and neck cancer. Saudi J Anaesth. 2018;12:35–41.

18. el-Ganzouri AR, McCarthy RJ, Tuman KJ, et al. Preoperative airway assessment: predictive value of a multivariate risk index. Anesth Analg. 1996; 82:1197–204.

19. Seo KS, Kim JH, Yang SM, et al. A new technique to reduce epistaxis and enhance navigability during nasotracheal intubation. Anesth Analg. 2007; 105:1420–4.

20. Takahata O, Kubota M, Mamiya K, et al. The efficacy of the "BURP" maneuver during a difficult laryngoscopy. Anesth Analg. 1997;84:419–21.

21. Eichhorn L, Erdfelder F, Kessler F, et al. Influence of apnea-induced hypoxia on catecholamine release and cardiovascular dynamics. Int J Sports Med. 2017;38:85–91.

22. Jones PM, Armstrong KP, Armstrong PM, et al. A comparison of glidescope videolaryngoscopy to direct laryngoscopy for nasotracheal intubation. Anesth Analg. 2008;107:144–8.

23. Bamgbade OA, Onaolapo MH, Zuokumor PA. Nasotracheal intubation with the McGrath videolaryngoscope in patients with difficult airway. Eur J Anaesthesiol. 2011;28:673–4.

24. Taylor AM, Peck M, Launcelott S, et al. The McGrath(R) series 5 videolaryngoscope vs the Macintosh laryngoscope: a randomised, controlled trial in patients with a simulated difficult airway. Anaesthesia. 2013;68:142–7.

25. Jones PM, Turkstra TP, Armstrong KP, et al. Effect of stylet angulation and endotracheal tube camber on time to intubation with the GlideScope. Can J Anaesth. 2007;54:21–7.

26. Eberhart LH, Arndt C, Aust HJ, et al. A simplified risk score to predict difficult intubation: development and prospective evaluation in 3763 patients. Eur J Anaesthesiol. 2010;27:935–40.

27. Cortellazzi P, Minati L, Falcone C, et al. Predictive value of the El-Ganzouri multivariate risk index for difficult tracheal intubation: a comparison of Glidescope videolaryngoscopy and conventional Macintosh laryngoscopy. Br J Anaesth. 2007;99:906–11.

28. Sgalambro F, Sorbello M. Videolaryngoscopy and the search for the holy grail. Br J Anaesth. 2017;118:471–2.

29. Singh S, Smith JE. Cardiovascular changes after the three stages of nasotracheal intubation. Br J Anaesth. 2003;91:667–71.

30. Carassiti M, Zanzonico R, Cecchini S, et al. Force and pressure distribution using Macintosh and GlideScope laryngoscopes in normal and difficult airways: a manikin study. Br J Anaesth. 2012;108:146–51.

31. Gaszynski T, Jakubiak J. Muscle activity during endotracheal intubation using 4 laryngoscopes (Macintosh laryngoscope, Intubrite, TruView Evo2 and king vision) - a comparative study. Med Pr. 2016;67:155–62.

32. Cortellazzi P, Caldiroli D, Byrne A, et al. Defining and developing expertise in tracheal intubation using a GlideScope((R)) for anaesthetists with expertise in Macintosh direct laryngoscopy: an in-vivo longitudinal study. Anaesthesia. 2015;70:290–5.

33. Herbstreit F, Fassbender P, Haberl H, et al. Learning endotracheal intubation using a novel videolaryngoscope improves intubation skills of medical students. Anesth Analg. 2011;113:586–90.

24

A data review of airway management in patients with oral cavity or oropharyngeal cancer

Gang Zheng[1]* ⓘD, Lei Feng[2] and Carol M. Lewis[3]

Abstract

Background: Oral cavity and oropharyngeal cancer impose significant threat to airway management. Head and neck radiotherapy (HNRT) may further increase the difficulty of tracheal intubation. We hypothesized that a history of HNRT would be associated with a high rate of difficult tracheal intubation.

Methods: Adult patients with a history of HNRT were identified. Non-HNRT controls were case-matched by age, sex and body mass index. The tracheal intubation status between the two patient groups (treated vs. untreated with HNRT) was compared. The t test was used to evaluate differences in continuous variables between the 2 groups. Fisher's exact test or a chi-square test was used to test for associations between radiation status and patient characteristics that may be associated with difficult tracheal intubation. Odds ratio and its confidence interval were used to assess the effect of radiation status on intubation status.

Results: The final cohort of 472 matched patients in age, sex and body mass index consisted of 236 patients who had HNRT before surgery and 236 who had upfront surgery without HNRT. The percentage of patients who had restricted neck range of motion in the HNRT group was significantly higher than in the control group (22.3% vs. 11.0%; $p = 0.001$). The proportion of patients with trismus ($p = 0.11$) or difficult tracheal intubation ($p = 0.73$) did not differ significantly between the 2 groups. 12.7% patients in the study had difficult tracheal intubation. Patients who had mallampati scores of 3 or 4 had significantly higher rate of difficult tracheal intubation than did patients with mallampati scores of 1 or 2 (17.8% vs. 8.7%; $p = 0.004$). Multivariate logistic regression model showed no difference between HNRT and intubation status after adjusting neck range of motion and mallampati score (OR = 0.91, 95% CI: 0.510 to1.612).

Conclusions: Previous treatment with HNRT was not associated with additional risk of difficult tracheal intubation. Mallampati score may be a sensitive measurement for difficult tracheal intubation in this patient population.

Keywords: Radiotherapy, Cancer, Trismus, Upper aerodigestive track, Airway

Background

In the United States, an estimated 41,000 oral cavity and oropharyngeal malignancies are diagnosed each year [1]. The anatomic sites of oral cavity cancer (OCC) cover the lips, anterior two-thirds of tongue, gingiva, retromolar trigone, buccal mucosa, hard palate and the floor of mouth; whereas, the sites of oropharyngeal cancer (OPC) are located in the posterior one-third of the tongue, palatine or lingual tonsils, soft palate, and posterior pharyngeal wall [2].

With the technologic improvement, radiotherapy, depending the subsite of a disease, has become a primary treatment for many head and neck malignancies in order to maximally maintain functionality of the upper aerodigestive track. Approximately 75% of patients with head and neck squamous cell carcinoma can benefit from head and neck radiation therapy (HNRT) [3, 4]. Although previous receipt of HNRT is a recognized risk factor for difficult airway management, the mechanisms of HNRT- related airway pathologic changes and the

* Correspondence: gzheng@mdanderson.org
[1]Department of Anesthesiology and Perioperative Medicine, The University of Texas MD Anderson Cancer Center, 1515 Holcombe Boulevard, Faculty Center – Unit 409, Houston, TX 77030, USA

overall influences of previous HNRT on the outcomes of tracheal intubation remain unclear.

In this retrospective study, we reviewed the performance and outcomes of tracheal intubation in patients who were undergoing surgery to resect primary OCC or OPC of any stage. The primary goal of the study was to determine if previous HNRT adds additional risk to the airway management in the patients with OCC and OPC disregarding the technique applied. In addition, the factors potentially associated with difficult tracheal intubation (DTI) were also analyzed.

Methods
Patient selection
The Institutional Review Board (IRB) at The University of Texas MD Anderson Cancer Center approved this study (IRB No. PA12–0699). The informed consent was waived by IRB because this is a retrospective study. A cancer registry including records of 4011 adult (age ≥ 18 y at the time of surgery) patients with primary diagnoses of OCC or OPC who subsequently underwent resection of the primary OCC or OPC tumor at MD Anderson from 2007 to 2012 was used as the primary study database. Patients who underwent tonsillectomy for positive cervical lymphadenopathy with unclear primary disease, whose cases had been used for teaching of flexible endoscopy for tracheal intubation and patients who were < 18 years of age at the time of HNRT were excluded from this study. In addition, because the majority of the patients in the registry received intensity modulated radiation therapy, those who underwent brachytherapy or proton therapy were excluded in order to ensure the uniformity of the sample.

All the patients in the registry who qualified for the study were assigned into 1 of 2 groups according to whether they had received HNRT: the HNRT group, which consisted of patients who received HNRT before tumor resection, and the non-HNRT group, who underwent upfront resection without having received HNRT. Because some of the data for this study were embedded in the notes describing tracheal intubation in patients' medical records, requiring a manual search, we used a matching strategy to avoid having to hand-search the entire registry. We first identified the HNRT group as described above; then, we used the exact matching method to select matched controls from the non-HNRT group. The control patients were selected according to age, sex, and body mass index (BMI) to match the patients in the HNRT group at a ratio of 1:1. The matching range for age was ±5 y. For BMI, the 2 groups were matched at 6 levels: ≤ 18.5 kg/m^2, 18.6–25.0 kg/m^2, 25.1–30.0 kg/m^2, 30.1–35.0 kg/m^2, 35.1–40.0 kg/m^2 and ≥ 40.1 kg/m^2. Each patient in the HNRT group was successfully matched with a non-HNRT control patient.

Data collection
The following data were electronically retrieved from the patients' medical records: age, sex, BMI, American Society of Anesthesiologists physical status score (ASA score), airway assessment (mouth opening, neck range of motion, edentulous and MP scores), cancer diagnosis, type of surgery, and whether the patient had a history of HNRT. Data on radiotherapy and on the method of tracheal intubation were manually retrieved from the records after matching. The missing data in the primary data sets were manually searched for and placed in the corresponding data set. When a patient had multiple surgeries after HNRT, the data for the first surgery with tracheal intubation after HNRT were used. For airway assessment, most anesthesia providers in our practice considered patients to have trismus if their inter-incisional distance was < 2 finger breadths (typically < 3.5 cm). However, no standardized criteria were used to measure neck extension, so the neck range of motion was based on providers' subjective judgment. In this study, edentulous referred to a patient with complete upper, lower, or whole-mouth removable dentures. We included the grade of laryngeal view during tracheal intubation in the analysis to reflect the intubation effort according to the Cormack-Lehane system [5]. The grade of laryngeal view mainly applied to the patients who had been intubated via either direct laryngoscopy or video laryngoscopy of any type. For flexible endoscopy trachea intubation, grade I was used for data analysis.

Statistical analysis
Summary statistics, including mean, standard deviation, median, and range, were calculated for continuous variables, such as age, BMI, and the interval between radiotherapy and surgery. Frequencies and percentages were used to summarize data for categorical variables, such as sex, BMI, Mallampati (MP) score, mouth opening, neck range of motion, cancer stage, radiation status, and airway intubation status. The t test was used to evaluate differences in continuous variables between the 2 patient groups. Fisher's exact test or a chi-square test was used to test for associations between radiation status (HNRT or control) and patient characteristics that may be associated with difficulty of tracheal intubation, including sex, BMI, MP score, mouth opening, neck range of motion, cancer stage, intubation difficulty status (difficult or easy) and patient characteristics. Odds ratio and its confidence interval were used to assess the effect of radiation status on intubation difficulty status. A P value of less than 0.05 was considered statistically significant.

The statistical software SAS 9.3 (SAS, Cary, NC) was used for all the analyses.

Results
Patient characteristics
Of the 4011 records of eligible patients included in the cancer registry database, 3999 records were eligible for inclusion in this study; 8 patients whose procedures had been used for teaching airway management and 4 patients who had received proton therapy were excluded. The final study cohort of 472 matched patients consisted of 236 patients who had HNRT before surgery and 236 who had upfront surgery without HNRT. The mean (± standard deviation) age of the included patients was 58.7 (± 9.1) years, and their mean BMI was 25.5 (± 4.5) kg/m². The mean interval between completion of HNRT and surgery in the HNRT group was 330.3 (± 474.5) days. Eight primary cancer locations were found in 447 patients. The characteristics of the study cohort are detailed in Table 1.

Data on intubation difficulty status (easy or difficult) were available for 456 of the 472 patients. Among them, 12.7% ($n = 58$) were described as having had DTI with the corresponding intubation technique used for each case. Intubation with the primary technique failed in 8 patients, whose airways were then managed using either the AirTraq technique ($n = 4$) or asleep intubation with flexible endoscopy ($n = 4$). The airways of 189 (40.0%) patients had been intubated with advanced techniques; the corresponding notes described 6 reasons for use of advanced techniques instead of direct laryngoscopy, including poor mandibular mobility (adequate mouth opening during assessment, but difficulty achieving full mouth opening after anesthetic induction; $n = 37$; 19.6%), cancer growth in the hypopharynx ($n = 35$; 18.5%), trismus (restricted mouth opening at assessment prior to anesthetic induction, $n = 31$; 16.4%), distorted airway anatomy from previous surgery ($n = 14$; 7.4%), short thyromental distance ($n = 10$; 5.3%), and a large tongue ($n = 10$; 5.3%). These 6 reasons accounted for 72.5% of the airways managed by advanced techniques; the reasons for use of advanced airway management techniques in the remaining 52 patients were not specified. Six patients who had initially been scheduled for cancer resection under general anesthesia were found to require tracheostomy before anesthetic induction owing to rapid cancer progression; therefore, airway intubation was not attempted in these patients. No cases of airway loss (cannot intubate and cannot ventilate) were found in the study population.

Radiation status and airway management characteristics
The mean (± standard deviation) age and BMI in the HNRT group were 58.3 (± 9.2) y and 25.5 (± 4.4) kg/

m², respectively. In the control group, the mean age and BMI were 59.1 (± 9.0) y and 25.5 (± 4.5) kg/m². The differences in age ($p = 0.37$) and BMI ($p = 0.83$) between the 2 patient groups were not statistically significant. Table 2 shows associations between radiation status and other covariates. The percentage of patients who had restricted neck range of motion in the HNRT group was significantly higher than in the control group (22.3% vs. 11.0%; $p = 0.001$). In addition, significantly more patients in the HNRT group had advanced-stage cancer than in the control group (51.2% vs. 40.8%; $p = 0.029$). However, the proportion of patients with trismus ($p = 0.11$) and with DAI ($p = 0.73$) did not differ significantly between the 2 groups. Finally, no significant differences were found between the 2 groups in the grade of laryngeal view during tracheal intubation.

The mean (± standard deviation) time interval between completion of HNRT and surgery was 330 ± 475 days and median interval was 134 days. The time interval from HNRT to surgery was not associated with the difficult tracheal intubation ($p = 0.9363$).

Ease of intubation and patient characteristics
Table 3 displays associations between intubation status and patient characteristics. Data on the intubation status were found for 456 of 472 patients; of these 456 patients, 58 (12.7%) had DTI. The mean (± standard deviation) age of patients who had DTI was 58.2 (± 8.8) y, and the mean age of patients who did not have DTI was 58.8 (± 9.2) y. The mean BMI of patients with DTI was 24.7 (± 4.3) kg/m², and the mean BMI of patients without DTI was 25.6 (± 4.5) kg/m². The 2 groups did not differ significantly in age ($p = 0.61$) or in BMI ($p = 0.13$). Patients who had MP scores of 3 or 4 had significantly higher rates of DTI than did patients with MP scores of 1 or 2 (17.8% vs. 8.7%; $p = 0.004$).

A multivariate logistic regression model was fitted to assess associations between radiation and intubation status after adjustment for neck range of motion and MP score. This analysis revealed no statistically significant association between receiving HNRT and having DTI (Table 4).

Discussion
The finding in this study did not reveal the correlation between previous HNRT and DTI in patients with OCC or OPC in spite of significant association between HNRT and restriction of neck range of motion. This can be explained by broadly using flexible endoscopy (35.5%) for tracheal intubation in the studied population, which effectively overcame the influences of restriction of neck range of motion to the performance of tracheal intubation. Nevertheless, our

Table 1 Characteristics of 472 patients with oral cavity or oropharyngeal cancer

Characteristic	No. of patients	%
Head/neck radiation		
No	236	50.0
Yes	236	50.0
Sex		
Female	60	12.71
Male	412	87.29
Body mass index (kg/m^2)		
≤ 18.5	17	3.6
18.6–25.0	228	48.3
25.1–30.0	157	33.26
30.1–35.0	51	10.81
35.1–40.0	16	3.39
≥ 40.1	3	0.64
Mallampati score		
Data missing [a]	16	
1	63	13.82
2	205	44.96
3	130	28.51
4	58	12.72
Mouth opening		
Data missing	3	
Full	367	78.25
Limited	102	21.75
Thyromental distance (≈ cm)		
Data missing	391	
< 5	20	24.69
≥ 5	61	75.31
Edentulous Removable denture		
Data missing	1	
Yes	101	21.44
No	370	78.56
Neck movement		
Data missing	3	
Full range of motion	391	83.37
Restricted	78	16.63
Cancer location		
Tongue	218	46.19
Tonsil	98	20.76
Floor of mouth	49	10.38
Mandible	26	5.51
Retromolar region	24	5.08
Buccal mucosa	22	4.66
Maxilla gingiva	5	1.06

Table 1 Characteristics of 472 patients with oral cavity or oropharyngeal cancer *(Continued)*

Characteristic	No. of patients	%
Soft palate	5	1.06
Multiple locations	25	5.30
Cancer stage		
Data missing	3	
T1	84	17.91
T2	155	33.05
T3	92	19.62
VT4	110	23.45
TX	24	5.12
Not staged	4	0.85
Intubation status		
Data missing	16	
Difficult	58	12.72
Easy	398	87.28
Primary intubation technique		
Data missing	10	
Direct laryngoscopy	267	57.79
Asleep FOI	137	29.65
Awake FOI	27	5.84
AirTraq video laryngoscopy	15	3.25
C-MAC video laryngoscopy	7	1.52
LMA intubation	3	0.65
Tracheostomy	6	1.30
Secondary intubation technique		
AirTraq video laryngoscopy	4	50
Asleep FOI	4	50

Abbreviations: *FOI* fiber-optic intubation, *LMA* laryngeal mask airway
[a]Data missing = no data found in the database or the corresponding patient records. Where data are missing, percentages are calculated using the total number of available records

finding does not necessarily mean that the influence of HNRT on tracheal intubation should be underestimated. In this study, 22.3% of patients treated with HNRT had restricted neck movement, whereas only 11.0% of patients in the non-HNRT group did. In addition, although the difference was not statistically significant, more patients in the HNRT group (24.8%) than in the non-HNRT group (18.7%) had trismus. Both restricted neck range of motion and trismus are significant risk factors for difficult direct laryngoscopy. Furthermore, in our clinical experience, trismus and restricted neck range of motion often coexist in patients who develop tissue fibrosis after radiotherapy, posing a significant challenge for both direct

Table 2 Comparison of patient characteristics by head and neck radiation status

Characteristic	Control N (%)	HNRT N (%)	P value
Sex			1.0
Female	30 (12.7)	30 (12.7)	
Male	206 (87.3)	206 (87.3)	
Body mass index (kg/m²)			1.0
≤ 18.5	8 (3.4)	9 (3.8)	
18.6—25.0	113 (47.9)	115 (48.7)	
25.1—30.0	79 (33.5)	78 (33.1)	
30.1—35.0	26 (11.0)	25 (10.6)	
35.1—40.0	8 (3.4)	8 (3.4)	
≥ 40.1	2 (0.8)	1 (0.4)	
Mallampati score			0.048
1	42 (18.3)	21 (9.3)	
2	96 (41.7)	109 (48.2)	
3	63 (27.4)	67 (29.6)	
4	29 (12.6)	29 (12.8)	
Mallampati score (1/2 vs. 3/4)			0.59
1/2	138 (60.0)	130 (57.5)	
3/4	92 (40.0)	96 (42.5)	
Mouth opening			0.11
Full	191 (81.3)	176 (75.2)	
Limited	44 (18.7)	58 (24.8)	
Edentulous			0.59
Yes	53 (22.5)	48 (20.4)	
No	183 (77.5)	187 (79.6)	
Neck movement			0.001
Full range	210 (89.0)	181 (77.7)	
Restricted	26 (11.0)	52 (22.3)	
Cancer stage			< 0.0001
T1	28 (13.1)	56 (24.6)	
T2	76 (35.7)	79 (34.6)	
T3	34 (16.0)	58 (25.4)	
T4	75 (35.2)	35 (15.4)	
Intubation status			0.73
Difficult	31 (13.2)	27 (12.2)	
Easy	203 (86.8)	195 (87.8)	
Laryngeal view			0.26
1	80 (58.8)	70 (49.6)	
2	41 (30.1)	58 (41.1)	
3	10 (7.4)	10 (7.1)	
4	5 (3.7)	3 (2.1)	
Laryngeal view (1/2 vs. 3/4)			0.62
1/2	121 (89.0)	128 (90.8)	
3/4	15 (11.0)	13 (9.2)	

Abbreviation: *HNRT* head and neck radiation therapy
Column percentages are provided

laryngoscopy and video laryngoscopy. Because the components of radiation fibrosis syndrome result from the combination of tonic contraction and fibrosis of the muscles of mastication [6], trismus and limited neck range of motion caused by radiation cannot be improved with anesthetic induction or use of a muscle relaxant. This is unlike the trismus induced by cancer pain or inflammation commonly seen in patients who have not undergone radiotherapy, which can often be improved with anesthestics and muscle relaxants. Furthermore, restricted neck range of motion is unlikely to exist in patients without tissue fibrosis unless it is caused by neck-related comorbidities, such as having undergone a neck fusion procedure. No good estimates of the morbidity rate attributable to restriction of neck range of motion after radiotherapy are available, but radiation-induced trismus occurs in up to 45% of patients who receive curative doses of radiation to the head and neck [7]. Thus, having a back-up plan is important when dealing with airways in patients who have undergone HNRT, so that appropriate tools will be available to manage DTI if it arises.

Another significant finding in this study was that MP scores of 3 or 4 were associated with DTI regardless of the technique used. This result is different from a previous report indicating that MP score alone is not significantly correlated with DTI in patients with otherwise normal airway [8]. The discrepancy can likely be attributed to the study populations. The MP scores in our patients reflected the additive effects of oncopathology, radiation therapy and baseline condition. A previous study reported that up to 75% of patients developed edema in the head and neck after radiotherapy, and > 50% of patients had edema in the airway [9]. However, the existing grading systems for assessment of airway edema are unreliable and lack consistency [10, 11]. Thus, anesthesiologists who manage such patients' airways are unlikely to find clinical reports useful in planning airway management. Patterson et al. [11] developed an airway edema rating scale system by measuring intrarater consistency and interrater agreement on the level of airway edema at several anatomic sites. They found that the aryepiglottic folds and arytenoids were the regions most amenable to visual check (Fiber-laryngoscopy) and that intrarater consistency and interrater agreement were low for the base of the tongue. Because radiotherapy-induced airway edema is mostly diffused throughout the area of treatment, the level of edema found in laryngeal or supraglottic areas may reflect edema in the base of the tongue, pharyngeal well, and floor of the mouth. We speculate that moderate edema in any hypopharyngeal or laryngeal site

Table 3 Comparison of patient characteristics by intubation status

Characteristic	DTI N (%)	Non-DTI N (%)	P value
Sex			0.42
Female	9 (16.1)	47 (83.9)	
Male	49 (12.3)	351 (87.8)	
Body mass index (kg/m^2)			0.23
≤ 18.5	3 (17.6)	14 (82.4)	
18.6–25.0	32 (14.7)	185 (85.3)	
25.1–30.0	19 (12.3)	136 (87.7)	
30.1–35.0	2 (4.1)	47 (95.9)	
35.1–40.0	1 (6.7)	14 (93.3)	
≥ 40.1	1 (33.3)	2 (66.7)	
HNRT			0.73
No	31 (13.2)	203 (86.8)	
Yes	27 (12.2)	195 (87.8)	
Mallampati score			0.032
1	4 (6.5)	58 (93.5)	
2	19 (9.5)	182 (90.5)	
3	22 (17.1)	107 (82.9)	
4	11 (19.6)	45 (80.4)	
Mallampati score (1/2 vs. 3/4)			0.004
1/2	23 (8.7)	240 (91.3)	
3/4	33 (17.8)	152 (82.2)	
Mouth opening			0.53
Full	44 (12.3)	314 (87.7)	
Limited	14 (14.7)	81 (85.3)	
Edentulous			0.42
Yes	10 (10.3)	87 (89.7)	
No	48 (13.4)	310 (86.6)	
Neck movement			0.066
Full range	44 (11.5)	337 (88.5)	
Restricted	14 (19.4)	58 (80.6)	
Cancer stage			0.58
T1	8 (9.6)	75 (90.4)	
T2	23 (15.1)	129 (84.9)	
T3	10 (11.4)	78 (88.6)	
T4	11 (10.8)	91 (89.2)	

Abbreviations: *DTI* difficult tracheal intubation, *HNRT* head and neck radiation therapy
Row percentages are provided

combined with an MP score of 3 or 4 is highly suggestive of DTI. Therefore, a bedside flexible endoscopy airway assessment before anesthetic induction on a patient suspected of airway edema should be incorporated into the routine practice for the clinicians who manage high-risk airways.

It is worth mentioning that the intubation technique used in any given case is based not only on clinical indications but also on the personal preference and skill level of the provider. Therefore, the techniques used in the study might not always directly reflect clinical indications. Furthermore, the outcomes of intubation of difficult airways in patients with OCC or OPC are highly experience-dependent. The techniques and equipment used for intubation are also influenced by local culture or practice; similar cases may be managed differently in different institutions [12, 13]. In this study, the intubations were all performed or supervised by a group of head and neck anesthesiologists who routinely use the techniques described; thus, the results of this study might not be widely applicable to institutions with different practices.

In addition, although the history of HNRT is important to airway management, the anatomic site of the tumor may also affect the airway management. However, the majority of patients (75%) in this study had tumors with local or regional invasion beyond the primary anatomic sites so that grouping the patients by discrete anatomic margins was not feasible. In addition, these cancers induce tissue reaction or inflammation that often extends the mass effect to a much larger area than the tumor itself. Therefore, the causal relationship between primary cancer site and the airway management was not studied.

Conclusions

In conclusion, history of HNRT does not increase the overall incidences of DTI in patients with OCC or OPC. Mallampati airway assessment may be used as a sensitive tool to predict difficult tracheal intubation in these patients.

Table 4 Multivariate logistic regression model showing associations between HNRT and intubation status (DAI vs. non-DAI) adjusted for neck range of motion and Mallampati score

Effect	P value	Odds ratio estimate	95% CI[a]	
Treatment (HNRT vs. Control)	0.74	0.907	0.510	1.612
Neck motion (restricted vs. full range)	0.21	1.563	0.773	3.160
Mallampati score (1/2 vs. 3/4)	0.016	0.483	0.268	0.873

Abbreviations: *HNRT* head and neck radiation therapy, *CI* confidence interval
[a]Wald confidence interval

Abbreviations
ASA score: American Society of Anesthesiologists physical status score;
BMI: Body mass index; DTI: Difficult tracheal intubation; HNRT: Head and neck
radiation therapy; MP score: Mallampati score; OCC: Oral cavity cancer;
OPC: Oropharyngeal cancer

Acknowledgement
The authors in this article thank A Ninetto, Department of Scientific
Publications at MD Anderson Cancer Center for manuscript editing.

Authors' contributions
G Zheng helped study design, data analysis, manuscript writing and
revisions. L Feng helped study design, data analysis and manuscript writing.
CM Lewis helped study design, data preparation, manuscript editing and
revisions. All authors have read and approved the final manuscript, and
ensure that this is the case.

Author details
[1]Department of Anesthesiology and Perioperative Medicine, The University
of Texas MD Anderson Cancer Center, 1515 Holcombe Boulevard, Faculty
Center – Unit 409, Houston, TX 77030, USA. [2]Department of Biostatistics, The
University of Texas MD Anderson Cancer Center, FCT4.5047, T. Boone Pickens
Academic Tower, 1400 Pressler St, Houston, TX 77030-4008, USA.
[3]Department of Head and Neck Surgery, The University of Texas MD
Anderson Cancer Center, Unit 1445, T. Boone Pickens Academic Tower, 1515
Holcombe Blvd, Houston, TX 77030-4009, USA.

References
1. Weatherspoon DJ, Chattopadhyay A, Boroumand S, Garcia AI. Oral cavity
    and oropharyngeal cancer incidence trends and disparities in the United
    States: 2000-10. Cancer Epidemiol. 2015;39:497–504.
2. Cleveland JL, Junger ML, Saraiya M, Markowitz LE, Dunne EF, Epstein JB. The
    connection between human papillomavirus and oropharyngeal squamous
    cell carcinomas in the United States: implications for dentistry. J Am Dent
    Assoc. 2011;142:915–24.
3. Barton MB, Jacob S, Shafiq J, Wong K, et al. Estimating the demand for
    radiotherapy from the evidence: a review of changes from 2003 to 2012.
    Radiother Oncol. 2014;112:140–4.
4. Overgaard J. Improving radiotherapy of squamous cell carcinoma of the
    head and neck (HNSCC) through a continuous process of biological based
    clinical trials: a 30 year experience from the Danish head and neck group
    [AHNS/IFHNOS abstract S397]. JAMA Otolaryngol Head Neck Surg. 2014;
    140(suppl):S397.
5. Cormack RS, Lehane J. Difficult tracheal intubation in obstetrics. Anaesthesia.
    1984;39:1105–11.
6. Wang CJ, Huang EY, Hsu HC, Chen HC, Fang FM, Hsiung CY. The degree
    and time-course assessment of radiation-induced trismus occurring after
    radiotherapy for nasopharyngeal cancer. Laryngoscope. 2005;115:1458–60.
7. Rudat V, Dietz A, Nollert J, et al. Acute and late toxicity, tumor control and
    intrinsic radiosensitivity of primary fibroblasts in vitro of patients with
    advanced head and neck cancer after concomitant boost radiotherapy.
    Radiother Oncol. 1999;53:233–45.
8. Shiga T, Wajima Z, Onoue T, Sakamoto A. Predicting difficult intubation in
    apparently normal patients. Anesthesiology. 2005;103:429–37.
9. Deng J, Ridner SH, Dietrich MS, et al. Prevalence of secondary lymphedema
    in patients with head and neck cancer. J Pain Symptom Manag. 2012;43:44–
    252.
10. Branski RC, Bhattacharyya N, Shapiro J. The reliability of the assessment of
    endoscopic laryngeal findings associated with laryngopharyngeal reflux
    disease. Laryngoscope. 2002;112:1019–24.
11. Patterson JM, Hildreth A, Wilson JA. Measuring edema in irradiated head
    and neck cancer patients. Ann Otol Rhinol Laryngol. 2007;116:59–564.
12. Mishra S, Bhatnagar S, Jha RR, Sknghal AK. Airway management of patients
    undergoing oral cancer surgery: a retrospective study. Eur J Anaesthesiol.
    2005;22:510–4.
13. Nikhar SA, Sharma A, Ramdaspally M, Gopinath R. Airway management of
    patients undergoing oral cancer surgery: a retrospective analysis of 156
    patients. Turk J Anaesthesiol Reanim. 2017;45:108–11.

25

A comparison of blind intubation with the intubating laryngeal mask FASTRACH™ and the intubating laryngeal mask Ambu Aura-i™

R. Schiewe[1*] , M. Stoeck[1], M. Gruenewald[2], J. Hoecker[2] and B. Bein[1]

Abstract

Background: The intubating laryngeal mask Fastrach™ is considered a gold standard for blind intubation as well as for fibreoptic guided intubation via a laryngeal mask. Recently, a single use version of the mask has been introduced. We compared the Fastrach single use with the new, low-priced single use intubating laryngeal mask Ambu Aura-i™. We hypothesised that the LMA Ambu Aura-i and the LMA Fastrach are comparable with respect to success rates for mask placement and blind tracheal intubation through the LMA device.

Methods: A prospective, randomised clinical trial. University Hospital Schleswig-Holstein, Campus Kiel, from April 2011 to April 2012.

Eighty patients undergoing general anaesthesia with planned tracheal intubation were randomised and enrolled in the study. Blind intubation was performed with either laryngeal mask using two different tracheal tubes (Rüsch Super Safety Silk™ and LMA ETT™). A crossover-design was performed after an unsuccessful procedure.

Primary outcome measure was the overall success rate of blind intubation. Secondary outcome measures were the time to the first adequate ventilation, a subjective handling score, and a fibreoptic control of placement, as well as the success rate of mask placement, time for mask removal after successful intubation, differences in airway leak pressure, and the incidence of postoperative sore throat and hoarseness.

Results: The success rate of tracheal intubation with the Fastrach for the first and second attempt was significantly better compared with the Ambu Aura-i. Tracheal intubation was also significantly faster (14.1 s. ±4.4 versus 21.3 s. ±9.0; $p < 0.01$), and the time interval for mask removal after successful intubation was significantly shorter using the Fastrach device (24.0 s. ±8.2 versus 29.4 s. ±7.5; $p < 0.001$). There were no significant differences between groups regarding the incidence of postoperative sore throat and hoarseness.

Conclusion: Both laryngeal mask devices are suitable for ventilation and oxygenation. Blind intubation remains the domain of the LMA Fastrach, the Ambu Aura-i is not suitable for blind intubation.

Keywords: Laryngeal mask airway, Laryngeal mask guided tracheal intubation, Airway management, Fiberoptic intubation

* Correspondence: r.schiewe@asklepios.com
[1]Department of Anaesthesiology and Intensive Care Medicine, Asklepios Hospital St. Georg, Lohmuehlenstr. 5, D-20099 Hamburg, Germany

Background

After development of laryngeal masks (LMA) in the 1980s, there have been anecdotical reports on their use in difficult airway management and during "cannot intubate, cannot ventilate" situations. In 1997, the intubating laryngeal mask Fastrach™ was introduced [1]. LMA Fastrach™ was developed for placing tracheal tubes without fibreoptic assistance [2]. With reported rates for successful intubation of 75% on the first attempt, and 99,7% with fibreoptic assistance [3, 4], LMA Fastrach became the reference for LMA assisted tracheal intubation. Following the increasing demand for single use equipment due to cleaning and sterilisation issues, a single use Fastrach was developed and introduced into the market. However, high costs hamper a more widespread use in clinical routine. Recently, similar and lower-priced intubating LMAs have been developed, such as the LMA Ambu Aura-i™. With this study, we investigated the feasibility of blind intubation using the LMA Ambu Aura-i and compared it with the LMA Fastrach as contemporary reference.

We hypothesised that the LMA Ambu Aura-i and the LMA Fastrach are comparable with respect to success rates for mask placement and tracheal intubation. Also, we supposed that tracheal intubation would be more successful in both laryngeal masks using the endotracheal tube (ETT) specifically designed for use with the Fastrach.

Methods

After local ethics committee approval (Ethics committee of the Christian-Albrechts-University at Kiel, Chair: Prof. Dr. H.M. Mehdorn, study Ref. No. AZ 107/02, 26.04.2011) and written, informed consent, 80 patients undergoing general anaesthesia with planned tracheal intubation for elective surgical procedures were enrolled in the study, starting on 26.04.2011. Patients were randomised to the Ambu Aura-i group (n = 40), and the LMA Fastrach group (n = 40), respectively, using a sealed envelope which had been prepared after a randomisation procedure using the website Randomization.com (http://www.randomization.com). Further, each group was divided in two subgroups to investigate the influence of different tracheal tubes on the success of LMA assisted tracheal intubation. Either a Rüsch Super Safety Silk™ (ID 7,5 mm, Rüsch, Kernen, Germany) representing a standard PVC tracheal tube, or a LMA ETT™ (ID 7,5 mm, LMA, Bonn, Germany) as a tube specifically developed for the LMA Fastrach, were used. After intubation failure, a crossover-design was performed, using the other LMA or the other tracheal tube.

Primary endpoint was the overall success rate of blind intubation with either mask after maximum of two attempts. Secondary endpoints were the influence of the tracheal tubes, equivalence of the masks regarding fibreoptic visualisation, a subjective handling score, differences in airway leak pressure, and the incidence of postoperative sore throat and hoarseness.

Inclusion criteria were the presence of all of the following: general anaesthesia with planned tracheal intubation, elective surgery, written, informed consent.

Exclusion criteria were the presence of at least one of the following: ASA physical status IV and V, severe pulmonary comorbidity (COPD GOLD >III, bronchial asthma), indication for rapid-sequence induction, mouth opening (interincisor distance) < 3 cm, and morbid obesity (BMI > 35 kg.m^{-2}).

The study investigators were three anaesthesiologists very well experienced in using different kinds of laryngeal mask devices, including both LMA devices compared in this study (BB, MS, JH).

All patients enrolled in the study were pre-medicated with midazolam 7.5 mg p.o. 30 min before the procedure with a sip of water. Routine monitoring included 5 lead ECG, SpO$_2$ and heart rate, as well as non-invasive blood pressure measurement. Depth of anaesthesia was monitored with bispectral index (BIS 2000 XP™, Aspect Medical Systems, Wallingford, USA), neuromuscular monitoring was performed by relaxometry (GE Healthcare, Helsinki, Finland). Clinical predictors of difficult airway, such as Mallampati score, mouth opening, and thyromental distance, were recorded.

Patient's head was placed in a neutral position. Pre-oxygenation with oxygen 100% via face mask for 3 min. Was followed by a standardised induction of anaesthesia using propofol 2 mg.kg^{-1} lean body weight and remifentanil 0.3 µg.kg^{-1}.min^{-1} lean body weight. Neuromuscular blockade was achieved with rocuronium 0.6 mg.kg^{-1} ideal body weight and anaesthesia was maintained by propofol bolus and remifentanil infusion at 0.2 µg.kg^{-1}.min^{-1}. After induction of anaesthesia, the study was started by placing the laryngeal mask (appropriate size #4 or #5, depending on patients' body weight) into the hypopharynx when an adequate depth of anaesthesia was recorded (BIS between 40 and 60). Cuffs were inflated according to the manufacturers' instructions (30/40 ml air), and time (T1) was recorded between picking up the laryngeal mask and the first successful ventilation. Successful ventilation was defined as positive capnometry combined with thorax excursions. When the first attempt at mask placing failed, a second attempt was allowed, and total time was then documented as T1. After a failure with the second attempt, a crossover-design with the alternate device was performed.

A subjective handling score was recorded, graded in "excellent", "good", "fair", and "poor". Laryngeal mask airway leak pressure (cm H$_2$O) was recorded by setting the APL valve to 40 cm H$_2$O, and fresh gas flow at 3 l/min. The presence of audible leakage as well as the absence of corresponding pressure increase on the monitor was documented as leakage. A stethoscope was used to distinguish between oral or gastric leakage.

Next, a fibreoptic evaluation of LMA placement was performed. With a fibrescope (Karl Storz, Tuttlingen, Germany), the position of the larynx relative to the laryngeal cuff and mask-aperture was visualised and categorised as "correct", "lateral deviation", "epiglottic downfolding" or "not assessable". Additionally, the view on the larynx comparable to Cormack/Lehane score was recorded. After relaxometry detected a TOF ratio of 0, the tracheal tube was placed through the respective LMA without any optical assistance. Time (T2) was stopped from picking up the tracheal tube until the first successful ventilation. If the first attempt was unsuccessful, an immediate second attempt with optimised LMA positioning and patient's head reclination was performed, and the total time (T2a) was recorded. If also the second attempt of tracheal tube placement was unsuccessful, a crossover-design with the alternate tracheal tube was performed identical to the attempt with the first tracheal tube, yielding time T2b. If the alternate tracheal tube could also not be placed correctly, the attending anaesthesiologist placed the tube with fibreoptic assisted (time T2c). The attempt was terminated and the attempt classified as "failure" if total time exceeded 300 s or SpO_2 decreased to < 91%.

After successful intubation, time was stopped for mask removal over the tracheal tube, either using the removal bar developed specifically for the LMA ETT™ or with a conventional Magill forceps for the Rüsch tube. Time (T3) was recorded from removal of the tube connector until successful ventilation. Finally, tracheal tube position was evaluated by bilateral auscultation using a stethoscope. Unilateral ventilation or accidental extubation upon LMA removal were also recorded.

On the day after surgery patients were interviewed by an investigator blinded to group assignment, and the incidence and extent (none/moderate/severe) of postoperative sore throat and hoarseness were recorded.

Statistical analyses were performed using Graph Pad version 6.00 for Windows (GraphPad Software, La Jolla California USA, www.graphpad.com). Sample size was calculated using Stat Mate version 2.00 for Windows (GraphPad Software, La Jolla California USA, www.graphpad.com). An estimated success rate for blind intubation of 60% in the Aura-i group versus 90% in the Fastrach group yielded a sample size of $n = 38$ for $\alpha = 0.05$ and $\beta = 0.20$. To compensate for dropouts, $n = 40$ subjects were enrolled in each group. Data were analysed regarding normal distribution by D'Agostino and Pearson Test (omnibus normality test). Normally distributed data were analysed by one-way-ANOVA, followed by Bonferroni correction for multiple comparisons if appropriate. Non-normal data were analysed by Kruskal-Wallis test. Proportions were compared with Fisher's exact test or the Chi-square test, as appropriate. Study data are presented as mean (SD) or median (IQR).

The study was retrospectively registered on Clinicaltrials. gov, Identification Number NCT03109678.

Results

Eighty patients were enrolled in the study, and all patients were analysed (Fig. 1). There were no significant differences between groups with regard to demographic data, ASA physical status (Table 1), or clinical predictors of difficult airway, such as Mallampati score, mouth opening, and thyromental distance (Table 2)

LMA placement on the first attempt was successful in 87.5% (Ambu Aura-i 82.5%, Fastrach 92.5%), and in all patients (100%) on the second attempt. Therefore, a second attempt was required in 17.5% of the Ambu Aura-i, and in 7.5% of the Fastrach group ($p > 0.05$). No patient had to be assigned to the alternate device.

There was a significant difference regarding the time to the first successful ventilation (T1) between both groups. The LMA Fastrach could be placed after 15.9 s (SD ± 7.0) on the first attempt, the LMA Ambu Aura-i after 18.8 s (SD ± 7.6) ($p = 0.017$). Mask size (#4 vs. #5) had no influence on time required for placement. There was no significant difference regarding the subjective handling score. Both masks were rated either "excellent" or "good" (Fig. 2).

Airway leak pressure was significantly lower ($p < 0.001$) in the Ambu Aura-i group (mean $19 cmH_2O$, SD ±6) compared to the LMA Fastrach group (mean $26 cmH_2O$, SD ±8), (Fig. 3).

Regarding the primary endpoint of the study, there was a significant difference between both LMA groups regarding successful blind intubation with the first tracheal tube:

Group Aura-i-Rüsch 9 (47%)/Fastrach-Rüsch 17 (81%), $p < 0.05$; group Aura-i-ETT 4 (81%)/Fastrach-Rüsch 17 (81%), $p < 0.01$; group Aura-i-Rüsch 9 (47%)/Fastrach-ETT 17 (90%), $p < 0.01$; group Aura-i-ETT 4 (19%)/Fastrach-ETT 17 (90%), $p < 0.01$; group Aura-i-Rüsch 9 (47%) + Aura-i-ETT 4 (19%)/Fastrach-Rüsch 17 (81%) + Fastrach-ETT 17 (90%), $p < 0.01$.

There was no significant difference on success of blind intubation with the first tracheal tube within either LMA-group (group Aura-i-Rüsch 9 (47%)/Aura-i-ETT 4 (19%), $p = 0.092$; Fastrach-Rüsch 17 (81%)/Fastrach-ETT 17 (90%), $p = 1.000$).

Tracheal tubes had no significant influence on success of blind intubation (group Aura-i-Rüsch + Fastrach-Rüsch/Aura-i-ETT + Fastrach-ETT, $p = 0.268$). Regarding the crossover attempts, Table 3 clarifies the poorer performance of the LMA Aura-i.

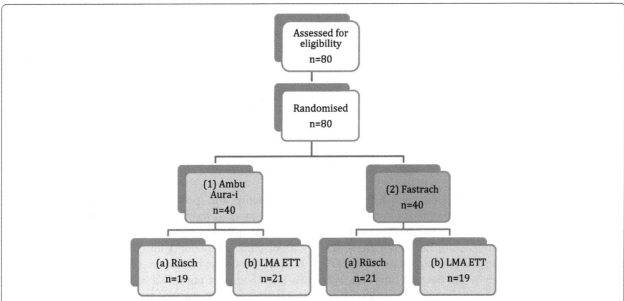

Fig. 1 *Flow chart study design.* 80 patients randomised; two laryngeal mask device groups (Ambu Aura-i™ and Fastrach™) with two subgroups each using two different tracheal tubes (Rüsch Super Safety Silk™ and LMA ETT™)

Fibreoptical tracheal tube placement was necessary more often in group 1 ($n = 23$) compared with group 2 ($n = 3$), $p = 0.0005$.

Using the Ambu Aura-i compared to LMA Fastrach leads to more cases of laryngeal lateralization (4/40 (10%) versus 1/40 (25%), $p = 0.17$), as well as significant more cases of epiglottic downfolding (13/40 (33%) versus 4/40 (10%), $p < 0.02$).

There was a significant difference between the groups regarding the time for tracheal intubation (T2). The combination of LMA Fastrach/LMA ETT showed the best results regarding overall success rates and regarding the time for tracheal intubation (Fig. 4; group 1a/2a, $p = 0.966$; group 1a/2b, $p < 0.05$; group 2a/2b, $p < 0.01$).

Regarding the time interval for mask removal (T3), using the LMA ETT removal bar was significantly faster than using the Magill forceps with the Rüsch tube (24 s. ±7.5, versus 29.4 s. ±8.2; $p < 0.001$). No influence of the LMA device on removal time could be detected.

Tracheal tube displacement occurred only once in the Ambu Aura-i/LMA ETT subgroup.

Postoperative interviews did not reveal any significant difference between either group regarding the occurrence of patient discomfort (Table 4).

Discussion

Introducing the intubating laryngeal mask Fastrach in 1997 was a milestone in modern airway management.

Table 1 Demographic data and ASA status

Combination LMA/tube	Subgroup 1a) Aura-i/Rüsch	Subgroup 1b) Aura-i/ETT	Subgroup 2a) Fastrach/Rüsch	Subgroup 2b) Fastrach/ETT	Total
Number	$n = 19$	$n = 21$	$n = 21$	$n = 19$	$n = 80$
Height [cm]	170 ± 12.9	172 ± 10.9	175 ± 10.8	169 ± 13.5	172 ± 12.0
	[147–200]	[152–198]	[160–197]	[154–200]	[147–200]
Weight [kg]	80 ± 18,5	76 ± 13.3	76 ± 12.1	70 ± 14.6	75 ± 14.8
	[47–105]	[57–105]	[58–100]	[46–110]	[46–110]
Age [years]	59 ± 15.1	58 ± 16.9	60 ± 12.6	57 ± 19	58 ± 15.7
	[32–90]	[25–83]	[37–82]	[15–81]	[15–90]
Sex [w:m (%)]	8: 11	10: 11	7: 14	12: 7	37: 43
	(42: 58)	(47: 53)	(33: 67)	(63: 37)	(46: 54)
ASA I/II/III (%)	2/12/5	5/12/4	4/15/2	3/10/6	14/49/17
	(10/64/26)	(24/57/19)	(19/71/10)	(16/52/32)	(17/61/21)

Values are median ± SD [minimum – maximum] or number (percent). No significant differences

Table 2 Clinical predictors of difficult airway

Combination LMA/tube	Subgroup 1a) Aura-i/Rüsch	Subgroup 1b) Aura-i/ETT	Subgroup 2a) Fastrach/Rüsch	Subgroup 2b) Fastrach/ETT	Total
Mallampati I/II/III	7/9/3 (37%/47%/16%)	11/8/2 (52%/38%/10%)	13/7/1 (62%/33%/5%)	10/5/4 (53%/26%/21%)	41/29/10 (51%/36%/13%)
Interincisor distance [cm]	4.3 ± 0.7 [3.5–6.2]	4.2 ± 0.5 [3.2–5.5]	4.4 ± 0.7 [3.2–6.0]	4.3 ± 0.7 [3.5–5.8]	4.3 ± 0.6 [3.2–6.2]
Thyromental dist. (Patil) [cm]	7.8 ± 1.9 [4–11]	7.5 ± 1.1 [4.8–10]	8.2 ± 1.1 [5.5–10]	7.6 ± 1.5 [4.5–11]	7.8 ± 1.4 [4–11]

Values are absolute values (percent) and mean ± SD [minimum – maximum]. No significant differences

While LMAs had been anecdotically used for difficult airway situations so far, now a secure airway could be easily established over the laryngeal mask airway [5]. Blind intubation procedures using the intubating LMA could be performed with success rates of more than 90% [1]. A fibreoptic guidance of the tracheal tube was usually not necessary for a successful intubation [3]. Subsequent studies confirmed these results, and the LMA Fastrach was considered as "gold standard" for laryngeal mask guided intubation. Some authors even suggested LMA guided intubation not only as a backup procedure, but also for primary usage in specific patient populations [6], as well as an alternative in preclinical emergency medicine [7]. Despite the benefits of intubating laryngeal masks, there were also limitations and disadvantages. Ulcerations of the laryngeal mucous membrane [8] were reported, and the LMA ETT was not suitable for long-term mechanical ventilation due to its cuff design [9]. Also, relatively high acquisition costs of the LMA Fastrach device and its corresponding specific tracheal tube encouraged the search for alternatives. However, their quality and performance in comparison to the existing standard has to be evaluated carefully [10].

Primary endpoint of our study was the overall success rate of blind intubation with either mask within two attempts. While high success rates regarding the LMA Fastrach had been published before [11, 12].

A recent study compared tracheal intubation using the Ambu Aura-i and a flexible intubating scope with blind intubation using LMA Fastrach. The data suggest that intubation with the LMA Fastrach is faster but that first-attempt and overall intubation success rates were comparable in both groups [13].

There were no data for the Ambu Aura-i mask regarding blind tracheal intubation available so far.

Our data confirm the efficiency of the LMA Fastrach.

Blind intubation success rates were significantly lower using the Ambu Aura-i mask, both regarding overall success rates as well as regarding the success rates in the predefined subgroups. Using the Ambu Aura-i with the Rüsch Super Safety Silk showed a success rate of 42% with the first attempt, while the success rate decreased

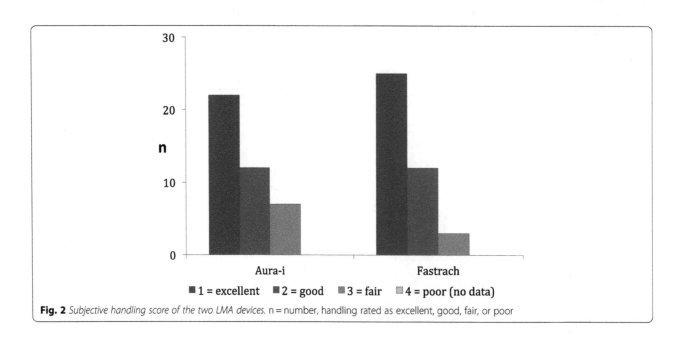

Fig. 2 *Subjective handling score of the two LMA devices.* n = number, handling rated as excellent, good, fair, or poor

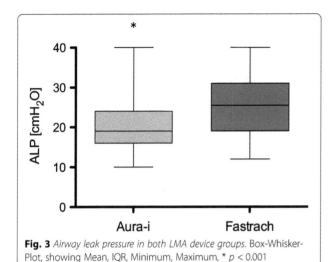

Fig. 3 *Airway leak pressure in both LMA device groups.* Box-Whisker-Plot, showing Mean, IQR, Minimum, Maximum, * $p < 0.001$

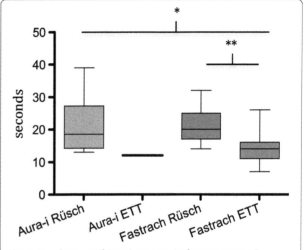

Fig. 4 *Time for successful intubation on the first attempt in all subgroups, in seconds.* Box-Whisker-Plot, showing Mean, IQR, Minimum, Maximum, * $p < 0.05$, ** $p < 0.01$

to only 5% with the LMA ETT. An optimised LMA position was not able to improve these results.

The Rüsch tube performed better with respect to overall success rates. Nevertheless, blind intubation with the Ambu Aura-i mask was successful in only a third of the patients, and is therefore not recommended for clinical use.

We suspect the less curvature of the Ambu Aura-i compared to the LMA Fastrach as well as the lack of tube guidance through the Ambu Aura-i as the two main reasons for the less success rate in blind tracheal intubation with this device.

For more than 50% of the patients ($n = 23/40$) in the Ambu Aura-i group, a fibreoptic assisted intubation was necessary. Overall success rate for intubation with the Ambu Aura-i mask was approximately 90%.

Even though there was a significant difference regarding fibreoptic control after placing the masks, with a better fit of the LMA Fastrach, this evaluation is limited due to different mask designs.

Regarding the fibreoptic control of LMA placement and differing descriptions in the literature [14], there is yet no definitive consensus regarding the evaluation of

the mask position with the fibrescope. Our data should be interpreted with caution, because we changed the fiberscope device during the study (after a few measured patients in both LMA groups), using a small diagnostic one at first and switching to a larger therapeutic one later to get a better lightning and a better overview. Nevertheless, using the Ambu Aura-i compared to LMA Fastrach leads to more cases of laryngeal lateralization, as well as epiglottic downfolding. Though these differences did not reach statistical significance in our study, they could be meaningful in individual subjects.

Both laryngeal mask devices could be placed at least with the second attempt, and therefore qualify for clinical use. Even though in our study the LMA Fastrach could be placed significantly faster than the Ambu Aura-i (16 s. versus 19 s.), we consider this time difference as negligible in a clinical context. Our results confirm previously reported ranges [15]. Furthermore, both devices were rated "excellent" or "good" by the investigators.

Airway leak pressure (ALP) is a commonly used method to quantify the efficiency of the airway seal [16]. In our study, we inflated cuffs with manufacturer recommended volumes to get comparable data. Furthermore, our study should not detect the smallest possible cuff volume, but the highest possible ALP. In a study with the LMA Unique, ALP was highest when the cuff was completely inflated [17]. Our analysis of the ALP showed significant differences between both devices (Ambu Aura-i 19 cmH_2O versus LMA Fastrach 26 cmH_2O) in favour of the LMA Fastrach, confirming existing data with ALP ranging from 25 to 30 cmH_2O [18]. Our study did not investigate the possibility of adverse events caused by higher ALP values. However, the LMA Fastrach group presented more cases of gastric insufflation

Table 3 Failed attempts of blind intubation in each subgroup, including attempts of *crossover-design*

	Subgroup 1a)	Subgroup 1b)	Subgroup 2a)	Subgroup 2b)
	Aura-i/Rüsch	Aura-i/ETT	Fastrach/Rüsch	Fastrach/ETT
Number	$n = 36$	$n = 31$	$n = 23$	$n = 23$
Attempts	62	61	29	29
Failed	49	57	11	10
Failed (%)	79%	93%	38%	34%
	*, **, ***	$, §		

* $p = 0.03$ compared to 1b, ** $p = 0.0003$ compared to 2a, *** $p < 0.0001$ compared to 2b
$ $p < 0.0001$ compared to 2a, § $p < 0.0001$ compared to 2b
Values are absolute values

Table 4 Postoperative interview about the intensity (none, moderate, severe) of different types of patient discomfort (sore throat, difficulty swallowing, hoarseness) in each subgroup

Subgroup	Sore throat				Difficulty swallowing				Hoarseness			
	1a	1b	2a	2b	1a	1b	2a	2b	1a	1b	2a	2b
None	14	14	15	16	15	17	17	16	15	16	16	16
%	74%	67%	71%	84%	79%	81%	81%	84%	79%	76%	76%	84%
Moderate	4	5	4	3	1	3	1	3	3	4	2	3
%	21%	24%	19%	16%	5%	14%	5%	14%	16%	19%	10%	16%
Severe	0	1	0	0	2	0	1	0	0	0	1	0
%	0%	5%	0%	0%	11%	0%	5%	0%	0%	0%	5%	0%

Values are absolute values and percent. No significant differences

(12/40 versus 7/39), possibly due to the ALP being higher than the lower oesophageal sphincter tone. Neither mask provides a drainage channel for gastric tube placement [19].

Regarding laryngeal mask removal over the tracheal tube, we compared two different procedures depending on which laryngeal mask was used: either using the removal bar specifically designed for the LMA ETT or a conventional Magill forceps for the Rüsch tube. Recorded times were significantly shorter using the LMA ETT system (24 s. ±8 versus 29 s. ±7). In our opinion, this difference is not due to the laryngeal mask used, but rather due to the large pilot-cuff of the Rüsch tube that needs to be fully deflated to pass it through the laryngeal mask.

Concerning airway discomfort after the procedure, about one third of the patients reported discomfort, but most of the patients were devoid of any symptoms. There were no significant differences between both groups, regarding the different types of discomfort, even though there were more (unsuccessful) attempts of intubation in the Ambu Aura-i group.

Our study has some limitations. (1) There were no patients with a difficult airway in each group. (2) The design of the study does not allow any statement about the equivalence of LMA guided placement compared to primary fibreoptic guided intubation (3) The fibreoptic evaluation of the laryngeal view analogous to the Cormack/Lehane score was not diagnostically conclusive.

Conclusion

In conclusion, the results of our study suggest that both laryngeal mask devices are suitable for ventilation and oxygenation. Blind intubation using an intubating LMA remains the domain of the LMA Fastrach device because of its high success rates. The success rate does not differ with respect to the tube used. The Ambu Aura-i device is not suitable for blind intubation. Tracheal intubation using this device should be performed with fibreoptic assistance, as recommended by the manufacturer.

Abbreviations
ALP: Airway leak pressure; APL: Valve adjustable pressure-limiting valve; BIS: Bispectral index; BMI: Body mass index; COPD: Chronic obstructive pulmonary disease; ETT: Endotracheal tube; LMA: Laryngeal mask

Acknowledgements
Assistance with the article: We would like to thank the nursing staff of the Department of Anaesthesiology of the University Hospital at Kiel for their assistance and outstanding patient care.

Authors' contributions
Data was collected by MS, BB and JH. Data was analysed and interpreted by RS, MS, MG, JH and BB. All authors have substantially contributed to the manuscript and take full responsibility for its content, RS was a major contributor in writing the manuscript. All authors gave read the final manuscript and gave their approval for publishment.

Author details
[1]Department of Anaesthesiology and Intensive Care Medicine, Asklepios Hospital St. Georg, Lohmuehlenstr. 5, D-20099 Hamburg, Germany.
[2]Department of Anaesthesiology and Intensive Care Medicine, University Hospital Schleswig-Holstein, Campus Kiel, Schwanenweg 21, D-24105 Kiel, Germany.

References
1. Brain AI, Verghese C, Addy EV, Kapila A. The intubating laryngeal mask. Development of a new device for intubation of the trachea. Br J Anaesth. 1997;79:699–703.
2. Brimacombe JR. Difficult airway management with the intubating laryngeal mask. Anesth Analg. 1997;85:1173–5.
3. Joo HS, Rose DK. The intubating laryngeal mask airway with and without fiberoptic guidance. Anesth Analg. 1999;88:662–6.
4. Combes X, Sauvat S, Leroux B, Dumerat M, Sherrer E, Motamed C, Brain A, D'honneur G. Intubating laryngeal mask airway in morbidly obese and lean patients: a comparative study. Anesthesiology. 2005;102:1106–9.
5. Brain AI, Verghese C, Addy EV, Kapila A, Brimacombe J. The intubating laryngeal mask. II: a preliminary clinical report of a new means of intubating the trachea. Br J Anaesth. 1997;79:704–9.
6. Asai T, Shingu K. Tracheal intubation through the intubating laryngeal mask in patients with unstable necks. Acta Anaesthesiol Scand. 2001;45:818–22.
7. Doerges V, Paschen HR. Management des schwierigen Atemwegs: Springer-Verlag Berlin Heidelberg; 2004.
8. Ulrich-Pur H, Hrska F, Krafft P, Friehs H, Wulkersdorfer B, Kostler WJ, Rabitsch W, Staudinger T, Schuster E, Frass M. Comparison of mucosal pressures induced by cuffs of different airway devices. Anesthesiology. 2006;104:933–8.
9. Suneel PR, Koshy T, Unnikrishnan KP. High cuff pressure in the silicone endotracheal tube of the LMA-Fastrach: implications for patient safety. J Clin Anesth. 2011;23:666–7.
10. Bein B, Francksen H, Steinfath M. Supraglottic airway devices. Anasthesiol Intensivmed Notfallmed Schmerzther. 2011;46:598–607.

11. Gerstein NS, Braude DA, Hung O, Sanders JC, Murphy MF. The Fastrach intubating laryngeal mask airway: an overview and update. Can J Anaesth. 2010;57:588–601.

12. Lu PP, Yang CH, Ho AC, Shyr MH. The intubating LMA: a comparison of insertion techniques with conventional tracheal tubes. Can J Anaesth. 2000;47:849–53.

13. Artime CA, Altamirano A, Normand KC, Ferrario L, Aijazi H, Cattano D, Hagberg CA. Flexible optical intubation via the Ambu Aura-i vs blind intubation via the single-use LMA Fastrach: a prospective randomized clinical trial. J Clin Anesth. 2016;33:41–6.

14. Mcneillis NJ, Timberlake C, Avidan MS, Sarang K, Choyce A, Radcliffe JJ. Fibreoptic views through the laryngeal mask and the intubating laryngeal mask. Eur J Anaesthesiol. 2001;18:471–5.

15. Francksen H, Renner J, Hanss R, Scholz J, Doerges V, Bein B. A comparison of the i-gel with the LMA-unique in non-paralysed anaesthetised adult patients. Anaesthesia. 2009;64:1118–24.

16. Keller C, Brimacombe J. Pharyngeal mucosal pressures, airway sealing pressures, and fiberoptic position with the intubating versus the standard laryngeal mask airway. Anesthesiology. 1999;90:001–6.

17. Francksen H, Bein B, Cavus E, Renner J, Scholz J, Steinfath M, Tonner PH, Doerges V. Comparison of LMA unique, Ambu laryngeal mask and soft seal laryngeal mask during routine surgical procedures. Eur J Anaesthesiol. 2007;24:134–40.

18. Keller C, Brimacombe JR, Keller K, Morris R. Comparison of four methods for assessing airway sealing pressure with the laryngeal mask airway in adult patients. Br J Anaesth. 1999;82:286–7.

19. Hernandez MR, Klock PA Jr, Ovassapian A. Evolution of the extraglottic airway: a review of its history, applications, and practical tips for success. Anesth Analg. 2012;114:349–68.

26

Conversion of I-gel to definitive airway in a cervical immobilized manikin: Aintree intubation catheter vs long endotracheal tube

Yun Jeong Chae[1], Heirim Lee[2], Bokyeong Jun[1] and In Kyong Yi[1]*

Abstract

Background: After prehospital insertion of i-gel, a popular supraglottic airway (SGA), fiberoptic-guided intubation through i-gel is often required to switch the i-gel to a definitive airway for anticipated difficult airway. The Aintree intubation catheter (AIC) was developed for this purpose yet it requires many procedural steps during which maintenance of adequate ventilation is difficult. We custom-made a long endotracheal tube (LET) which may facilitate this procedure and compared the efficacy of the AIC and LET in a cervical immobilized manikin.

Methods: In this 2 × 2 crossover manikin-based trial, 20 anaesthesiologists and residents performed both methods in random order. Total intubation time, fiberoptic time, and procedure time were recorded. The ease of insertion, procedure failure rate, difficulty score, and participants' preference were recorded.

Results: Total intubation time was significantly shorter for the LET than the AIC group (70.8 ± 16.4 s vs 94.0 ± 28.4 s, $P = 0.001$). The procedure time was significantly shorter in the LET group (51.9 ± 13.8 s vs 76.5 ± 25.4 s, $P < 0.001$). The ease of insertion score was lower, i.e., easier, in the AIC than the LET group (2.0 [1.0–2.75] vs 1.0 [1.0–1.0], $P < 0.001$). Fiberoptic time (19.0 ± 6.9 s vs 17.5 ± 12.3 s) and subjective difficulty (4.0 [3.0–6.0] vs 4.0 [3.0–5.75]) were similar between groups. Fourteen participants preferred the LET method (70%) due to its fewer procedural steps.

Conclusions: LET resulted in a shorter intubation time than the AIC during fiberoptic-guided intubation through the i-gel, possibly due to the less procedural steps compared to AIC.

Keywords: Airway management, Fiberoptic, Intratracheal intubation, Manikin, Supraglottic airway device

Background

Supraglottic airway (SGA) has become a common method of airway management for out-of-hospital cardiac arrest [1–3]. The I-gel (Intersurgical, Berkshire, United Kingdom), a second generation SGA, has shown higher success rates in prehospital setting than first generation SGAs and endotracheal intubation [1, 2, 4]. As utilization of i-gel continues to increase, there is also an increasing clinical need for an easy yet reliable conversion method to a definitive airway after prehospital i-gel insertion. Currently, there are two non-surgical options for the conversion: intubation using a laryngoscopy after pre-existing i-gel removal or intubation through i-gel [5, 6]. If a difficult airway is expected in a well-functioning i-gel, intubation through i-gel is recommended [7] as its removal could make the situation worse.

* Correspondence: lyrin01@gmail.com
[1]Department of Anaesthesiology and Pain Medicine, Ajou University School of Medicine, 164, World cup-ro, Yeongtong-gu, Suwon 16499, South Korea

When using a conventional endotracheal tube with the i-gel during conversion, however, there is a risk of dislodgement of the endotracheal tube due to the different lengths of the endotracheal tube and the i-gel [8]. Devices such as Aintree Intubation Catheter (AIC; Cook Critical Care, Bloomington, IN, USA) were developed to facilitate conversion, but it requires many procedural steps during which maintenance of adequate ventilation is difficult [9].

To compensate for the shortcomings, we custom-made a long endotracheal tube (LET) that facilitates removal of a SGA, especially when combined with an i-gel [10–12]. The LET was designed to not only have a longer tube length, but also avoid impingement of the cuff inflation line and cuff pilot balloon during conversion (Fig. 1). The aim of this study was to compare the clinical efficacy of the AIC and LET in the conversion from i-gel to ETT in a cervical immobilized manikin.

Methods

The study protocol was approved by Ajou Institutional Review Board at Aug, 13, 2018 (AJIRB-MED-OBS-18-226). The current study was also registered in ClinicalTrials.gov (NCT03645174). Participants were anaesthesiologists and anaesthesia residents recruited from our university hospital; the eligibility criterion was not having previous experience of AIC or LET placement. Written informed consent was obtained from all participants.

This study was designed as a 2 × 2 crossover trial, in which each participant performed two types of procedures in a sequence of AB or BA. The first trial was performed in the sequence AB or BA, as allocated by randomization. Previous studies using the AIC reported a mean intubation time of 69.9 s, with a standard deviation of 26.1 s [13]. Therefore, an intubation time difference exceeding 20 s was considered clinically significant; thus, we calculated that at least 16 participants were required ($\alpha = 0.05$, $\beta = 0.2$). Considering potential drop-out rates, 20 participants were recruited.

A two-way analysis of variance was used for data analysis with the AB and BA sequences as the grouping factor and the primary endpoint being the procedural time. Parametric data were analyzed using a paired t-test and nonparametric data, using the Wilcoxon signed-rank test. Categorical variables were analyzed using the McNemar test.

All participants were educated to perform fiberoptic-guided endotracheal intubation through a SGA using two methods by means of an educational video. The rationale behind choosing fiberoptic-guided intubation instead of blind intubation for this study is the overall higher success rate of fiberoptic-guided intubation compared to the blind method in a difficult airway situation (98.6% vs 85.3%) [6]. The first method of intubation involved using the AIC, and the second method involved using the LET developed by our group. Each participant used both methods, in a random order, as determined by a random number table (http://www.random.org).

The manikin (Laerdal Airway Management Trainer; Laerdal Medical, Stavanger, Norway) was fit with a rigid neck collar (Philadelphia, West Deptford, NJ, USA) producing a simulated difficult airway. Prior to the trial, a size 4 i-gel was inserted into the manikin and the position confirmed as a grade 1 laryngeal view using a fiberoptic endoscope. A flexible intubation video-endoscope (KARL STORZ, Tuttlingen, Germany) was used as the fiberoptic endoscope during the procedure.

All participants followed the same intubation protocols. For the AIC method, the catheter was first

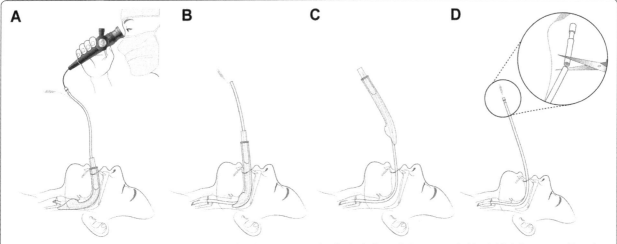

Fig. 1 a Fiberoptic-guided LET insertion, **(b)** Removal of i-gel, **(c)** Position of cuff pilot balloon during removal of i-gel, **(d)** Adjustment of length of the LET. Abbreviation: LET, long endotracheal tube. Abbreviations: LET, long endotracheal tube

connected to the fiberoptic device and inserted within the i-gel lumen. The i-gel was removed after confirming the catheter position within the trachea, after which an ETT of ID 7.0 mm (Shiley™ Endotracheal Tubes with TaperGuard™ Cuff; Medtronic, Minneapolis, MN, USA) was inserted using the catheter as a guide. Finally, inflation of the manikin's lungs was confirmed by artificial manual breathing unit (ambu) bagging. For the LET method, an LET of ID 7.0 mm was fitted to the fiberoptic endoscope and inserted within the i-gel lumen. After confirmation of the LET insertion into the trachea, the fiberoptic endoscope and subsequently the i-gel were removed. Inflation of the manikin's lungs was confirmed in the same manner as for the AIC method.

The primary performance parameter was the total intubation time, measured by a separate observer using a timer. 'Total intubation time' was defined as the time from when the tip of the fiberoptic endoscope was inserted into the i-gel lumen up to inflation of the manikin's lungs after ambu bagging. 'Fiberoptic time' was defined as the time from the entrance of the fiberoptic endoscope into the i-gel lumen to its passage of the vocal cords. 'Procedural time' was the difference between the total intubation and fiberoptic times, and reflected the actual time required for each method independent of the participant's fiberoptic skill level. 'Intubation failure' was defined as failure of lung inflation after ambu bagging. This occurred from oesophageal intubation or situations requiring i-gel reinsertion for various reasons, such as dislodgement of the ETT or AIC, or moving of the fiberoptic endoscope away from the vocal cords. The ease of insertion for vocal cord passage of the ETT was scored during each procedure by a separate observer as follows: 1; excellent, no resistance, 2; good, moderate resistance, 3; difficult, remarkable resistance, and 4; insertion impossible in three attempts. After each procedure, the participants rated intubation difficulty using a numeric scale from 1 (extremely easy) to 10 (extremely difficult). Each participant also recorded their preference between the two methods and the reason for their preference [14].

We set the length of LET to 45 cm. The length was based on previous studies and our experiments. Takenaka et al. [11] showed that if removal of SGA is not considered, the optimal length of ETT for adequate endotracheal insertion through SGA was the sum of the length of the SGA, the distance between the SGA mask aperture and the vocal cords, and the distance between the upper border of the ETT cuff and ETT tip. The length thus derived was approximately 33 cm considering the length of SGA being 22 cm [11]. This was similar or somewhat greater than the conventional ETT length. In addition to this length, the proximal end of the ETT

above the proximal end of the SGA after endotracheal insertion should be long enough if SGA removal is necessary to prevent dislodgement of the ETT [12]. The distance from the teeth to the proximal end of the ETT should be longer than the length of the SGA, so that during removal of the SGA, the ETT can be caught and prevented from coming out altogether. Assuming that the depth of ETT fixed at the teeth is 23 cm, and the SGA length is 22 cm, at least 45 cm is needed for LET. In addition, the length of the ETT should be shorter than 55 cm so that the LET does not interfere with the distal flexible portion of the fiberoptic endoscope (65 cm long). The cuff inflation line was also kept long enough such that the cuff pilot balloon would not get caught during tube change. Therefore, the range of length for LET was 45–55 cm. Accordingly, we chose the shortest length, 45 cm, to keep the length of the cuff inflation line as short as possible. The branching point of the cuff inflation line from the body of the ETT was the same as that of a conventional tube, so that after the procedure, the device could be cut to a similar length as a conventional ETT without damaging the inflation line (Fig. 1). Both the LET and the Shiley™ Endotracheal Tubes with TaperGuard™ Cuff are made of polyvinyl chloride.

Results

Demographics

Twenty participants were enrolled (Fig. 2), of whom eight were anaesthesia specialists and 12, anaesthesia residents. The mean age of the participants was 32.7 ± 2.6 years. The mean experience with fiberoptic-assisted intubation other than with AIC or LET was 12.9 ± 12.6 times. All the participants completed the study training (Table 1).

Primary outcomes of intubation time

The total intubation time for the AIC group was 94.0 ± 28.4 s, which was significantly longer than that for the LET group (70.8 ± 16.4 s) ($P = 0.001$). The fiberoptic time was not different between the two groups (AIC: 17.5 ± 12.3 s, LET: 19.0 ± 6.9 s, $p = 0.61$). The procedural time, which was the difference between the total intubation time and fiberoptic time, was significantly longer in the AIC group (76.5 ± 25.4 s) than in the LET group (51.9 ± 13.8 s) ($P < 0.001$) (Fig. 3). One participant failed one time due to dislodgement of the AIC.

Subjective outcomes

The score of ease of insertion was lower for the AIC (AIC 1.0 [1.0–1.0] vs LET 2.0 [1.0–2.75], $P < 0.001$), but no difference in subjective difficulty was found between the two groups (AIC 4.0 [3.0–5.75] vs LET 4.0 [3.0–6.0], $P = 1.000$) (Table 2). Overall analysis of preference between the two methods showed that six participants

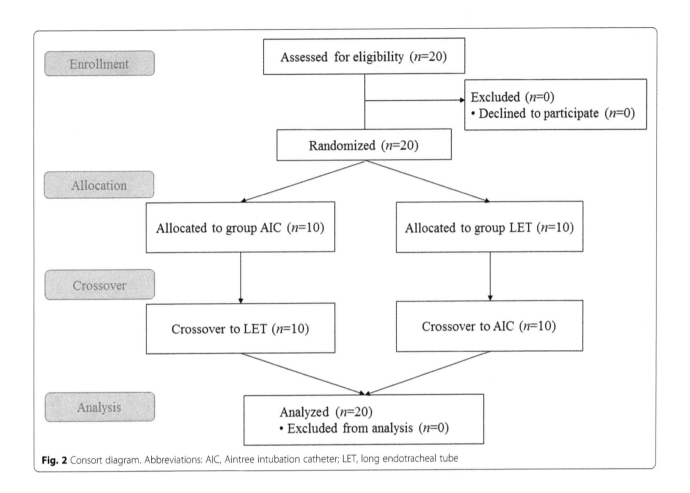

Fig. 2 Consort diagram. Abbreviations: AIC, Aintree intubation catheter; LET, long endotracheal tube

preferred the AIC method (30.0%) and 14 preferred the LET method (70.0%). Among those who preferred the AIC method, four described it as having easier vocal cord passage, and two felt that the LET was more difficult to maneuver due to its reduced rigidity. The 14 participants who preferred the LET method described the reason for their preference as the reduced number of procedure steps compared to the AIC method.

Discussion

In our comparison of using the AIC or LET method for fiberoptic-guided endotracheal intubation through i-gel in a difficult airway manikin, the LET resulted in shorter intubation and procedural times. The score for ease of vocal cord passage of the ETT was higher by approximately 1 point (in a range of 1 to 4 points) compared with that for LET, but there was no difference in the subjective difficulty. Seventy percent of participants preferred the LET method due to its reduced number of procedure steps.

Previous studies using the AIC method report that the intubation time excluding the SGA insertion time was 67–90 s [15, 16]. In our study, the mean intubation time was longer (94.0 s), probably because none of the participants had previous experience with the AIC or the LET. Nevertheless, the LET method had shorter intubation times than the AIC (70.8 s). Even when considering the procedural time, excluding the time required for locating the vocal cords with the fiberoptic device, there was a significant difference between the two methods (AIC: 76.5 s vs LET: 51.9 s). Intubation time and procedure time are of clinical significance since the patients are in apnea condition during the procedure.

When using the AIC, the ETT is inserted after removal of the SGA, and the patient remains in apnea until the ETT is in place. Although connecting the AIC to Rapi-Fit® adaptors (Cook Critical Care, Bloomington, IN, USA) allows jet ventilation for a while, reinsertion of the SGA may eventually be needed. In the LET method, however, ventilation is more secure because the SGA is not removed before ETT placement is confirmed. If procedural problems occur, ventilation can be performed by connecting the ETT to the circuit or through the SGA in situ. This ensures safety against apnea in case of prolonged procedures. Hence, the LET has clinical value in that it decreases the intubation time and provides a ventilation tool at hand. Another significant finding was the high user-preference for the LET due to the fewer

Table 1 Demographics

No.	Position	Sex	Age	Experiences			
				Anesthesiology (years)	Fiberoptic intubation (times)	AIC (times)	LET (times)
1	Resident	M	30	3	20	0	0
2	Resident	F	35	4	20	0	0
3	Fellow	M	37	5	16	0	0
4	Resident	M	28	1	0	0	0
5	Resident	F	31	1	0	0	0
6	Fellow	M	34	5	20	0	0
7	Resident	M	32	1	0	0	0
8	Resident	F	31	2	10	0	0
9	Resident	F	30	3	15	0	0
10	Resident	F	33	4	20	0	0
11	Resident	F	33	4	10	0	0
12	Resident	F	28	3	15	0	0
13	Fellow	F	32	5	20	0	0
14	Resident	F	32	2	15	0	0
15	Resident	F	32	2	23	0	0
16	Attending	M	36	10	50	0	0
17	Attending	F	35	9	20	0	0
18	Fellow	F	34	5	15	0	0
19	Fellow	M	36	5	3	0	0
20	Fellow	M	35	6	25	0	0

Abbreviations: *AIC* Aintree intubation catheter, *LET* long endotracheal tube

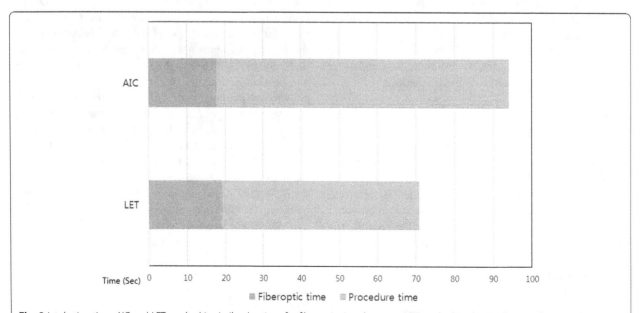

Fig. 3 Intubation time. AIC and LET resulted in similar durations for fiberoptic time, however, LET resulted in shorter duration for procedure time. Total intubation time was shorter in LET. Abbreviations: AIC, Aintree intubation catheter; LET, long endotracheal tube.

Table 2 Intubation profile

Parameter	AIC (n = 20)	LET (n = 20)	P value
Total intubation time, sec	94.0 ± 28.4	70.8 ± 16.4	0.001
Fiberoptic time, sec	17.5 ± 12.3	19.0 ± 6.9	0.612
Procedure time, sec	76.5 ± 25.4	51.9 ± 13.8	< 0.001
Success, n (%)	19 (95)	20 (100)	1.000
Ease of insertion	1.0 [1.0–1.0]	2.0 [1.0–2.75]	< 0.001
Difficulty	4.0 [3.0–5.75]	4.0 [3.0–6.0]	1.000

Values are mean ± standard deviation or median [interquartile range] or
number (%)

Abbreviations: *AIC* Aintree intubation catheter, *LET* long endotracheal tube

procedural steps. Overall, the LET method showed advantages over the AIC method in terms of decreased intubation time, simplicity of the procedure, and safety.

A small number of studies have utilised a similar concept during intubation through SGA. Knoshita et al. [10] reported using a longer tube to facilitate conversion of an LMA Fastrach™ (Laryngeal Mask Company, Henley-on-Thames, UK) but did not compare it to other methods. Similar to our concept, Weiss et al. [17] reported on a method in paediatric patients that used two separate uncuffed ETTs connected to each other. They reported that ventilation was possible during LMA removal; hence, there was no need to rush the procedure [17]. This is not only related to the psychological stability of the intubator but is also clinically significant because most paediatric patients intubated through SGAs have difficult airway situations. Unfortunately, this cannot be applied to adults as they require the use of cuffed ETTs. When using the Weiss method, the cuff pilot balloon is impinged due to the lack of space within the SGA lumen, resulting in an obstacle during SGA removal and possible damage to the balloon. The LET used for this study has several advantages in terms of tube design. The cuff inflation line is longer than the total length of the tube, so that the cuff pilot balloon is positioned distal to the tube end and does not interfere with SGA removal. Balloon inflation can be performed before SGA removal, if required.

Direct insertion of ETTs into the SGA has been studied, such as with the use of an intubating laryngeal mask airway (iLMA). The iLMA has a stiff angled shank and a wide internal diameter for ETT insertion, as does the LMA Fastrach™. It is also shorter than other LMAs and has a stabiliser rod that pushes the ETT [14]. A previous study compared the efficacy of the iLMA with that of a combination of the AIC and classic LMA (cLMA) during insertion of a 7.0 mm ID ETT. They reported that not only was iLMA insertion more difficult than cLMA, but it also resulted in a poor glottis view in 26% of cases, even after insertion [14]. Furthermore, the iLMA is less widely available than the cLMA [9] and has a steeper

learning curve, hampering its routine use [18] Thus, the iLMA does not appear to improve upon the combination of the AIC and cLMA [14, 19]. The i-gel and LET combination used in this study shares conceptual similarities with the iLMA, but compensates for iLMA shortcomings. Several studies have shown that i-gel yields a higher insertion success rate, the best fiberoptic view, and superior results in intubation through SGAs than those with other SGAs [16, 20, 21]. The i-gel and LET combination used in this study shares conceptual similarities with the iLMA, but compensates for iLMA shortcomings. The i-gel and LET combination is therefore a potentially better option than iLMA, but further study is definitely warranted.

In the AIC method, resistance during vocal cord passing ("railroading") was reported in 24% of cases [15]. A previous study utilising iLMA and a 7.0-mm ID ETT as a fiberoptic guide, without the AIC, reported intubation failure in three of eight cases due to railroading [19]. This problem occurs due to the difference in diameter between the outer and inner layers. In this case, the difference is between the outer diameter of the AIC and internal diameter of the ETT. In the LET method, the difference in diameter is larger than in the AIC method; therefore, impediment at the glottis may be greater than that with the AIC [19, 22]. In our study, we described this phenomenon as 'ease of insertion'. We found that both methods had acceptable ease of insertion scores; however, the LET group showed slightly more resistance than the AIC group, without any difference in the subjective difficulty. Three cases showed marked resistance (grade 3) during LET insertion, but railroading was finally possible in all cases in our study, possibly because it was performed within the established SGA path. A different tube tip design [23] or a thicker fiberoptic device may be useful to facilitate railroading. Nevertheless, further investigations are required.

This study has some limitations. It was performed at a single center, used a manikin, and only included situations with proper positioning of the SGA and good laryngeal view by the fiberoptic. Additional clinical trials are warranted, including situations with a poor laryngeal view through the SGA. Furthermore, combinations of the LET with other commercially available SGAs should be compared. Finally, further studies and possible design modifications are required to test the incorporation of blind method intubation through SGA.

Conclusions

The LET designed by our group resulted in a shorter intubation time for residents and anaesthesiologists than did the AIC during fiberoptic-guided intubation through an i-gel. This is possibly due to its more concise procedural steps. The LET appears to be a useful tool during exchange from i-gel to definitive airway in anticipated difficult airway situations.

Abbreviations
AIC: Aintree intubation catheter; LET: Long endotracheal tube; LMA: Laryngeal mask airway; SGA: Supraglottic airway

Acknowledgements
We would like to thank Editage (www.editage.com) for English language editing. We used Adobe Illustrator C2020 to generate the Fig. 1.

Authors' contributions
Study design; data analysis; HL, IKY, YJC. Education of the participants, data collection; BJ, IKY. Writing the paper; IKY, YJC. Supervision of the investigation; IKY. The author(s) read and approved the final manuscript.

Author details
[1]Department of Anaesthesiology and Pain Medicine, Ajou University School of Medicine, 164, World cup-ro, Yeongtong-gu, Suwon 16499, South Korea. [2]Office of Biostatics, Ajou Research Institute for Innovative Medicine, Ajou University Medical Center, 164, World cup-ro, Yeongtong-gu, Suwon 16499, South Korea.

References
1. Middleton PM, Simpson PM, Thomas RE, Bendall JC. Higher insertion success with the i-gel supraglottic airway in out-of-hospital cardiac arrest: a randomised controlled trial. Resuscitation. 2014;85:893–7.
2. Duckett J, Fell P, Han K, Kimber C, Taylor C. Introduction of the I-gel supraglottic airway device for prehospital airway management in a UK ambulance service. Emerg Med J. 2014;31:505–7.
3. Taylor J, Black S, JB S, Kirby K, Nolan JP, Reeves BC, et al. Design and implementation of the AIRWAYS-2 trial: A multi-centre cluster randomised controlled trial of the clinical and cost effectiveness of the i-gel supraglottic airway device versus tracheal intubation in the initial airway management of out of hospital cardiac arrest. Resuscitation. 2016;109:25–32.
4. Bielski A, Rivas E, Ruetzler K, Smereka J, Puslecki M, Dabrowski M, et al. Comparison of blind intubation via supraglottic airway devices versus standard intubation during different airway emergency scenarios in inexperienced hand: Randomized, crossover manikin trial. Medicine (Baltimore). 2018;97:e12593.
5. Hernandez MC, Aho JM, Zielinski MD, Zietlow SP, Kim BD, Morris DS. Definitive airway management after pre-hospital supraglottic airway insertion: outcomes and a management algorithm for trauma patients. Am J Emerg Med. 2018;36:114–9.
6. Michalek P, Donaldson W, Graham C, Hinds JD. A comparison of the I-gel supraglottic airway as a conduit for tracheal intubation with the intubating laryngeal mask airway: a manikin study. Resuscitation. 2010;81:74–7.
7. Frerk C, Mitchell VS, McNarry AF, Mendonca C, Bhagrath R, Patel A, et al. Difficult airway society 2015 guidelines for management of unanticipated difficult intubation in adults. Br J Anaesth. 2015;115:827–48.
8. Alfery DD. Laryngeal mask airway and the ASA difficult airway algorithm. Anesthesiology. 1996;85:685 author reply 7–8.
9. Higgs A, Clark E, Premraj K. Low-skill fibreoptic intubation: use of the Aintree catheter with the classic LMA. Anaesthesia. 2005;60:915–20.
10. Kinoshita H, Nakahata K, Iranami H, Yamada S, Hironaka Y, Hatano Y. A long endotracheal tube to facilitate intubation via the Fastrach™ laryngeal mask airway. Can J Anaesth. 2006;53:210–1.
11. Takenaka I, Aoyama K. Optimizing endotracheal tube size and length for tracheal intubation through single-use supraglottic airway devices. Can J Anaesth. 2010;57:389–90.
12. Xue FS, Xiong J, Yuan YJ, Wang Q. Optimal size and length of the endotracheal tube for tracheal intubation via supraglottic airway devices. Can J Anaesth. 2010;57:624–5 author reply 5.
13. Olesnicky BL, Rehak A, Bestic WB, Brock JT, Watterson L. A cadaver study comparing three fibreoptic-assisted techniques for converting a supraglottic airway to a cuffed tracheal tube. Anaesthesia. 2017;72:223–9.
14. Malcharek MJ, Rockmann K, Zumpe R, Sorge O, Winter V, Sablotzki A, et al. Comparison of Aintree and Fastrach techniques for low-skill fibreoptic intubation in patients at risk of secondary cervical injury: a randomised controlled trial. Eur J Anaesthesiol. 2014;31:153–8.
15. Blair EJ, Mihai R, Cook TM. Tracheal intubation via the classic™ and Proseal™ laryngeal mask airways: a manikin study using the Aintree intubating catheter. Anaesthesia. 2007;62:385–7.
16. Dhimar AA, Sangada BR, Upadhyay MR, Patel SH. I-gel versus laryngeal mask airway (LMA) classic as a conduit for tracheal intubation using ventilating bougie. J Anaesthesiol Clin Pharmacol. 2017;33:467–72.
17. Weiss M, Gerber AC, Schmitz A. Continuous ventilation technique for laryngeal mask airway (LMA) removal after fiberoptic intubation in children. Paediatr Anaesth. 2004;14:936–40.
18. Chan YW, Kong CF, Kong CS, Hwang NC, Ip-Yam PC. The intubating laryngeal mask airway (ILMA): initial experience in Singapore. Br J Anaesth. 1998;81:610–1.
19. Heard AM, Lacquiere DA, Riley RH. Manikin study of fibreoptic-guided intubation through the classic laryngeal mask airway with the Aintree intubating catheter vs the intubating laryngeal mask airway in the simulated difficult airway. Anaesthesia. 2010;65:841–7.
20. Lopez NT, McCoy SK, Carroll C, Jones E, Miller JA. Non-conventional utilization of the Aintree intubating catheter to facilitate exchange between three supraglottic airways and an endotracheal tube: a cadaveric trial. Mil Med. 2019;184:e222–8.
21. Izakson A, Cherniavsky G, Lazutkin A, Ezri T. The i-gel as a conduit for the Aintree intubation catheter for subsequent fiberoptic intubation. Rom J Anaesth Intensive Care. 2014;21:131–3.
22. Ayoub CM, Rizk MS, Yaacoub CI, Baraka AS, Lteif AM. Advancing the tracheal tube over a flexible fiberoptic bronchoscope by a sleeve mounted on the insertion cord. Anesth Analg. 2003;96:290–2.
23. Greer JR, Smith SP, Strang T. A comparison of tracheal tube tip designs on the passage of an endotracheal tube during oral fiberoptic intubation. Anesthesiology. 2001;94:729–31.

27

Ultrasonographic identification of the cricothyroid membrane in a patient with a difficult airway as a result of cervical hematoma caused by hemophilia

Ippei Jimbo, Kohji Uzawa[*] ⓘ, Joho Tokumine, Shingo Mitsuda, Kunitaro Watanabe and Tomoko Yorozu

Abstract

Background: Surgical cricothyroidotomy is a last resort in patients with an anticipated difficult airway, but without any guarantee of success. Identification of the cricothyroid membrane may be the key to successful cricothyrotomy. Ultrasonographic identification of the cricothyroid membrane has been reported to be more useful than the conventional palpation technique. However, ultrasonographic identification techniques are not yet fully characterized.

Case presentation: A 28-year-old man with hemophilia and poor adherence to medication. He was brought to the emergency department with a large cervical hematoma and respiratory difficulty. An otolaryngologist decided to insert a tracheal tube to maintain his airway. However, emergent laryngoscopy indicated an anticipated difficult airway. A backup plan that included awake intubation by the anesthesiologists and surgical cricothyroidotomy by an otolaryngologist was devised. The cricothyroid membrane could not be identified by palpation but was detected by ultrasonographic identification with a longitudinal approach. Awake fiberoptic intubation was successfully performed.

Conclusions: In this case, the cricothyroid membrane could be identified using the longitudinal approach but not the transverse approach. It may be ideal to know which ultrasound technique can be applied for each patient.

Keywords: Cricothyroid membrane, Cricothyroidotomy, Ultrasonography, Difficult airway, Hemophilia

Background

Management of worsening respiratory distress in a patient with a difficult airway is problematic. When a difficult airway is anticipated, the decision regarding whether or not to perform awake intubation or surgical cricothyroidotomy is challenging. Furthermore, there is no guarantee of success using either procedure and there is an ever-present possibility of "cannot intubate cannot oxygenate" (CICO) [1]. Guidelines for the management of a difficult airway, as followed in the US [2], UK [3], Canada [1], and Japan [4], recommend securing of the airway by surgical incision or puncture of the cricothyroid membrane (CTM) as a last resort in a CICO situation. Preparation for both less invasive awake fiberoptic intubation and invasive cricothyroidotomy is known as the "double standby" strategy [1]. However, an anesthesiologist is unlikely to be able to palpate the cricothyroid membrane accurately [5]. Misidentification of the cricothyroid membrane is a major reason for tube misplacement resulting in failed cricothyroidotomy, and in a CICO situation, serious complications, such as tension pneumothorax and pneumomediastinum [6, 7]. We have encountered a patient in whom a difficult airway was anticipated as a result of cervical hematoma caused by untreated hemophilia in whom we elected to use the double standby method. The CTM could not be identified by the conventional palpation technique but could be identified on ultrasonographic examination.

* Correspondence: kohji.fentanyl@gmail.com
Department of Anesthesiology , Kyorin University, School of Medicine 6-20-2 Shinkawa, Mitaka City, Tokyo 181-0004, Japan

Case presentation

A 28-year-old man (height 165 cm, body weight 80 kg, body mass index 29) with congenital hemophilia A was admitted to hospital with cervical swelling, difficulty vocalizing, and stridor during inspiration (Fig. 1). The patient had complied poorly with medication and discontinued treatment 6 months earlier. Laboratory tests revealed impaired coagulation (activated partial thromboplastin time 95.8 s, prothrombin time-international normalized ratio 1.04).

The patient's SpO₂ was 97% in room air and his respiratory rate was 10 breaths/min. One hour later, his respiratory distress had progressed to orthopnea and his SpO₂ had decreased to 92%. An otolaryngologist performed a transnasal endoscopic examination that revealed severe swelling and a large mass around the vocal cords (Fig. 2). These findings suggested the possibility of imminent suffocation and a need for urgent securing of the airway.

The attending otolaryngologist and anesthesiologists discussed how to secure the airway and agreed to prepare for double standby. However, the otolaryngologist could not identify the CTM by conventional palpation, so an anesthesiologist searched for the CTM using ultrasonographic examination. The search was started from just above the jugular notch of the sternal manubrium because this site looked anatomically normal. However, although the thyroid cartilage could be identified easily on a transverse view, no clear picture of the CTM could be obtained. The anesthesiologist subsequently identified the CTM on a longitudinal view (Fig. 3) and marked its location for surgical cricothyroidotomy.

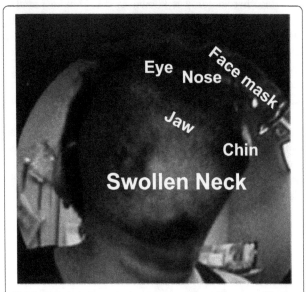

Fig. 1 Clinical photograph showing the neck swelling caused by the large hematoma

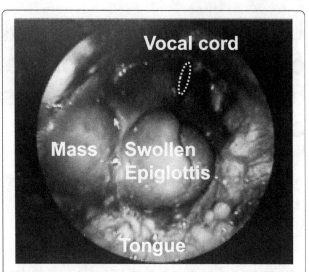

Fig. 2 Transnasal endoscopic findings in the laryngeal cavity. The image shows a swollen epiglottis with a mass on the right side of the epiglottis. The vocal cords can be seen under the swollen epiglottis

Awake fiberoptic intubation was successfully performed via an oral approach under topical anesthesia with 8% lidocaine spray and intravenous administration of fentanyl 100 μg. The patient's hypoxia did not worsen during the procedure. The patient was treated with steroid replacement therapy and coagulation factor VIII, and his glottic edema gradually resolved. The patient was extubated on day 6 and discharged without complications on day 13.

Discussion and conclusion

The guidelines for management of a difficult airway recommend incision or puncture of the CTM in a CICO situation. However, the fourth National Audit Project [8] reported that surgical securing of the airway under anesthesia in such circumstances had a 43% risk of serious complications.

Cricothyroidotomy by incision of the CTM is more reliable than puncture, and its success depends on correct identification of the CTM [9]. However, the CTM may be difficult to identify by the conventional palpation technique if it is not in the normal anatomical location [10]. In the present case, the otolaryngologist could not identify the superior thyroid notch by palpation because of the overlying hematoma. The conventional palpation technique is usually started from the superior thyroid notch as an anatomical landmark. Ultrasonographic guidance may have an advantage over conventional palpation for identifying the CTM in the event of an anatomical abnormality [10].

In our case, the CTM could not be identified by the widely used transverse ultrasound approach [5] because the patient's hematoma extended from the mandible to

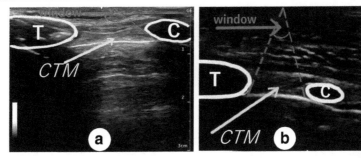

Fig. 3 Cervical ultrasonographic images obtained using the longitudinal approach. Either the transverse or longitudinal approach can be used for ultrasonographic identification of the cricothyroid membrane (CTM). Using the transverse approach, the operator manipulates the ultrasound probe while tilting it up and down on the patient's neck to locate the CTM; if the operator is attempting to locate a deeply positioned CTM (a), the angle of tilt of the probe may be restricted, and is shown as a window (a, red lettering). In contrast, if the CTM is in a shallow position (b), the angle of tilt of the probe may be wider using the transverse approach. However, there is no need to tilt the probe when using the longitudinal approach. **a** An ultrasonographic image of the patient's neck using the longitudinal approach. **b** An ultrasonographic image of the first author's neck using the longitudinal approach. The first author is a healthy male adult with a standard physique (height 174 cm, body weight 68 kg). T, thyroid cartilage; C, cricoid cartilage; CTM, cricothyroid membrane

the upper neck. The superior thyroid notch could not be identified by palpation, so the anesthesiologist started to scan from the patient's lower neck. A longitudinal ultrasound approach has been described but its efficacy is thought to be limited because the ultrasound probe cannot be positioned correctly on the skin surface in a patient with a short neck or severe cervical flexion deformity [5]. Kristensen et al. reported that the transverse and longitudinal approaches for ultrasonographic identification of the CTM in obese female subjects had a 90% success rate for identifying the CTM [7]. Interestingly, they found that neither approach was inferior to the other for identification of the CTM in obese patients [7]. The anesthesiologists' first choice in the report by Kristensen et al. was a transverse approach because they were familiar with it and unfamiliar with the longitudinal approach. However, our anesthesiologists could identify the CTM using the longitudinal approach but not the transverse approach. In our patient, the CTM was deep below the skin surface, which made it difficult to locate using the transverse approach because of the narrow searching space between the thyroid cartilage and the cricoid cartilage (Fig. 3).

Siddiqui et al. reported that ultrasonography successfully identified the CTM even in cadavers with poorly defined neck anatomy and speculated that ultrasonographic identification may reduce complications and improve the success rate of cricothyroidotomy [11]. The 2015 UK Difficult Airway Society guidelines recommend preoperative use of ultrasonography for identification of the CTM to ensure successful cricothyroidotomy in patients anticipated to have a difficult airway [3] but not otherwise, and with the caveat that ultrasonographic identification of the CTM might be unnecessarily time-consuming when the airway needs to be surgically secured in an emergency. We believe that ultrasonographic

identification of the CTM is not time-consuming when performed by a skilled operator. It has been reported that competence can be achieved by a short period of hands-on training [7, 12]. Therefore, training should make reliable identification of the CTM easier and ensure successful cricothyroidotomy.

The CTM could not be found by palpation in our patient but could be identified by ultrasonography. Fortunately, awake intubation was successful in this case. However, we cannot state with certainty that cricothyroidotomy would be successful using the method described here in a patient approaching CICO after awake intubation has failed. It is difficult to conduct high-quality clinical research on the success rate of cricothyroidotomy under ultrasonographic guidance, so the efficacy of identification of the CMT using this modality is still a matter of debate. However, it was recently found that ultrasound-guided identification of the cricothyroid membrane [6, 13] is highly effective and is comparable to a CT-scan as the accepted standard [14] in patients with abnormal neck anatomy. This strongly indicates that this technique can be applied for patients such as the one described in this report.

Abbreviations
CICO: "cannot intubate cannot oxygenate"; CTM: cricothyroid membrane

Acknowledgements
Not applicable.

Authors' contributions
JI: original draft writing. UK: conceptualization and draft writing. TJ: conceptualization, and editing. MS: procedure and draft writing. WK: procedure and conceptualization. YT: supervision and validation. All authors read and approved the final manuscript.

Authors' information
JI: Clinical Fellow.
UK: Assistant Professor.
TJ: Clinical Professor.

MS: Assistant Professor.
WK: Assistant Professor.
YT: Chief Professor.

References
1. Law JA, Broemling N, Cooper RM, Drolet P, Duggan LV, Griesdale DE, Hung OR, Jones PM, Kovacs G, Massey S, Morris IR, Mullen T, Murphy MF, Preston R, Naik VN, Scott J, Stacey S, Turkstra TP, Wong DT; Canadian Airway Focus Group. The difficult airway with recommendations for management--part 2--the anticipated difficult airway. Can J Anaesth. 2013;60:1119-38.
2. Apfelbaum JL, Hagberg CA, Caplan RA, Blitt CD, Connis RT, Nickinovich DG, Hagberg CA, Caplan RA, Benumof JL, Berry FA, Blitt CD, Bode RH, Cheney FW, Connis RT, Guidry OF, Nickinovich DG. Ovassapian A. American Society of Anesthesiologists Task Force on Management of the Difficult Airway Practice guidelines for management of the difficult airway: an updated report by the American Society of Anesthesiologists Task Force on Management of the Difficult Airway Anesthesiology. 2013;118:251-70.
3. Frerk C, Mitchell VS, McNarry AF, Mendonca C, Bhagrath R, Patel A, O'Sullivan EP, Woodall NM, Ahmad I; Difficult Airway Society intubation guidelines working group. Difficult Airway Society intubation guidelines working group. Difficult Airway Society 2015 guidelines for management of unanticipated difficult intubation in adults. Br J Anaesth. 2015;115:827-48.
4. Japanese Society of Anesthesiologists. JSA airway management guideline 2014: to improve the safety of induction of anesthesia. J Anesth. 2014;28: 482-93.
5. Kristensen MS, Teoh WH, Rudolph SS. Ultrasonographic identification of the cricothyroid membrane: best evidence, techniques, and clinical impact. Br J Anaesth. 2016;117(Suppl 1):i39-48.
6. Siddiqui N, Arzola C, Friedman Z, Guerina L, You-Ten KE. Ultrasound improves cricothyrotomy success in cadavers with poorly defined neck anatomy: a randomized control trial. Anesthesiology. 2015;123:1033-41.
7. Asai T. Surgical cricothyrotomy, rather than percutaneous cricothyrotomy, in "cannot intubate, cannot oxygenate" situation. Anesthesiology. 2016;125: 269-71.
8. Cook TM. Woodall N, Frerk C, fourth National Audit Project. Major complications of airway management in the UK: results of the fourth National Audit Project of the Royal College of Anaesthetists and the difficult airway society. Part 1: Anaesthesia. Br J Anaesth. 2011;106:617-31.
9. Okano H, Uzawa K, Watanabe K, Motoyasu A, Tokumine J, Lefor AK, Yorozu T. Ultrasound-guided identification of the cricothyroid membrane in a patient with a difficult airway: a case report. BMC Emerg Med. 2018;18:5.
10. Kristensen MS, Teoh WH, Rudolph SS, Hesselfeldt R, Børglum J, Tvede MF. A randomised cross-over comparison of the transverse and longitudinal techniques for ultrasound-guided identification of the cricothyroid membrane in morbidly obese subjects. Anaesthesia. 2016;71:675-83.
11. Oliveira KF, Arzola C, Ye XY, Clivatti J, Siddiqui N, You-Ten KE. Determining the amount of training needed for competency of anesthesia trainees in ultrasonographic identification of the cricothyroid membrane. BMC Anesthesiol. 2017;17:74.
12. Kristensen MS. Ultrasonography in the management of the airway. Acta Anaesthesiol Scand. 2011;55:1155-73.
13. Kristensen MS, Teoh WH, Rudolph SS, Hesselfeldt R, Borglum J, Tvede MF. A randomised cross-over comparison of the transverse and longitudinal techniques for ultrasound-guided identification of the cricothyroid membrane in morbidly obese subjects. Anaesthesia. 2016;71:675-83.
14. Siddiqui N, Yu E, Boulis S, You-Ten KE. Ultrasound is superior to palpation in identifying the cricothyroid membrane in subjects with poorly defined neck landmarks: a randomized clinical trial. Anesthesiology. 2018;129:1132-9.

28

Airway Management of the Right Anterior Segmentectomy through Uniportal video-assisted thoracoscopic surgery (VATS) after left pneumonectomy by an adapted double-lumen endobronchial tube (DLT)

Yang Gu[†], Ruowang Duan[†], Xin Lv and Jiong Song[*] ⓘ

Abstract

Background: Lung resection after previous contralateral pneumonectomy is rare. We present a case of right anterior segmentectomy despite previous left pneumonectomy, demanding special airway management strategy.

Case presentation: A 48-year-old woman who had left pneumonectomy 2 years ago was scheduled to have the right anterior segmentectomy through uniportal video-assisted thoracoscopy (VATS). A 32-French (Fr) left-sided double-lumen endobronchial tube (DLT) was chosen and adapted. The DLT was intubated into the bronchus intermedius. And the upper lobe can be isolated from the ventilation in the middle and lower lobes when the bronchial cuff's inflated. The perioperative period was uneventful and the pathological diagnosis was adenocarcinoma.

Conclusion: Lung cancer radical resection was discouraged after previous contralateral pneumonectomy partly due to the challenging ventilation and isolation. With this new DLT adapting and intubation technique showed in this case, the challenging ventilation and isolation that deter the implementation of the operation mentioned above could be solved.

Keywords: Double-lumen endobronchial tube, Pneumonectomy, Ventilation, Isolation

Background

Contralateral lung resection in postpneumonectomy patient is rare due to its significant perioperative mortality [1]. Thus, the experience in ventilation and isolation for this kind of operation is very limited. Double-lumen endobronchial tube (DLT) has been widely used in thoracic operations to acquire better surgical fields, and the left-sided DLTs are preferred over the right-sided DLTs, because of easier intubation, positioning and effective bilateral suctioning [2]. In postpneumonectomy patients, lung isolation with DLTs could be tricky due to one lung left only. Bronchial blockers (BB) are recommended in selective lobe blockade [3], however, BB is not omnipotent in selective lobe blockade, as in this case, selective right upper lobe blockade entails the balloon to be placed in the right upper lobe bronchus, however, the short right upper lobe bronchus and the angle of the right main bronchus and right upper lobe bronchus would make the placement even more difficult. We have obtained the approval from the Research Ethics Committee and a written patient consent for this report to be published.

* Correspondence: sw480@126.com; 896274362@qq.com
†Yang Gu and Ruowang Duan contributed equally to this work as first authors.
The Department of Anesthesiology, Tongji University Affiliated Shanghai Pulmonary Hospital, 507 Zhengmin Rd, Shanghai, China

Case presentation

A 48-year old woman (weight 52 kg, height 152 cm, ASA II) was admitted in Sept 18th 2016 because of a ground glass opacity (GGO) which had been detected in the right lung 2 years ago. She had her left pneumonectomy through uniportal VATS owing to the left upper lobe adenocarcinoma invasive to the left main bronchus in Mar 2014. Her pre-operative diagnoses were GGO in the right upper lobe, suspect for malignancy and left postpneumonectomy (Fig. 1). No abnormal findings were detected among other tests, and some of the important figures in the arterial blood gas test were showed as follows: pH 7.44, $PaCO_2$ 37 mmHg, PaO_2 84 mmHg, SaO_2 97.7%. Her pulmonary function test showed FEV1 46.9%, FEV1/FVC 83.3%, and her predicted postoperative $FEV_1\%$ would be close to 44.7%. Although other tests of evaluating cardiopulmonary reserve function and lung parenchymal function were not performed, her regular 3-floor climbing activity was not compromised. The operation was scheduled as right anterior segmentectomy through uniportal VATS under general anesthesia. Routine monitoring was applied and the first data were recorded as follows: body temperature 36.7 °C, blood pressure 123/70 mmHg, heart rate 86/min and SpO_2 98% when the patient was placed in a supine position in the operation room. After the insertion of an 18-gauge intravenous cannula and the right internal jugular vein catheter, intravenous induction was carried out with an injection of midazolam 0.03 mg/kg, sufentanil 0.6 µg/kg, propofol 1 mg/kg, and rocuronium 0.8 mg/kg. Intubation preparation: the patient was scheduled to have the right anterior segmentectomy through VATS after the left pneumonectomy, which entailed us to make a good balance between ventilation and collapse on the right lung only, to make good use of ventilation in the lower and middle lobes, and to produce an effective collapse in the upper lobar. After a prudent study of

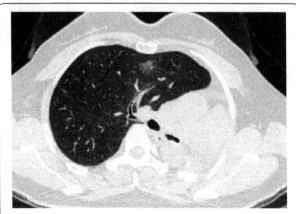

Fig. 1 CT (computed tomography) scan of the right anterior GGO (ground glass opacity) and postpneumonectomy

the following parameters, the diameter of the narrowest part of the tracheal is 11.9 mm, the length of right upper lobe bronchus is 6.2 mm, the angle of the right main bronchus and right upper lobe bronchus is close to 90 degree, the diameter of the bronchus intermedius is 8.8 mm, and the length of bronchus intermedius is about 15 mm, a 32 Fr left-sided DLT was chosen and adapted (Fig. 2). Permission was granted by our hospital ethical committee to adapt the DLTs. The cutting edge of the tube should be smooth and clean, only in this way can we make sure that it won't do any harm to the airways. One cut (cut just for once) would be best in adapting. Whether the cutting edge is qualified or not can be detected by our sensitive finger tips. And this technique has been proved safe from our experience in tracheal and bronchial operations. The 32Fr left-sided DLTs have been used among short women for left thoracic operations in our facility, and its external diameter is about 10.7 mm, the bronchial internal diameter is about 3.5 mm. But it's our first time to insert the left-sided DLT to the right for the right lung surgery. As we can see from Fig. 1, the mediastinum has shifted to the left, the intubation should be gentle and carried out by an experienced anesthesiologist in case of any possible injury or even perforation to the former carina. After induction, we performed a FOB (3.0 mm diameter) guided endobronchial intubation with the bronchial cuff into the right bronchus intermedius, and the tracheal cuff's orifice up against the upper bronchial port (Fig. 3), in this way, the ventilation of the dependent right middle and lower lobes and the collapse of the upper lobar were guaranteed (Fig. 4), thus an appropriate balance between surgical field and oxygenation was achieved, and the blood and sputum from the upper lobe bronchial port can be sucked out. An automatic infusion of propofol and sufentanil combined with manual administration of rocuronium maintained the anesthesia for the operation. And a lung protective mechanical ventilation strategy was taken, positive end-expiratory pressure (PEEP) 5 cmH_2O, tidal volume (Vt) 4–6 ml/kg, frequency 15–18/min. In the meantime, end tidal CO_2 and arterial blood gas analysis were recorded to adjust ventilation. The lung recruitment, air leak test and sputum suction went well throughout the operation and the surgery was completed as planned. The patient recovered well after the surgery, so she was extubated in the operation room and sent to the postanesthesia care unit (PACU) for transition, where a routine oxygen supplementation was applied. Oxygenation, ventilation, and circulation were all strictly monitored and no adverse events were recorded in the PACU. She recovered better on the next day follow-up and was discharged from the hospital 6 days later. The pathological diagnosis was invasive adenocarcinoma.

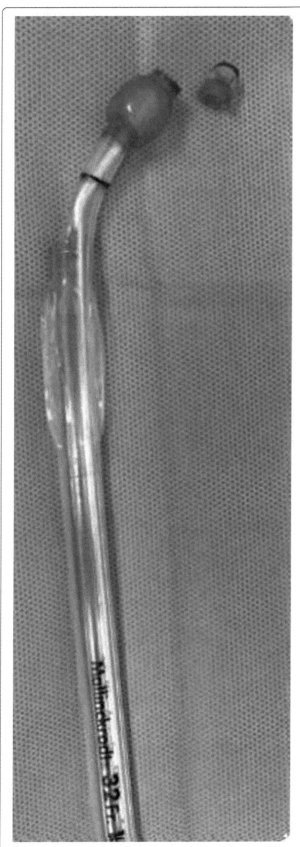

Fig. 2 The adapted DLT (double-lumen endobronchial tube)

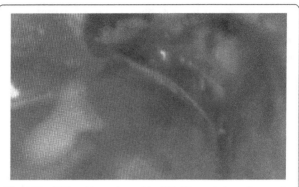

Fig. 3 The DLT position achieved by FOB (fiberoptic bronchoscopy)

Discussion and conclusion

It is a case of right lung surgery with previous left pneumonectomy, which entails the resection to be least impairment to the respiratory function and least trauma as well. Uniportal VATS right anterior segmentectomy should be the optimal choice because of its complete removal of the tumor while maximally functional lung kept, and smallest intercostal incision left.

However, this procedure is very challenging in lung ventilation, isolation and maintenance throughout the operation. Except for the way we have successfully implemented, other options could be recommended. First, a single-lumen tracheal tube (SLT) could be intubated into the right bronchus intermedius, this could make use of the ventilation in the middle and lower lobes, yet it also would lead to the upper lobar inflation, unless a detachment of the SLT with the cuff deflated and the ventilator was made before the establishment of pneumothorax. Besides, the blood and sputum from the

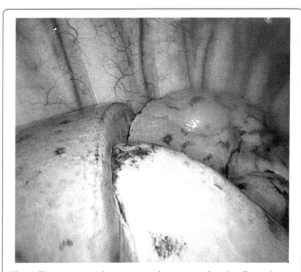

Fig. 4 The moment when pneumothorax completed, collapsed upper lobe and ventilated middle and lower lobes

upper lobe would be a problem since the export would have been blocked by the SLT. Another approach is BB. BB can be served for the purpose of one lung ventilation and selective lobar blockade in VATS, and also its advantages in children and difficult airway placement are widely-accepted [4]. As for this case, however, if BB were chosen, it should be placed into the right upper lobe bronchus, given the knowledge of the anatomical features, it would be more likely placed into some segmental bronchus of the right upper lobe, resulting in inflation in the right upper lobar; besides, even if by any chance, BB were suitably placed, it would have a great probability of being dispositioned given the thought of the short right upper lobe bronchus and the surgical intervention. Although DLT has rarely been taken in selective lobar blockade for lung resections [5], there was a precedent in partial sternotomy [6]. Comparing to partial sternotomy, we believe that lung resection, as in this case segmentectomy is more challenging in ventilation, isolation and drainage. First, we have to make sure the bronchial cuff is intubated into the bronchus intermedius, and it can protect the middle and lower lobes from the upper lobe contamination when inflated, and the bronchial orifice should be above the middle lobe bronchial port to guarantee the ventilation in the middle and lower lobes. But the length of bronchus intermedius varies, and that length was only about 15 mm in this woman while the length of bronchial cuff and the tip included was about 30 mm, so we cut off the tip (about 10 mm without damage to the cuff) and made it clean and smooth without any possible damage to the human body. Still, our approach has some limitations too, the bronchial cuff of this modified DLT was meant to be positioned in the bronchus intermedius, however, the shorter, the easier to be dispositioned; also, skilled adapting and intubation technique, and the recognition of the bronchial anatomy are needed.

But putting the DLT in the expected position doesn't guarantee a safe oxygenation, considering the middle and lower lobes only for ventilation. Although we assumed it would do, based on her preoperative arterial blood gas results and her daily exercise tolerance, still we asked for ECMO (extracorporeal membrane oxygenation) as an emergent plan in case of extreme low oxygenation. Our lung protective ventilation strategy was a combination of low Vt, high respiratory rate and a small PEEP. It's been showed in a meta-analysis that in patients without ARDS (acute respiratory distress syndrome), lower Vt is associated with better outcomes, including fewer lung injuries and less pulmonary infection [7]. However, Vt can't be too low to cause small and distal airways earlier closing and alveoli collapsing, leading to atelectasis, decreased ventilation/perfusion (V/Q) and increased intrapulmonary shunt. It's been demonstrated that a low Vt combined with an adequate PEEP could promote oxygenation, improve the desaturation status, and decrease the hypoxic lung injury [8].

In conclusion, we have succeeded in managing the ventilation in right middle and lower lobes and the upper lobar isolation by the adapted DLT, enlightening a new technique in selective lobar blockade, and the promotion of radical lung resection after previous pneumonectomy could be benefited.

Abbreviations

BB: Bronchial blocker; CT: Computed tomography; DLT: Double-lumen endobronchial tube; FOB: Fiberoptic bronchoscope; GGO: ground glass opacity; PACU: Postanesthesia care unit; PEEP: Positive end-expiratory pressure; SLT: Single-lumen tracheal tube; Tidal volume: Vt; V/Q: Ventilation/Perfusion; VATS: Video-assisted thoracoscopic surgery

Acknowledgements

All contributors for this study are those included in the authors.

Authors' contributions

GY and DRW contributed equally to the drafting and revision of the manuscript, LX revised the manuscript, SJ collected, analyzed and interpreted the patient data, reviewed the literature and revised the manuscript. All authors have critically revised the manuscript for important content, read, and approved the final manuscript.

References

1. Ayub A, Rehmani SS, Al-Ayoubi AM, Raad W, Flores RM, Bhora FY. Pulmonary resection for second lung Cancer after pneumonectomy: a population-based study. Ann Thorac Surg. 2017;104(4):1131–7.
2. Seo JH, Bae JY, Kim HJ, Hong DM, Jeon Y, Bahk JH. Misplacement of left-sided double-lumen tubes into the right mainstem bronchus: incidence, risk factors and blind repositioning techniques. BMC Anesthesiol. 2015;15:157.
3. Valencia Orgaz O, Real Navacerrada MI, Cortes Guerrero M, Garcia Gutierrez AF, Marron Fernandez C, Perez-Cerda Silvestre F. Lung isolation in patients with previous lung resections: selective sequential lobar blockade using a Fuji Uniblocker((R)) endobronchial blocker. Rev Esp Anestesiol Reanim. 2016;63(9):539–43.
4. Granell M, Parra MJ, Jimenez MJ, Gallart L, Villalonga A, Valencia O, Unzueta MC, Planas A, Calvo JM. Review of difficult airway management in thoracic surgery. Rev Esp Anestesiol Reanim. 2018;65(1):31–40.
5. Campos JH. Update on selective lobar blockade during pulmonary resections. Curr Opin Anaesthesiol. 2009;22(1):18–22.
6. Ng JM, Hartigan PM. Selective lobar bronchial blockade following contralateral pneumonectomy. Anesthesiology. 2003;98(1):268–70.
7. Serpa Neto A, Cardoso SO, Manetta JA, Pereira VG, Esposito DC, Pasqualucci Mde O, Damasceno MC, Schultz MJ. Association between use of lung-protective ventilation with lower tidal volumes and clinical outcomes among patients without acute respiratory distress syndrome: a meta-analysis. Jama. 2012;308(16):1651–9.
8. Vegh T, Juhasz M, Szatmari S, Enyedi A, Sessler DI, Szegedi LL, Fulesdi B. Effects of different tidal volumes for one-lung ventilation on oxygenation with open chest condition and surgical manipulation: a randomised cross-over trial. Minerva Anestesiol. 2013;79(1):24–32.

29

Effect of neck extension on the advancement of tracheal tubes from the nasal cavity to the oropharynx in nasotracheal intubation

Hyerim Kim[1], Jung-Man Lee[1]*⃝, Jiwon Lee[2], Jin-Young Hwang[1,3], Jee-Eun Chang[1], Hyun-Joung No[4], Dongwook Won[1], Hyung Sang Row[5] and Seong-Won Min[1,3]

Abstract

Background: Clinicians sometimes encounter resistance in advancing a tracheal tube, which is inserted via a nostril, from the nasal cavity into the oropharynx during nasotracheal intubation. The purpose of this study was to investigate the effect of neck extension on the advancement of tracheal tubes from the nasal cavity into the oropharynx during nasotracheal intubation.

Methods: Patients were randomized to the 'neck extension group (E group)' or 'neutral position group (N group)' for this randomized controlled trial. After induction of anesthesia, a nasal RAE tube was inserted via a nostril. For the E group, an anesthesiologist advanced the tube from the nasal cavity into the oropharynx with the patient's neck extended. For the N group, an anesthesiologist advanced the tube without neck extension. If the tube was successfully advanced into the oropharynx within two attempts by the same maneuver according to the assigned group, the case was defined as 'success.' We compared the success rate of tube advancement between the two groups.

Results: Thirty-two patients in the E group and 33 in the N group completed the trial. The success rate of tube passage during the first two attempts was significantly higher in the E group than in the N group (93.8% vs. 60.6%; odds ratio = 9.75, 95% CI = [1.98, 47.94], $p = 0.002$).

Conclusion: Neck extension during tube advancement from the nasal cavity to the oropharynx before laryngoscopy could be helpful in nasotracheal intubation.

Keywords: Intubation, Nasotracheal, Neck extension, Tracheal tube

* Correspondence: jungman007@gmail.com
[1]Department of Anesthesiology and Pain Medicine, Seoul Metropolitan Government Seoul National University Boramae Medical Center, 20 Boramae-ro 5-gil, Dongjak-gu, Seoul 07061, Republic of Korea

Background

Nasotracheal intubation is useful in some clinical situations, such as oral and maxillofacial surgery. Anesthesiologists sometimes encounter resistance in the advancement of a tracheal tube inserted via a nostril from the nasal cavity to the oropharynx before introducing a laryngoscope during nasotracheal intubation. This resistance might be caused by a large-sized tracheal tube compared to the nasal cavity [1] or blockage by the posterior wall of the nasopharynx. Clinicians can easily detect the former as a cause of resistance and resolve the problem by changing to a smaller tube. Regarding the latter cause, the blockage might be possibly due to that the angle between the nasal floor and posterior wall of the nasopharynx is about 90 degrees.

Previous review articles on nasotracheal intubation [2–4] have not addressed the role of neck extension in tracheal tube advancement from the nasal cavity to the oropharynx. A few previous articles introduced resistance in tube advancement from naso/oro-pharyngeal junctional space, and authors commented rotation of the tracheal tube inserted in the nasal cavity could help tube passage at the posterior nasopharynx [2, 3]. However, it has been not investigated yet. It is well known that neck extension is useful in laryngoscopy during tracheal intubation [5, 6]. However, this maneuver seems to be not well-acknowledged to most clinicians for tube advancement from the nasal cavity to the oropharynx in nasotracheal intubation.

Some previous studies presented that red rubber catheters or nasogastric tubes were helpful for safer nasotracheal intubation [7–9]. Even though these materials can help successful advancement of tracheal tubes from the nasal cavity to the oropharynx before laryngoscopy, the aid of them may need additional cost, time, and experienced assistants. If any method with significant efficiency for the advancement of tracheal tubes from the nasal cavity to the oropharynx will be introduced, that will be meaningful.

The aim of this study was to assess the effect of neck extension during the advancement of a tracheal tube from the nasal cavity to the oropharynx on the success of tube advancement. The primary hypothesis of this study was that neck extension could assist in the successful advancement of a tracheal tube from the nasal cavity to the oropharynx in nasotracheal intubation.

Methods

This prospective, randomized controlled study was approved by the institutional review board of the Seoul Metropolitan Government Seoul National University Boramae Medical Center (no: 16–2017-64), and written informed consent was obtained from all subjects. The trial was registered prior to patient enrollment at ClinicalTrials.gov (NCT03377114). This manuscript adheres to the applicable 2010 CONsolidated Standards of Reporting Trials guidelines. American Society of Anesthesiologists (ASA) physical status I-II adult patients (≥ 18 years old) requiring nasotracheal intubation were recruited between December 2017 and June 2018. Patients with cervical spine instability, coagulopathy, history of taking an anticoagulant, or those in need of awake intubation were excluded from this study.

Patients were randomly assigned to the neck extension group or the neutral position group with 1:1 ratio. An investigator who did not participate in this study generated the randomization allocation sequence using computer-generated block randomization (4-sized blocks, including letters A and B). Each generated letter was concealed in a sequentially numbered opaque envelope. Enrolled patients were allocated to the assigned groups depending on the letter (A to the neck extension group and B to the neutral position group) inside the envelope, and the concealed envelope was opened in an operating theatre by an assistant nurse on the operating day. We blinded the assigned group to each patient in the trial.

Patients were admitted to the operating theatre without any premedication. Patients were positioned on the operating table in a supine position with a standard pillow under the head. A preformed nasal RAE (Ring-Adair-Elwyn) tube (Mallinckrodt Preformed Nasal RAE tube; Covidien, Mansfield, MA) was softened in warm sterile saline at 45 °C prior to use (inner diameter (ID) 6.5 mm for females, 7.0 mm for males). Pulse oximetry, electrocardiography, and non-invasive arterial blood pressure were monitored in a standard manner. Anesthesia was induced with intravenous administration of glycopyrrolate (0.2 mg), lidocaine (30 mg), propofol (1.5 mg/kg), and fentanyl (100 μg). After confirming that patients became unconscious, patients' lungs were ventilated by manual bag/mask ventilation with oxygen and sevoflurane after the nares were topically pretreated with sterile cotton swabs soaked with a diluted solution of 0.01% epinephrine. Next, rocuronium (0.6 mg/kg) was administered to achieve muscle relaxation for tracheal intubation. During manual bagging, an investigator measured the distance from the midpoint of the nasal tip to the posterior wall of the nasopharynx using a fiberscope with an outer diameter of 4.1 mm (Olympus LE-P; Olympus Optical Co. Tokyo, Japan) with a brief pause in manual bagging. Immediately prior to nasotracheal intubation, the thermo-softened RAE tube was well lubricated with lidocaine jelly and gently inserted into the nostril that was determined to be most suitable for surgery with the nasal tip lifting maneuver [10]. When the tube was inserted into the nasal cavity approximately 3–4 cm, further advancement of it into the oropharynx was performed as followings in accordance with the assigned group. In the neck extension group, an anesthesiologist advanced the tube into the oropharynx after extending the patient's neck, as shown in Fig. 1a. Neck extension during tube advancement was performed with a routinely used manner, without any fixed angle, for tracheal intubation in common clinical situations. For patients in the neutral position group, the intubation performer continued to advance the tube to the oropharynx with the patient's head in a neutral position, as shown in Fig. 1b. During this advancement, the performer and the investigator checked the resistance by blockage at the posterior wall of the nasopharynx. In the case of blockage, the investigator measured the inserted length of the tube at the moment of blockage by using thread as in a previous study [11]. Following this measurement in the case of blockage, we attempted to advance the tube one more with the same maneuver after withdrawing the tube 1–2 cm. If tube advancement succeeded within the two attempts, we recorded the case as 'success.' Otherwise, we recorded the case as 'failure.' In the case of 'failure,' we tried to advance the tube into the oropharynx with alternative methods including change of neck position for tracheal intubation. After finally successful advancement of the tube into the oropharynx, standard nasotracheal intubation was performed using a laryngoscope with the

aid of Magill forceps. During this intubation procedure, a second investigator recorded the time from initiation of tube insertion via the nares to passage of the tube into the oropharynx and total intubation time. Individuals who performed tracheal intubation were board-certified anesthesiologists.

After completion of nasotracheal intubation, another investigator checked whether the tube had passed through the upper pathway or the lower pathway with the fiberscope as in a previous study [10]. Also, the investigator checked the presence and grade of epistaxis or nasopharyngeal bleeding. The severity of epistaxis or nasopharyngeal bleeding was classified as "no bleeding," "blood-tinged mucus," "mild bleeding," or "severe bleeding."

Statistical analysis

Patient characteristics and outcome measures, including patient age, height, weight, body mass index (BMI), and intubation time are presented as the mean ± standard deviation (SD). Numbers with percentages are presented for sex and the success in advancing a tracheal tube from the nasal cavity to the oropharynx in the first two attempts (the first and second attempts). Additionally,

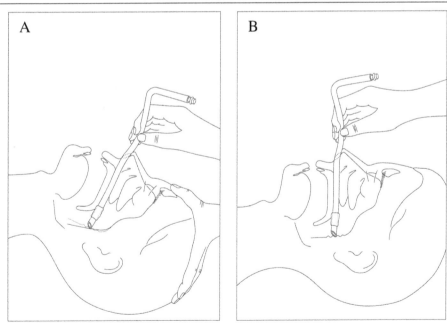

Fig. 1 Schematic diagram of two methods with or without neck extension for tube advancement from the nasal cavity into the oropharynx. **a** depicts advancement of a preformed nasal RAE tube with neck extension. With neck extension, the angle between the axis of the distal part of the tube and the posterior wall of the nasopharynx could be obtuse, and the wrinkled soft tissue might be spread, such as a change from dotted lines to solid lines. Based on our results, we hypothesized that these possible changes might aid smooth advancement of the tube. However, these hypotheses were not investigated in the study. **b** depicts advancement of a preformed nasal RAE tube without neck extension (neutral head position). Although not presented in the results, the angle between the nasal floor and the posterior wall of the nasopharynx, without neck extension, was measured as about 100 degrees in the sagittal view of maxillofacial computed tomography of 39 among the study subjects. Also, we observed the angle became widen with neck extension in 3 patients who were preoperatively examined about cervical spine mobility, when we reviewed radiologic findings of cervical spine series of flexion/neutral/extension postures. RAE indicates Ring-Adair-Elwyn

the incidence by which tracheal tubes passed through the lower pathway in the nasal cavity and the incidence of epistaxis or nasopharyngeal bleeding are presented as numbers with percentages.

We compared the success rate in advancing the inserted tube via a nostril from the nasal cavity to the oropharynx in the first two attempts between the two groups (primary outcome) with a χ^2 test. We compared the incidence of nasal bleeding between two groups with a χ^2 test. We assessed the incidence of tube passing pathway to verify the results of our previous study [10]. We also assessed the intubation times between two groups with Student's t-test. The odds ratio or mean difference was calculated for appropriate outcomes. A p-value < 0.05 was considered statistically significant. Statistical analyses were performed using SPSS Statistics 21.0 software (IBM Corporation, Chicago, IL, USA).

During a literature search, we could not find any previous study investigating the subject of our study. Therefore, we initially planned to perform this trial as a pilot study with a sample size of 66 (33 for each group). We hoped that we would obtain 80% power at the 0.05 significance level to determine that neck extension could help increase the success rate during the first two attempts by 30% compared with a neutral head position. If this goal was reached in this pilot study, we planned to represent the results as the final results of the study on this issue. Alternatively, we planned to perform an additional study with an appropriately calculated sample size on the basis of the results of the present study.

Results

Patient screening, enrollment, randomization, and analysis are shown in the CONSORT flow diagram in Fig. 2. Sixty-six patients requiring nasotracheal intubation for general anesthesia were enrolled in the study. Patients were randomly assigned to the two groups with a 1:1 ratio. Sixty-five patients completed the present study. One patient in the E group declined participation of the study after the assignment of a group. The demographic data of all patients, who completed the study in both groups, are presented in Table 1. Tracheal intubation was finally successful in all participants. There was no important harm or unintended effect in all participants.

The success rate of tube passage in the first two attempts was higher in the E group than in the N group (93.8% vs. 60.6%, odds ratio (OR) = 9.75; 95% confidence interval (CI) = [1.98, 47.94], $p = 0.002$). Additionally, the success rate of smooth advancement of the tube during the first attempt was significantly higher in the E group (87.5%) than in the N group (51.5%) (OR = 6.59, 95% CI = [1.89, 23.01], $p = 0.003$).

The mean insertion time from tube insertion via the nares to the tube passing into the oropharynx was shorter in the E group (10.3 ± 6.6 s) than the N group (16.5 ± 14.8 s) ($p = 0.035$). However, there was no significant difference among patients who were successfully intubated during the first attempt without any blockage between the two groups (9.3 ± 3.9 s in 28 patients of the E group, 8.2 ± 2.3 s in 17 patients of the N group, $p = 0.720$). The total intubation time was not significantly different between the two groups (61.2 ± 35.3 s in the E group, 69.6 ± 37.4 s in the N group, $p = 0.356$). There was no significant difference in the incidence of epistaxis or nasopharyngeal bleeding between the two groups (5/32 in the E group, 11/33 in the N group; OR = 0.40, 95% CI = [0.20, 2.15], $p = 0.150$). All patients who experienced nasal bleeding in both groups exhibited 'blood-tinged' mucus (Table 2).

For 20 patients who experienced tube blockage in the first attempt, the discrepancy between the distance from the midpoint of the nares to the posterior wall of the nasopharynx and the length of the inserted part of the tracheal tube, which was measured when the tube was blocked during advancement into the oropharynx, was not different (mean difference = 0.18 ± 0.48 cm, 95% CI = [− 0.41, 0.46]) ($p = 0.111$).

Tracheal tubes passed through the lower pathway of the nasal cavity in 47 patients when we inserted the tube via a nostril with nasal tip lifted in all patients of both groups (72.3, 95% CI = [61.3, 83.3%]) (Table 3).

Discussion

Our study demonstrated that neck extension during advancing a tracheal tube from the nasal cavity into the oropharyngeal space could assist in smooth passage of the tube. For successful nasotracheal intubation, some previous studies have focused on tube impingement and solutions [12–15]. However, these previous studies mentioned impingement at the hypopharyngeal and laryngeal space but not at the naso/oro-pharyngeal space in fiberoptic intubation. For example, the tube can be impinged at the arytenoid cartilage, vocal cord, epiglottis, or esophageal inlet in fiberoptic nasotracheal intubation, which can be solved by counter-clockwise tube rotation after withdrawal the tube 2–3 cm [14]. Also, if the block occurs due to small-sized nostril before advancing the tube, clinicians can easily realize and solve the problem with changing the nostril side or tube size. Even though there are not these two situations, clinicians commonly encounter resistance in the process of advancing the tube, when it reaches at the posterior wall of the naso-pharynx [3]. Our study presented the impingement of the tube in the naso/oro-pharyngeal space and the solution for this issue. Our results showed that the straight distance from the midpoint of the nares to the posterior wall of nasopharynx was very similar to the inserted tube length when the tube was blocked during advancement.

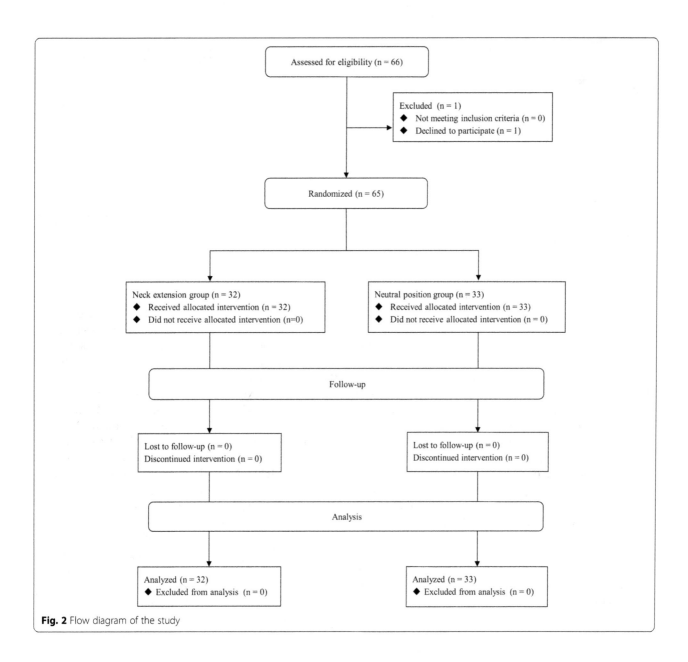

Fig. 2 Flow diagram of the study

Table 1 Patient characteristics

Patient characteristics	Neck extension group ($n = 32$)	Neutral position group ($n = 33$)
Gender (M / F)	17/ 15	21 / 12
Age (y)	42.3 ± 18.2	41.5 ± 18.6
Height (cm)	165.4 ± 10.4	167.2 ± 10.0
Weight (kg)	65.8 ± 13.9	66.5 ± 12.1
BMI (kg/m^2)	23.8 ± 3.6	23.7 ± 3.5
Nose-posterior wall of nasopharynx distance (cm)	9.6 ± 0.8	9.7 ± 0.8

BMI body mass index. Data are presented as the mean ± standard deviation or numbers

Table 2 Primary and secondary outcomes in the two groups

	Neck extension group (n = 32)	Neutral position group (n = 33)	OR or MD [95% CI]	P-value
Primary outcome				
Success rate in tube advancement at the first two attempts	30/32 (93.8%)	20/33 (60.6%)	9.75 [1.98, 47.94]	0.002
Secondary outcomes				
Nasal bleeding				
Incidence, n(%)	5 (15.6%)	11 (33.3%)	0.4 [0.20, 2.15]	0.150
Severity (no/tinged/mild/severe), n	27/ 5 / 0/ 0	22/ 11/ 0/ 0		
Intubation time				
Time from initiation of inserting tube to passing into oropharynx (s)	10.3 ± 6.6	16.5 ± 14.8	−6.2 [− 11.9, − 0.5]	0.035
Total intubation time (s)	61.2 ± 35.3	69.6 ± 37.4	−8.4 [− 26.4, 9.7]	0.356

OR odds ratio, MD mean difference, CI confidence interval

We hypothesized that the angle between the posterior wall of the nasopharynx and nasal floor was about 90 degrees. Although we could not find out any reference about the angle, the mean of the angle and SD was 100.3 ± 7.8 degree when we measured the angle in a sagittal view of preoperative computed tomography images of 39 subjects among all participants in our study. Wrinkles in the posterior nasopharyngeal wall might be a possible cause of blockage because the wall is covered by lymphoid tissue that often undergoes hypertrophy (adenoid) during the transition period to puberty [16]. There are some folds such as salpingopharyngeal fold, salpingopalatine fold, or torus tubarius [17].

For blockage in tube passing from the nasal cavity to the oropharynx, clinicians usually try re-advancing 2–3 times, which can increase the possibility of nasal bleeding. In extreme cases, the tube might perforate the posterior wall [18–22]. Therefore, some experienced clinicians gently rotate the shaft of the inserted tube in the nasal cavity or extend the patient's neck while advancing the tube like as our study protocol.

We supposed that neck extension could lead to the traction of naso/oro-pharyngeal soft tissue, as shown in Fig. 1a and b. That is, we hypothesized that the soft tissue could be tightened from Fig. 1b to Fig. 1a, which could make the angle between the posterior wall of the nasopharynx and nasal floor more obtuse than neutral position (about 100 degrees in 39 subjects of our study). Finally, this extension can force the tube tip to slide more smoothly across the surface of the posterior wall of the nasopharynx toward the oral cavity. Additionally, we hypothesized that these series of processes could help in spreading the wrinkles of the posterior pharyngeal wall, which can lead to smooth passage of the tube.

However, these hypotheses were not verified in our study. Nevertheless, we identified that the neck extension could increase the angle between the nasal floor and the posterior wall of the pharynx when we observe the cervical spine lateral view with the patient's neck flexed/neutral/extended in 3 of our study subjects. The angle changed 103.2–107.8-116.8, 84.6–92.4-102.4, and 89.6–93.8-99.3 degrees respectively in them. Also, we identified that soft tissue such as folds of the posterior nasopharyngeal wall of some patients widened and slightly stretched by neck extension when we observed the posterior wall of the nasopharynx with otolaryngologists using a rigid endoscope in clinical situation of endoscopic sinus surgeries.

Neck extension can lead to the alignment of the three axes, including the oral axis, pharyngeal axis, and tracheal axis [6]. Alignment provides physicians the best view of the glottic opening with a laryngoscope for tracheal intubation. Therefore, neck extension is a very familiar maneuver for clinicians in tracheal intubation. Moreover, this maneuver is very easy to perform and is acceptable for most patients except for those with cervical spine injury [23]. Therefore, this maneuver can easily reduce the spent on nasotracheal intubation and improve patient safety.

We evaluated the tube passing pathway to verify the results of our previous study [10]. Unfortunately, our previous study had a small sample size by mistake. Therefore, it had lower power than originally planned. In the present study, we initially inserted the tracheal tube via a nostril with a nasal tip lifted in all subjects. As

Table 3 The incidence of tracheal tube passage through the lower pathway in the nasal cavity

	Neck extension group (n = 32)	Neutral position group (n = 33)	Total (n = 65)
Lower pathway, n(%) [95% CI]	22 (68.8%)	25 (75.8%)	47 (72.3%) [61.3, 83.3%]

Lower pathway indicates the pathway below the inferior turbinate and above the nasal floor in the nasal cavity. CI confidence interval

a result, 72.3% of tubes passed the lower pathway in the nasal cavity. These results were similar to our previous data (78%) in the nasal tip lifting group [10]. Therefore, the results of our present study supported the results of our previous study.

Tube passage from the nasal cavity to the oropharynx was successfully achieved within the first two attempts in the majority of our study subjects. However, tube passage was attempted four times in 4 patients and five times in 1 patient in our study regardless of the group. We thought that the advancement of the inserted tube should be tried 2–3 times to minimize mucosal injury. According to Lim et al., the Levin tube is useful for guiding a tracheal tube for nasotracheal intubation [9]. Therefore, use of it should be considered after 2–3 times failed tube advancements.

In our study, the time was about 10 s on average for passing the tube into the oropharynx in the neck extension group. Considering a simple process of tube passing into the oropharynx from initiation of tube insertion via a nostril, 10 s may be considered a rather long time. To prevent any injury during nasotracheal intubation, clinicians usually perform thermosoftening and local vasoconstriction like as our practice in the study. Also, gentle advancement of the tube through the nasal pathway and naso/oro-pharyngeal junctional space must be important to minimize injury. However, clinicians tend to be tempted to apply a little more force for the advancement of it into the oral cavity during nasotracheal intubation. Additional force may be effective to shorten the required time for tube passing. However, that can cause mucosal injury in some cases. We focused the minimal mucosal injury and emphasized using minimal force to advance the tube in this trial. Therefore, we needed 10 s for tube passing in the extension group. Although the total of 16 patients experienced nasal bleeding, the severity of it was 'blood-tinged' for all of them in our study. They did not need any specific treatment for nasal bleeding. Also, gentle force could affect the success rate of tube passing in the first two attempts. If we had used additional force in tube passing, the success rate would have been higher than our results in both groups.

Our study had many limitations. First, our study had a small sample size. During the literature search, we found no previous studies focusing on our hypothesis. Therefore, we initially designed the present study as a pilot study because we could not calculate adequate sample size. However, when we calculated the sample size based on the hypothesized results of this trial, the required sample size was 64 (32 for each group) with 80% power at the 0.05 significance level. We assumed that the success rate for smooth tube passage into the oropharynx in the first two

attempts would be increased by 30% with neck extension compared with 60% with the neutral neck position based on our data (60.6%). Therefore, according to our sample size calculation, we decided that the trial should be terminated without increasing the sample size. Second, our study did not overcome the influence of confounding covariates from personal difference in terms of anatomy. If we performed this randomized controlled study with larger sample size or planned a randomized crossover design study for our interest, we could have minimized the confounding effect. However, we did this study with small sample size, and we could not perform a crossover design study due to ethical reason. If we designed this study with a crossover manner, we had to retry to pass the tube with an alternative method (neck extension or neutral) for a patient after pulling back the tube even though the tube passed successfully into the oropharynx with the first maneuver. Third, we could not thoroughly blind the study protocol to intubation performers because it was difficult to blind anesthesiologists for our study design, including tracheal intubation. Although the outcomes of this study such as success rate were objective variables, there still might be bias from that. However, we believed that intubation performers tried to do their best to pass the tube smoothly from the nasal cavity to oropharynx in all cases of the two groups. Finally, we could not found the exact reason why the neck extension could be helpful for smooth advancing the tube from the nasal cavity to the oropharynx. We just conjectured the angle could become slightly widen by neck extension from cervical spine radiologic series of only three subjects. And, we just observed soft tissue of the posterior nasopharyngeal wall became widen and slightly stretched by neck extension in some patients. Therefore, further study should be necessary to investigate our hypotheses.

Conclusions
Neck extension during tube advancement from the nasal cavity to the oropharynx may facilitate the tube advancement in nasotracheal intubation. We suggest that this maneuver should be standard for tube advancement for nasotracheal intubation.

Abbreviations
ASA: American Society of Anesthesiologists; BMI: body mass index; ID: Inner diameter; OR: Odds ratio; RAE: Ring-Adair-Elwyn; SD: Standard deviation

Acknowledgements
The authors would like to thank Sohee Oh, Ph.D. (Medical Statistician, Department of Biostatistics in SMG-SNU Boramae Medical Center), for statistical advice and analysis.

Authors' contributions

HK participated in data acquisition, statistical analysis, data interpretation, revised and drafted the manuscript. JML participated in study design, data acquisition, statistical analysis, data interpretation, revised and drafted the manuscript. JL participated in data interpretation and drafted the manuscript. JYH participated in data acquisition and data interpretation. JEC participated in data acquisition and data interpretation. HJN participated in data acquisition and data interpretation. DW participated in data acquisition and data interpretation. HSR participated in data acquisition. SWM participated in data acquisition. All authors read and approved the final manuscript.

Author details

¹Department of Anesthesiology and Pain Medicine, Seoul Metropolitan Government Seoul National University Boramae Medical Center, 20 Boramae-ro 5-gil, Dongjak-gu, Seoul 07061, Republic of Korea. ²Department of Anesthesiology and Pain Medicine, Keimyung University Dongsan Medical Center, Keimyung University School of Medicine, 1095 Dalgubeol-daero, Dalseo-gu, Daegu 42601, Republic of Korea. ³Department of Anesthesiology and Pain Medicine, Seoul National University College of Medicine, 101 Daehak-ro, Jongno-gu, Seoul 03080, Republic of Korea. ⁴Department of Anesthesiology and Pain Medicine, Anesthesia and Pain Research Institute, Yonsei University College of Medicine, 50-1 Yonsei-ro, Seodaemun-gu, Seoul 03722, Republic of Korea. ⁵Department of Anesthesiology and Pain Medicine, Seoul National University Hospital, 101 Daehak-ro, Jongno-gu, Seoul 03080, Republic of Korea.

References

1. Futagawa K, Takasugi Y, Kobayashi T, Morishita S, Okuda T. Role of tube size and intranasal compression of the nasotracheal tube in respiratory pressure loss during nasotracheal intubation: a laboratory study. BMC Anesthesiol. 2017;17(1):141.
2. Hall CE, Shutt LE. Nasotracheal intubation for head and neck surgery. Anaesthesia. 2003;58(3):249–56.
3. Prasanna D, Bhat S. Nasotracheal intubation: an overview. J Maxillofac Oral Surg. 2014;13(4):366–72.
4. Chauhan V, Acharya G. Nasal intubation: a comprehensive review. Indian J Crit Care Med. 2016;20(11):662–7.
5. Horton WA, Fahy L, Charters P. Defining a standard intubating position using "angle finder". Br J Anaesth. 1989;62(1):6–12.
6. Matsumoto T, de Carvalho WB. Tracheal intubation. J Pediatr. 2007;83(2 Suppl):S83–90.
7. Wong A, Subar P, Witherell H, Ovodov KJ. Reducing nasopharyngeal trauma: the urethral catheter-assisted nasotracheal intubation technique. Anesth Prog. 2011;58(1):26–30.
8. Garside M, Hatfield A. Using Jaques Nelaton catheter as an introducer for nasotracheal intubation. Anaesthesia. 2014;69(12):1399–401.
9. Lim CW, Min SW, Kim CS, Chang JE, Park JE, Hwang JY. The use of a nasogastric tube to facilitate nasotracheal intubation: a randomised controlled trial. Anaesthesia. 2014;69(6):591–7.
10. Kim H, Lee JM, Lee J, Hwang JY, Chang JE, No HJ, Won D, Choi S, Min SW. Influence of nasal tip lifting on the incidence of the tracheal tube pathway passing through the nostril during Nasotracheal intubation: a randomized controlled trial. Anesth Analg. 2018;127(6):1421–6.
11. Lee J, Lee JM, Min JJ, Koo CH, Kim HJ. Optimal length of the pre-inserted tracheal tube for excellent view in nasal fiberoptic intubation. J Anesth. 2016;30(2):187–92.
12. Dogra S, Falconer R, Latto IP. Successful difficult intubation. Tracheal tube placement over a gum-elastic bougie. Anaesthesia. 1990;45(9):774–6.
13. Katsnelson T, Frost EA, Farcon E, Goldiner PL. When the endotracheal tube will not pass over the flexible fiberoptic bronchoscope. Anesthesiology. 1992;76(1):151–2.
14. Asai T, Shingu K. Difficulty in advancing a tracheal tube over a fibreoptic bronchoscope: incidence, causes and solutions. Br J Anaesth. 2004;92(6):870–81.
15. Solanki SL, Kaur J. "two-hand-manoeuver" during nasotracheal intubation. Saudi J Anaesth. 2017;11(4):512.
16. Vilella Bde S, Vilella Ode V, Koch HA. Growth of the nasopharynx and adenoidal development in Brazilian subjects. Braz Oral Res. 2006;20(1):70–5.

17. Simkins CS. Functional anatomy of the eustachian tube. Arch Otolaryngol. 1943;38(5):476–84.
18. Kras JF, Marchmont-Robinson H. Pharyngeal perforation during intubation in a patient with Crohn's disease. J Oral Maxillofac Surg. 1989;47(4):405–7.
19. Bozdogan N, Sener M, Yavuz H, Yilmazer C, Turkoz A, Arslan G. Retropharyngeal submucosal dissection due to nasotracheal intubation. B-ENT. 2008;4(3):179–81.
20. Ersoy B, Gursoy T, Celebiler O, Umuroglu T. A complication of nasotracheal intubation after mandibular subcondylar fracture. J Craniofac Surg. 2011;22(4):1527–9.
21. Kamatani T, Kohzuka Y, Kondo S, Shirota T, Iijima T, Shintani S. Retropharyngeal dissection: a case report of cervicofacial subcutaneous emphysema and mediastinal emphysema during attempted nasotracheal intubation. J Anesth. 2013;27(5):785–6.
22. Hakim M, Cartabuke RS, Krishna SG, Veneziano G, Syed A, Lind MN, Tobias QD. Submucosal dissection of the retropharyngeal space during nasal intubation. Middle East J Anaesthesiol. 2015;23(3):309–14.
23. Durga P, Sahu BP. Neurological deterioration during intubation in cervical spine disorders. Indian J Anaesth. 2014;58(6):684–92.

30

Supreme™ laryngeal mask airway insertion requires a lower concentration of sevoflurane than ProSeal™ laryngeal mask airway insertion during target-controlled remifentanil infusion

Cristina Monteserín-Matesanz[1], Tatiana González[1], María José Anadón-Baselga[2] and Matilde Zaballos[1,2]*

Abstract

Background: ProSeal (PLMA) and Supreme (SLMA) laryngeal mask airways are effective ventilator devices with distinctive designs that may require different anaesthetics for insertion. Sevoflurane induction provides acceptable conditions for laryngeal mask insertion, and remifentanil significantly decreases the minimum alveolar concentration of sevoflurane required for that insertion. The study aimed to evaluate the optimal end-tidal (ET) sevoflurane concentration for successful insertion of PLMA versus SLMA in patients receiving a remifentanil infusion without a neuromuscular blocking agent.

Methods: Altogether, 45 patients ASA (American Society Anaesthesiologists) physical status I–II, aged 18–60 years were scheduled for elective ambulatory surgery. Exclusion criteria were a difficult airway, recent respiratory infection, reactive airway, obstructive sleep apnoea syndrome, gastric aspiration's risk factors, pregnancy, and lactation. Patients were randomly allocated to receive the SLMA or the PLMA. Sevoflurane induction with co-administration of remifentanil was performed at an effect-site concentration of $4\,ng\,mL^{-1}$. ET_{50} was calculated with a modified Dixon's up-and-down method (starting at 2.5% in steps of 0.5%). Predetermined sevoflurane concentration was kept constant during the 10 min before LMA insertion. Patient's response to LMA insertion was classified as "movement" or "no movement". Sevoflurane ET_{50} was determined as the midpoint concentration of all the independent pairs that manifested crossover from "movement" to "no movement".

Results: The ET_{50} sevoflurane concentration co-administered with remifentanil required for PLMA insertion was $1.20 \pm 0.41\%$ (95% confidence interval 0.76 to 1.63%). For SLMA insertion, it was $0.55 \pm 0.38\%$ (95% confidence interval 0.14 to 0.95%) ($p = 0.019$).

Conclusions: The end-tidal sevoflurane concentration with co-administered remifentanil required to allow insertion of the SLMA was 54% lower than that needed for inserting the PLMA.

(Continued on next page)

* Correspondence: mati@plagaro.net
[1]Anaesthesia department, Hospital General Universitario Gregorio Marañón, C/ Doctor Esquerdo, N° 46, 28007 Madrid, Spain
[2]Department of Legal Medicine, Psychiatry and Pathology Universidad Complutense, Madrid, Spain

(Continued from previous page)

Keywords: End-tidal sevoflurane concentration, Supraglottic airway devices, Remifentanil effect-site concentration, Laryngeal mask airway supreme, Laryngeal mask airway Proseal

Background

The ProSeal™ laryngeal mask airway (PLMA) (Teleflex, Teleflex Medical Europe, Westmeath, Ireland) was the first second-generation reusable device designed to separate the gastrointestinal and respiratory tracts. It exhibited safety and efficacy as an instrument for providing adequate ventilation during general anaesthesia even for advanced clinical uses [1]. The Supreme™ laryngeal mask airway (SLMA) (Teleflex, Teleflex Medical Europe, Westmeath, Ireland) was developed in 2007 as a modified single-use second-generation device that combines the design of the Fastrach™ laryngeal mask airway (Teleflex, Teleflex Medical Europe, Westmeath, Ireland) and the PLMA. The gastric tube of the SLMA is incorporated within an oval airway tube designed to match the shape of the mouth and oropharyngeal inlet and facilitate its insertion [2].

The two devices have differences in their structure, design, and components, which means different compression in the pharyngeal structures during the placement phase and thus influencing the anaesthetic requirements. The anaesthetic strategy commonly used for insertion of LMAs relies on administration of an intravenous (propofol) or a volatile (sevoflurane) induction agent with or without a co-induction agent such as an opioid (fentanyl, alfentanil, remifentanil), midazolam, or lidocaine [3–6]. The use of a co-induction agent could facilitate and significantly reduce the dose of induction agent required for LMA insertion.

Previous studies have compared the effectiveness and safety of the PLMA and SLMA in different clinical scenarios, showing differences regarding the oropharyngeal leak pressure, success rate, insertion time, and airway complications [7–10]. In contrast, little information is available regarding the optimal end-tidal sevoflurane concentration when used for co-induction with remifentanil to ensure successful LMA insertion.

Because of the features of the SLMA and its ease of insertion, we hypothesised that the predicted end-tidal (ET) concentration of sevoflurane during co-induction with a target-controlled infusion of remifentanil (4 ng/ml) without neuromuscular blocking drugs in adult patients would be lower than that for PLMA.

Methods
Study design
We conducted a single-centre, double-blind, randomised controlled trial registered at www.clinicaltrials.gov (number

NCT03003377). Ethical approval for this study (Ethical Committee code FIBHGM-ECNC002–2013) was provided by the Ethics Committee of Hospital General Universitario Gregorio Marañón, Madrid, Spain (Chairman Dr. Fernando Díaz Otero) on 12 June 2013. Patient were consecutively enrolled in the study from November 2014, to October 2015. This study is reported in accordance with the CONSORT-Statement.

Participants
We enrolled 55 patients (ASA physical class I–II, aged 18–60 years) scheduled for elective ambulatory surgery under general anaesthesia and in whom the use of a supraglottic airway was indicated. We excluded patients with more than three criteria for a difficult airway [Mallampati III–IV, thyromental distance < 6 cm, limited mouth opening (≤3 cm), cervical spine disease], increased risk of aspiration, recent upper respiratory tract infection, pregnancy, lactation, body mass index exceeding $35 \, kg.m^2$ and/or patient refusal to participate in the study. Patients in psychiatric treatment, abuse of alcohol or use any medication that could interfere with the study were also excluded. All participants provided written informed consent prior to study entry.

Randomisation and blinding
Participants were randomly assigned to the PLMA or SLMA group according to a computer-generated block randomisation sequence using the Research-Randomizer program, version 4.0 (http://www.randomizer.org/). The sequence was stored in sealed opaque envelopes kept by the study coordinator (MZ). A single study investigator (CM) had access to the randomisation code and opened the envelope before the scheduled case at which time the patient was assigned to his or her study group.

Intervention
Routine monitoring, including pulse oximetry, heart rate, and non-invasive arterial blood pressure, were applied (Datex-Ohmeda Cardiocap™/5, Louisville, CO, USA). In addition to standard monitoring, the Bispectral Index (BIS VISTA™ Monitoring System, Aspect Medical Systems, Inc., Mansfield, MA, USA) was used in all patients. Inhaled and exhaled concentrations of O_2, CO_2, and sevoflurane were monitored breath by breath (Datex-Ohmeda Cardiocap™/5).

The patients were given midazolam 1 mg IV 20 min before anaesthesia induction. All patients were preoxygenated with 100% oxygen for 3 min. The anaesthetic circuit was then filled with 5% sevoflurane at a fresh gas flow of $6 \, l \, min^{-1}$ for 3 min. Inhalational anaesthesia started with simultaneous target-controlled infusion (TCI) of remifentanil with the pharmacokinetic model of Minto through a commercial TCI pump (Alaris® PK, Cardinal Health, 1180 Rolle, Switzerland) adjusted to an effect-site concentration of $4 \, ng \, ml^{-1}$ [11].

Patients were manually ventilated, if needed, to maintain normal PCO_2 values (35–40 mmHg). After loss of consciousness, the inspired sevoflurane concentration was adjusted in each participant to obtain the predetermined ET concentration of sevoflurane using the modified sequential Dixon's up-and-down methodology [12]. Thus, each patient's response determined the sevoflurane concentration used in the next patient. The first patient's predetermined ET concentration of sevoflurane was 2.5% delivered in steps of 0.5% (although below the limit of sevoflurane 0.5%, the step size was 0.1%). In each participant, the predetermined sevoflurane concentration was maintained for more than 10 min to ensure equilibration between the alveolar gas tension, blood, and cerebral tissue before attempting any device insertion. An anaesthesiologist (MZ) experienced in the use of LMA (> 200 cases) inserted the randomly allocated device following the manufacturer's recommendations without using neuromuscular blocking agents. The digital insertion technique was performed with the PLMA. The LMA size was chosen according to the patient's sex (size 4 for women, size 5 for men), although size 3 was inserted for subjects weighing ≤50 kg. However, a change in the size or in the LMA device was permitted according to the judgement of the attending anaesthetist. The LMA cuff was inflated to 60 cm H_2O after insertion. Once stable ventilation with oxygen in air was established, the oropharyngeal leak pressure (OLP) was measured closing the expiratory valve to 40 cm H_2O and maintaining fresh gas flow at $3 \, l \, min^{-1}$. The rising pressure within the system was measured with a pressure gauge and was allowed to increase until it reached equilibration, which was considered the OLP.

The participant's response to the LMA insertion was classified as "failure" or "success" by the surgeon and/or nurse, who were blinded to the sevoflurane concentration. Failure was defined as the presence of coughing, bucking, laryngospasm, or gross purposeful withdrawal movement of the extremities within 1 min of insertion. The presence of laryngospasm should be confirmed by the anesthesiologist performing the LMA insertion. The absence of verbal contact before SADs insertion were classified as 'movement'. The presence of minor finger movement or hiccup was not classified as failure. Jaw

relaxation was evaluated and graded according to Muzi's score [13]—that is, 1: fully relaxed, 2: mild resistance, 3: tight but could be opened, 4: closed requiring a dose of propofol. To guarantee patient comfort, an intravenous bolus dose of propofol $1–2 \, mg \, kg^{-1}$ was administered to each subject experiencing a positive response during LMA insertion. A single measurement was obtained from each participant.

Haemodynamic data, respiratory parameters, and BIS values were recorded at baseline immediately before LMA insertion and 1 and 6 min after LMA insertion. Hypotension was defined as mean arterial pressure < 50 mmHg and was treated with ephedrine 3 mg. Bradycardia was defined as heart rate < 45 bpm and was treated with atropine $0.1 \, mg \, kg^{-1}$.

All study subjects were interviewed in the recovery room to assess memory recall by a blinded observer.

Statistical analysis

The sevoflurane ET_{50} co-administered with remifentanil required for PLMA and SLMA insertions was determined by calculating the midpoint concentration of all the independent pairs of patients who manifested crossover from a movement response to a non-movement response. The standard deviation of the sevoflurane ET_{50} represented the standard deviation of the crossover midpoint of each group.

Dose–response curves were assessed to determine the probability of no movement relative to the sevoflurane concentration and to obtain a sevoflurane concentration where 50% (ET_{50}) and 95% (ET_{95}) of the device attempts were successful in both groups and the maximum likelihood estimators of the model parameters. Goodness of fit was obtained using logistic regression curves [14].

Sevoflurane ET_{50} values in the PLMA and the SLMA groups were compared using Student's t-test. Haemodynamic data and the BIS value were compared by repeated measures analysis of variance. The ^{2} test, with Fisher's exact probability test, when appropriate, was used to compare jaw relaxation. The OLP was compared using the unpaired Student's t-test.

A value of $P < 0.05$ was considered to indicate statistical significance.

Statistical analyses were performed using SPSS 22.0 software for Windows (IBM Corp., Armonk, NY, USA).

Simple size calculation

We applied the Dixon approach for simple size calculation for the up-and-down method design. In similar studies in the field of anaesthesia, the number of crossovers varies between six and eight with six crossovers being most common. For this study's purposes, the allocation sequence continued until the six crossovers points from "failure" to "success" were obtained in each group [12, 15].

Results

Participants' flow during the study is shown in Fig. 1. Forty-five subjects were randomised to either the PLMA ($n = 23$) or the SLMA ($n = 22$) group. There were no significant differences in terms of patients' characteristics although general surgery was performed more frequently in the PLMA group and vascular surgery in the SLMA group (Table 1).

Individual dose–response data obtained by Dixon's up-and-down method are shown in Fig. 2 (PLMA) and Fig. 3 (SLMA). The predicted ET_{50} of sevoflurane was significantly higher for successful PLMA insertion ($1.20 \pm 0.41\%[95\%$ CI 0.76–1.63]) than for SLMA insertion ($0.55 \pm 0.38\%$ [95% CI 0.14–0.95] ($p = 0.019$). Using

logistic regression curves, the ET_{50} and the ET_{95} of sevoflurane required for PLMA insertion were 1.15% (95% CI 0.57–2.33) and 2.43% (95% CI 1.10–5.34), respectively. For SLMA insertion, they were 0.43% (95% CI 0.02–7.76) and 1.50% (95% CI 0.55–4.08) respectively (Fig. 4). Table 2 presents the estimated values from the logistic and goodness-of-fit analyses.

In two participants in the PLMA group, we changed the size of the LMA (size 4 to a size 3). In three patients in the SLMA group, we changed the SLMA to a PLMA because of inadequate ventilation. Overall, we found a higher incidence of patients with resistance to jaw relaxation and requiring propofol in the PLMA group but without statistical significance ($p = 0.30$) (Table 3).

Baseline BIS and haemodynamic data did not differ between the two groups (Table 4). In both groups, the heart rate, systolic and diastolic pressures, and BIS

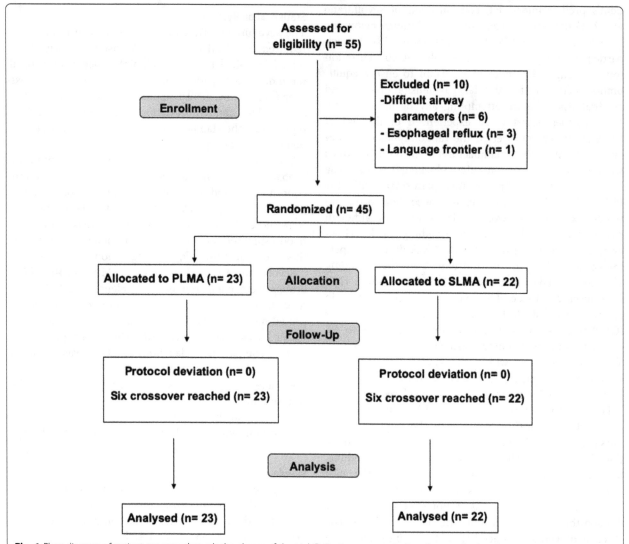

Fig. 1 Flow-diagram of patient progress through the phases of the trial. Patients were recruited until a sample size of seven crossovers was reached in each group

Table 1 Demographic data of patients and surgical procedures

	PLMA ($n = 23$)	SLMA ($n = 22$)
Patients	23	22
Age (yr)	43 ± 13	46 ± 11
Female/Male	15/8	15/7
Weight (kg)	72 ± 13	75 ± 16
Height (cm)	169 ± 8	168 ± 9
BMI	24.98 ± 3.61	26.32 ± 4.63
Mallampati classification		
I	12	11
II	10	7
III	1	4
ASA I / ASA II	13/10	11/11
Surgical procedure*		
Vascular (varicose veins)	6	12
Orthopaedic	3	3
General	14	7

Data are expressed as mean ± SD or number.
PLMA Laryngeal mask airway ProSeal™, *SLMA* Laryngeal mask airway
Supreme™, *BMI* Body mass index, *ASA* American Society of Anaesthesiologists´
physical status, *SD* Standard deviation.
* $p = 0.04$ for surgical procedure

significantly decreased relative to baseline values. The number of subjects who required atropine or ephedrine did not differ significantly.

The BIS value significantly differed between the two groups, being higher in the SLMA group than in the PLMA group (Table 4). Nevertheless, no participant manifested intraoperative recall during recovery.

No episodes of laryngospasm were described, although three subjects experienced peripheral oxygen desaturation of < 90% during LMA insertion (one patient in the PLMA group and two in the SLMA group). In all cases, it recovered after the LMA was in place and working.

The mean OLP was higher in the PLMA group (24.42 cm ± 4.9 cm H_2O) than in the SLMA group (22.55 cm ± 3.97 cm H_2O), but the difference was not statistically significant.

Discussion

To our knowledge, this is the first randomised study designed to compare the ET_{50} of the sevoflurane concentration during co-induction with remifentanil TCI at 4 ng mL^{-1}, which is required for successful insertion of the PLMA and SLMA in adult patients. The results of the present study show that the SLMA can be inserted at a lower sevoflurane concentration than that required for the PLMA. (The ET_{50} value of sevoflurane for SLMA insertion was 54% less than that for PLMA.)

Previous reports found that insertion of a PLMA may take longer and require more attempts than the SLMA requires [7, 9]. This finding might be attributed to several factors such as the insertion technique of each LMA because of the design variations between the devices. The anatomically shaped airway tube and thin wedge-shaped leading edge of the SLMA have been purported to permit smoother, successful insertion with a simple circular movement. In contrast, during placement, the posterior aspect of the PLMA is pressed up against the hard palate with a finger maintaining a constant backward pressure to

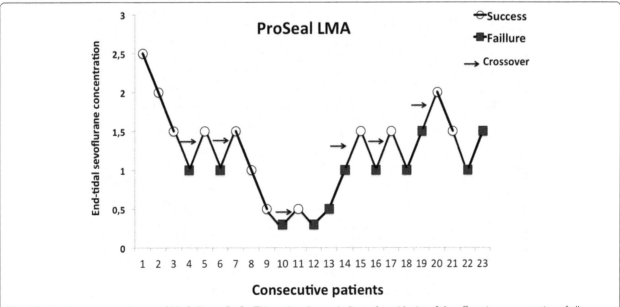

Fig. 2 Patients' responses to Laryngeal Mask Airway ProSeal™ insertion. Arrows indicate the midpoint of the effect-site concentration of all independent pairs of patients involving crossover from device insertion failure to successful Laryngeal Mask Airway Airway ProSeal™ insertion

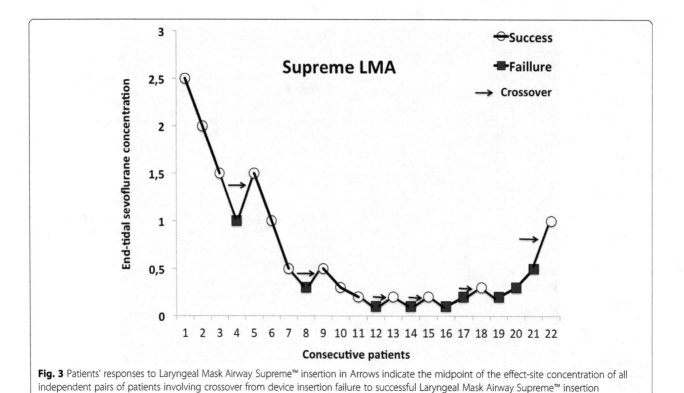

Fig. 3 Patients' responses to Laryngeal Mask Airway Supreme™ insertion in Arrows indicate the midpoint of the effect-site concentration of all independent pairs of patients involving crossover from device insertion failure to successful Laryngeal Mask Airway Supreme™ insertion

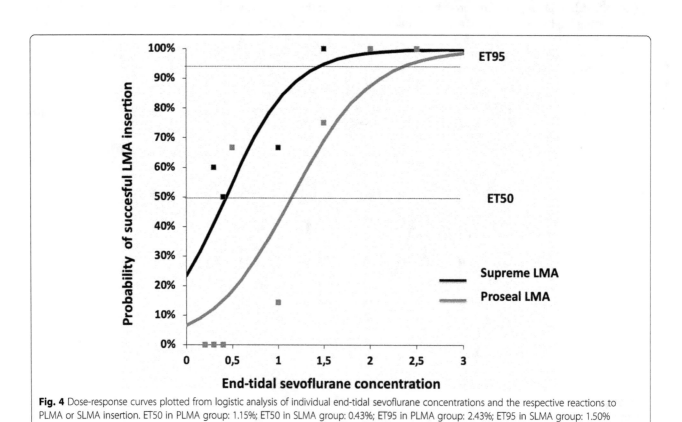

Fig. 4 Dose-response curves plotted from logistic analysis of individual end-tidal sevoflurane concentrations and the respective reactions to PLMA or SLMA insertion. ET50 in PLMA group: 1.15%; ET50 in SLMA group: 0.43%; ET95 in PLMA group: 2.43%; ET95 in SLMA group: 1.50%

Table 2 Estimated values of the of the logit coefficients

	PLMA	SLMA
ET-50% LMA (CI)	1.15 (0.57–2,33)	0.43 (0.02–7.76)
ET 95% LMA (CI)	2.43(1.10–5.34)	1.50(0.55–4.08)
B0	−2.647	−1.188
B1	2.304	2.749
p Value	0.106	0.676
Goodness of fit chi-squared	7.634	3.170

CI: 95% confidence interval.
$p/(1 − p) = B_0 + B_{1X}$.
B0 = intercept; B1 = slope; X = end-tidal concentration (%).

facilitate its passage around the posterior pharyngeal wall. These differences in insertion technique can affect the pattern and intensity of stimulation and thus the anaesthetic needs of the devices. A greater proportion of patients in the PLMA group showed resistance regarding relaxation of the jaw.

Kodaka et al. [3] compared the ET_{50} of sevoflurane required for CLMA and PLMA insertions and observed that the ET_{50} of sevoflurane for PLMA placement was 20% higher ($2.82 \pm 0.45\%$) than that for CLMA placement ($2.36 \pm 0.22\%$). Our results show that adding remifentanil induces a significant reduction in the sevoflurane requirement. In fact, the ET_{50} of sevoflurane for PLMA placement ($1.20 \pm 0.41\%$) was nearly 60% less than that reported by Kodaka [3]. Zaballos et al. [4], using the up-and-down method, showed that the ET_{50} of sevoflurane for SLMA placement was $3.03 \pm 0.75\%$ in patients premedicated with 1 mg of midazolam. The results of the present study showed an even greater reduction of the sevoflurane concentration (82%) needed for SLMA insertion ($0.55 \pm 0.38\%$) when remifentanil was added.

Adding a potent, short-acting opioid such as remifentanil during sevoflurane inhalation induction has been reported to improve conditions for LMA insertion or tracheal intubation, decreasing the incidence of excitatory movements during induction [5, 6, 16, 17]. This effect of remifentanil may be due to blockade of afferent nerve impulses resulting from stimulation of the laryngopharynx during LMA insertion and cuff inflation. Although adequate induction for LMA placement can be achieved using sevoflurane alone, an opioid analgesic is

Table 3 Assessment of jaw relaxation according to Muzi score

	PLMA (n = 23)	SLMA (n = 22)
Fully relaxed.	12	13
Mild resistance.	2	3
Resistance but could be opened.	2	4
Resistance requiring a dose of propofol (mg)	7 111 ± 12	2 110 ± 14

Data are expressed as number of patients or mean ± SD.

Table 4 Haemodynamic and BIS data at different times in the two groups

	PLMA (n = 23)	SLMA (n = 22)
Systolic arterial pressure		
Baseline	138 ± 16	135 ± 20
Before insertion	98 ± 13 [29%]	96 ± 15 [29%]
1st min post-insertion*	101 ± 13 [27%]	108 ± 17 [20%]
6th min post-insertion*	98 ± 13 [29%]	97 ± 14 [28%]
Diastolic arterial pressure		
Baseline	80 ± 12	79 ± 11
Before insertion*	56 ± 9 [30%]	53 ± 9 [33%]
1st min post-insertion*	58 ± 13 [30%]	60 ± 12 [24%]
6th min post-insertion*	55 ± 11 [31%]	57 ± 8 [28%]
Heart rate		
Baseline	73 ± 17	73 ± 13
Before insertion*	56 ± 11 [23%]	54 ± 9 [26%]
1st min post-insertion*	57 ± 10 [22%]	59 ± 11 [19%]
6th min post-insertion*	56 ± 12 [23%]	60 ± 11 [18%]
BIS value		
Baseline	95 ± 4	96 ± 5
Before insertion*†	60 ± 8 [37%]	63 ± 9 [35%]
1st min post-insertion*†	56 ± 13 [41%]	64 ± 14 [34%]
6th min post-insertion*†	41 ± 15 [57%]	43 ± 16 [55%]

Data are expressed as mean ± SD [% difference from baseline].
PLMA Laryngeal mask airway ProSeal™, SLMA Laryngeal mask airway Supreme™, BIS Bispectral index, SD Standard deviation.
* $p < 0.05$ for significant differences from baseline (difference within the group) by repeated measures ANOVA
† $p < 0.05$ for significant differences between the PLMA and the SLMA groups by repeated measures ANOVA.

commonly co-administered to increase synergistically the clinical anaesthetic level, thereby facilitating the LMA placement [5, 17].

Other studies are in agreement that the ET_{50} of sevoflurane needed for PLMA insertion is higher than that required for other first-generation devices. To our knowledge, however, no studies have compared the sevoflurane requirement for PLMA insertion with that for other second-generation devices [3, 18].

>BIS values were significantly higher in the SLMA group, which is consistent with the lower sevoflurane administration in this group. However, no patient reported recall when questioned in the recovery room. Manyam et al. [19] investigated the impact on BIS values when adding remifentanil to sevoflurane in doses sufficient to change the clinical level of sedation. Although clinical sedation increased significantly with the addition of remifentanil to a sevoflurane anaesthetic, the BIS was insensitive to the change in the clinical level of sedation. The authors suggested that during sevoflurane-remifentanil anaesthesia,

targeting a BIS < 60 may result in an excessively deep anaesthetic state.

Our data support this finding as the addition of remifentanil at an effect-site concentration of $4\,ng\,mL^{-1}$ to the different sevoflurane concentrations generated a mean BIS value of 61 ± 9 before insertion of the LMA without significant differences between subjects who showed a "movement" response and those who did not (64 ± 8 vs. 60 ± 10, respectively; $p = 0.16$).

Oropharyngeal leak pressure was higher in the PLMA group, which is consistent with the results of previous publications [7]. This finding may be related to a deeper anaesthetic plane, which could influence the tone of the pharyngeal muscles.

This study had some limitations. First, our main objective was to determine the sevoflurane ET_{50} for co-administration with remifentanil that was required for successful insertion of the PLMA and the SLMA according to Dixon's up-and-down method. A minimum amount of time is required to guarantee drug concentration equilibration between phases (10 min in the present study). This prolonged time is not representative of the clinical experience. Second, according to Dixon's design, the sample size is limited when a specific number of crossovers (4–10) between up-and-down steps have been achieved. It is typically limited to 20–40 patients. Because the effect of varying the number of crossovers can induce bias in the estimation, there is agreement that six crossovers are sufficient [15, 20]. Third, an expert anaesthesiologist on regular use of supraglottic airway devices in clinical practice inserted all the devices. Our results therefore cannot be extrapolated to the insertion of LMAs by novice users.

Conclusion

The end-tidal sevoflurane concentration during remifentanil co-administration needed to allow insertion of the SLMA is 54% lower than that needed for insertion of the PLMA. Both devices are effective for applying positive-pressure ventilation to patients undergoing ambulatory surgery with few adverse effects.

Abbreviations

ASA: American society anesthesiologist; BIS: Bispectral index; ET: End-tidal; ET_{50}: ET concentration in 50%; ET_{95}: ET concentration in 95%; MAC: Minimal alveolar concentration; OLP: Oropharyngeal leak pressure; PLMA: ProSeal laryngeal mask airway; SLMA: Supreme laryngeal mask airway; TCI: Target controlled infusion

Acknowledgements

We thank Nancy Schatken, BS, MT(ASCP), from Edanz Group (www.edanzediting.com/ac), for editing a draft of this manuscript.

Authors' contributions

MZ designed and conducted the study, analysed the data, and wrote the text. CMM contributed to design of the study, analysis of the data and helped to write the main text. TG contributed to the design and conduction of the study. MJAB contributed to conduction of the study and analysis of the results. All authors have read and approved the final manuscript.

References

1. Cook TM, Lee G, Nolan JP. The proseal™laryngeal mask airway: a review of the literature. Can J Anaesth. 2005;52:739–60.
2. Cook TM, Gatward JJ, Handel J, et al. Evaluation of the LMA supreme™ in 100 non-paralysed patients. Anaesthesia. 2009;64:555–62.
3. Kodaka M, Okamoto Y, Koyama K, et al. Predicted values of propofol EC50 and sevoflurane concentration for insertion of laryngeal mask classic and ProSeal. Br J Anaesth. 2004;92:242–5.
4. Zaballos M, Bastida E, Jiménez C, et al. Predicted end-tidal sevoflurane concentration for insertion of a laryngeal mask supreme. Eur J Anaesthesiol. 2013;30:170–4.
5. Ganatra SB. D'Mello J, Butani M et al. conditions for insertion of the laryngeal mask airway: comparisons between sevoflurane and propofol using fentanyl as a co-induction agent. A pilot study. Eur J Anaesthesiol. 2002;19:371–5.
6. Sivalingam P, Kandasamy R, Madhavan G, et al. Conditions for laryngeal mask insertion. A comparison of propofol versus sevoflurane with or without alfentanil. Anaesthesia. 1999;54:271–6.
7. Maitra S, Khanna P, Baidya DK. Comparison of laryngeal mask airway supreme and laryngeal mask airway pro-seal for controlled ventilation during general anaesthesia in adult patients: systematic review with meta-analysis. Eur J Anaesthesiol. 2014;31:266–73.
8. Timmermann A, Cremer S, Eich C, et al. Prospective clinical and fiberoptic evaluation of the supreme laryngeal mask airway. Anesthesiology. 2009;110:262–5.
9. Eschertzhuber S, Brimacombe J, Hohlrieder M, et al. The laryngeal mask airway supreme--a single use laryngeal mask airway with an oesophageal vent. A randomised, cross-over study with the laryngeal mask airway ProSeal in paralysed, anaesthetised patients. Anaesthesia. 2009;64:79–83.
10. Seet E, Rajeev S, Firoz T, et al. Safety and efficacy of laryngeal mask airway supreme versus laryngeal mask airway ProSeal: a randomized controlled trial. Eur J Anaesthesiol. 2010;27:602–7.
11. Minto CF, Schnider TW, Shafer SL. Pharmacokinetics and pharmacodynamics of remifentanil. II Model application. Anesthesiology. 1997;86:24–33.
12. Dixon WJ. Staircase bioassay: the up-and-down method. Neurosci Biobehav Rev. 1991;15:47–50.
13. Muzi M, Robinson BJ, Ebert TJ, et al. Induction of anesthesia and tracheal intubation with sevoflurane in adults. Anesthesiology. 1996;85:536–43.
14. de Jong RH, Eger EI. MAC expanded: AD50 and AD95 values of common inhalation anesthetics in man. Anesthesiology. 1975;42:384–9.
15. Paul M, Fisher DM. Are estimates of MAC reliable? Anesthesiology. 2001;95:1362–70.
16. Cros AM, Lopez C, Kandel T, et al. Determination of sevoflurane alveolar concentration for tracheal intubation with remifentanil, and no muscle relaxant. Anaesthesia. 2000;55:965–9.
17. Kwak HJ, Chae YJ, Lee KC, et al. Target-controlled infusion of remifentanil for laryngeal mask airway insertion during sevoflurane induction in adults. J Int Med Res. 2012;40:1476–82.
18. Ghai B, Jain K, Bansal D, et al. End-tidal sevoflurane concentration for ProSeal™ versus classic™ laryngeal mask airway insertion in unpremedicated anaesthetized adult females. Anaesth Intensive Care. 2016;44:221–6.
19. Manyam SC, Gupta DK, Johnson KB, et al. When is a bispectral index of 60 too low?: rational processed electroencephalographic targets are dependent on the sedative-opioid ratio. Anesthesiology. 2007;106:472–83.
20. Pace NL, Stylianou MP. Advances in and limitations of up-and-down methodology: a précis of clinical use, study design, and dose estimation in anesthesia research. Anesthesiology. 2007;107:144–52.

31

The evaluation of a better intubation strategy when only the epiglottis is visible

Tzu-Yao Hung[1,2,3], Li-Wei Lin[3,4,5], Yu-Hang Yeh[2], Yung-Cheng Su[6,7], Chieh-Hung Lin[2] and Ten-Fang Yang[1,8*] ⓘ

Abstract

Background: The Cormack-Lehane (C-L) grade III airway is considered to be a challenging airway to intubate and is associated with a poor intubation success rate. The purpose of this study was to investigate whether the holding position, shapes, bend angles of the endotracheal tube (ET) and the stylet-assisted lifting of the epiglottis could improve the success rate of intubation.

Methods: Thirty-two participants, 26 physicians, 2 residents, and 4 nurse practitioners, with 12.09 ± 5.38 years of work experience in the emergency department and more than 150 annual intubation events, were enrolled in this randomized, cross-over mannequin study. We investigated the effects of straight-to-cuff ET shapes with 35° and 50° bend angles, banana-shaped ET with longitudinal distances of 28 cm and 26 cm, two methods of holding the ET (either on the top or in the middle), and lifting or not the epiglottis, on the intubation duration, its success rate, and its subjective difficulty. The aim of the study is to provide optimized intubation strategies for difficult airway with C-L IIb or III grades, when the inlet of the trachea cannot be visualized.

Results: The two groups that lifted the epiglottis using the stylets, in bend angles of 35° and 50°, had the shortest duration of intubation (23.75 ± 14.24 s and 20.72 ± 6.90 s, hazard ratios 1.54 and 1.85 with 95% confidence intervals [95% CI] of 1.01–2.34 and 1.23–2.78, respectively) and a 100% success rate in intubations. In the survival analysis, lifting of the epiglottis was the only significant factor ($p < 0.0001$, 95% CI 1.34–2.11) associated with the success rate of intubation.

Conclusions: The use of the epiglottic lift as an adjunctive technique can facilitate the intubation and improve its success rate without increasing procedure difficulty, in C-L III airway, when only the epiglottis is seen.

Keywords: Difficult airway, Intubation technique, Stylet shapes, Lifting of epiglottis, Bend angles, Cormack-Lehane grade

Background

When the vocal cords are visible using the laryngoscope, such as in C-L grades I and IIa, successful intubation is usually anticipated. However, among C-L grades IIb–IV, blind intubations (without seeing the endotracheal tube pass through the vocal cords) are more difficult because the distances between the tip of the ET and the epiglottis

or other landmarks are obscured [1, 2]. Under such circumstances, if the practitioner can keep the tip of the ET moving along and just beneath the epiglottis (anterior part of the larynx), the ET would slip from the larynx into the trachea. Compared with holding the middle part of the ET and hooking an imaginary target - the tracheal inlet – that is outside of the visual field, two techniques might help. In the first method, managing and using the stylet as a Trachway intubating stylet (Biotronic Instrument Enterprise Ltd., Tai-Chung, Taiwan) could be of benefit. This involves holding the top of the ET with the right hand so that the ET can be levered immediately after the cuff passes the incisors, with the elbow bending to the chest. Such a technique may provide greater torque with which

* Correspondence: taipeicityer@gmail.com; tfy@tmu.edu.tw; tfy2008@mail.nctu.edu.tw
[1]Department of Biological Science and Technology, College of Biological science and Technology, National Chiao Tung University, NO.75 Po-Ai Street, Hsinchu 30068, Taiwan
[8]Graduate Institute of Medical Informatics and Cardiology, Taipei Medical University, Taipei, Taiwan

to hook and move the tip of the ET inferiorly and parallel to the epiglottis (Fig. 1a & b). This technique was initially introduced by James Ducanto (https://videopress.com/v/9dd9jIfN). The second method involves lifting the epiglottis with the tip of the stylet-equipped ET. We always use our left hands to manipulate the laryngoscope to obtain a better glottic view. When the glottic view is insufficient to perform intubation, we adjust the tip of the laryngoscope in the vallecula and try to lift more. However, Wasa et al. reported on a patient's case that lifting the epiglottis with the stylet may also improve the glottic view directly [3].

Levitan et al. proved that the shapes and bend angles of the stylet affect the success of intubation [4]. Although a hockey shape is widely used in emergency practice, the ways in which the different stylet shapes and curvatures might affect intubation remained unclear. This study was designed to optimise intubation strategies for difficult airway with higher modified C-L grades, namely, IIb or III, when the inlet of the trachea cannot be visualized.

Methods
Study design and participants
This study was approved on October 31st, 2017 by the Institutional Review Board (approval no.: TCHIRB-10610108-W) and registered in the ClinicalTrials Registry (https://clincaltrials.gov, identifier NCT03366311). This study was a randomized, cross-over study. The 32 participants were attending physicians, residents, and nurse practitioners (26, 2, and 4, respectively), having 12.09 ± 5.38 years of practice in the emergency department with more than 150 annual intubation events and at least three years of

clinical practice in the emergency department with more than 150 intubations. They were recruited from multiple medical centres in north and south Taiwan (Taipei City Hospital, Shin Kong Wu Ho-Su Memorial Hospital, Dalin Tzu Chi Buddhist Hospital, Shuang Ho Hospital, Taipei Municipal Wanfang Hospital, Chang Gung Memorial Hospital) during an airway training course (CATLAB, Critical Airway Training Laboratory). All participants were neither experienced in holding the top of the ET nor lifting the epiglottis with a stylet while intubating in their past practice. To successfully participate the study, they were instructed to perform these two methods and to complete at least three successful intubations on the AMBU Mannequin Intubation Airway (Ambu Enterprise Ltd., Ballerup, Denmark) before the study began.

Protocol
A direct laryngoscope (Macintosh #3 blade) was used in all the participants, and a conventional 7.0-mm internal diameter tracheal tube (Covidien, Mallinckrodt Pharmaceuticals Ltd., Surrey, United Kingdom) was used to intubate the mannequin without assistance. They were asked to lift the epiglottis with moderate force to avoid visualization of the vocal cord and intubate under C-L grade III (only the epiglottis is visible). All intubation processes were recorded and reviewed later to ensure the intubation processes were C-L grade IIb to III with a camera embedded on the blade (Fig. 1c). The full length of the Covidien Cuffed Mallinckrodt™ ET (7.0-mm internal diameter) from the tip to the adaptor was 32.5 cm. The estimated curvature with a longitudinal distance of 28

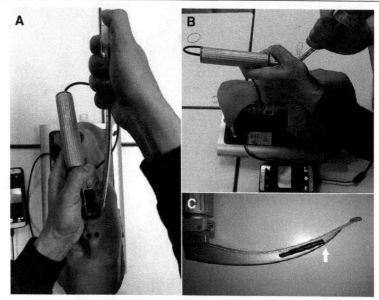

Fig. 1 a Holding the top of the endotracheal tube and (**b**) bending the elbow to the chest right after the cuff passed through the incisors to elevate the tip of the tube with greater torque. All processes were recorded with a video camera. (**c**) The camera was attached to the blade for recording purposes. The participants used the direct laryngoscope without watching the screen. The white arrow indicates the location of the camera

and 26 cm was 1/0.07 (ρ = 0.07 m) and 1/0.08 (ρ = 0.08 m), respectively. These curvatures were approximate to the bend angles of straight-to-cuff of 35° and 50° at the cuff level. When the practitioners had a proper view of the glottis under direct laryngoscopy, they would receive the ET equipped with standardized stylet shapes and curvatures (straight-to-cuff 35° or 50°; banana shape with a longitudinal distance of 26 cm and 28 cm) and be instructed to hold the ET on top or in the middle (Two different shapes with each shape of two different curvatures and two different holding positions formed 8 possible settings (Fig. 2). These were randomized using random.org before the study began, (https://www.random.org/lists/). The participants only knew the shape at the time when the glottic view fulfilled the study setting and were asked to keep the shape and holding position during the intubation. Intubation time exceeding 90 s was considered as failed attempt. A successful intubation was defined as one when the tube was passed through the vocal cords exceeding the vocal cords marker. After each intubation, the participants provided a subjective visual analogue scale (VAS) score to assess the difficulty (0, not difficult; 10: impossible to intubate). All the study processes were recorded by a video camera on the tip of blade (Fig. 1c). The time from inserting the laryngoscope in the mouth of the mannequin, the time of initial proper glottic view to initiate tracheal intubation, the time of withdrawal of the endotracheal tube, and success or failure of intubation were all determined retrospectively by viewing the video clips.

At the end of the study, the participants performed intubations by lifting the epiglottis and holding the middle part of the stylet-equipped ET, straight-to-cuff shape of 35° or 50°, in a randomized order (two possible settings with random.org, https://www.random.org/lists/) (Additional file 1: Video S1). All practitioners intubated the mannequin a total of ten times.

Measurements

The number of years of experience in the ED, the specialty of the participants (attending physicians, residents, or nurse practitioners), and height of the participants were all recorded. The primary outcome in our study was the total duration of the intubation process (laryngoscope blade in and out of the mouth of the mannequin) and intubation success rate. The secondary outcome was subjective difficulty scales. All the results were reviewed and calculated based on the recorded video clips and VAS records.

Statistical analysis

Study data was taken by convenience sampling from our airway training courses (CATLAB). The characteristics of the participants, glottis views during intubation, duration of intubation, success rate of intubation, and VAS scores were collected and analyzed in the study. We evaluated the time to successful intubation by plotting Kaplan-Meier survival curves to determine the trends. To cope with the correlated data from multiple intubation attempts by the same participants, we applied Cox regression models stratified by proportional hazard types. We used these models in the evaluation of the different manipulations of the hazard ratios (HRs) of successful intubation after adjusting for relevant confounding factors, namely duration of service in years, sex, height, type of participant, and different shapes and bend angles of the stylet.

Linear regression was used to evaluate intubation time and VAS score, while logistic regression was applied to evaluate the odds ratio of the success rate by using the VAS scores after adjusting for the confounding factors. The generalized estimate equation method was adapted to account for the clustering of the participants.

SAS statistical package version 9.4 (SAS Institute, Inc., Cary, NC, USA) and STATA version 11.2 (StataCorp, College Station, TX, USA) were used for data analysis. A two-tailed p value of < 0.05 was considered statistically significant.

Results

Table 1 shows the distribution of sex, class, height, and duration of practice in the emergency department of the 32 participants. Of the 32 participants, 26, 4, and 4, were attending physicians, residents, and nurse practitioners, respectively. After the video clips were reviewed, 96.87% of glottis views were C-L grade III, and the rest were grade IIb. The overall success rate of the intubation was 95.63%. The duration of the intubation with holding top

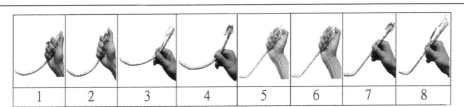

Fig. 2 Eight settings in the study including different shapes of stylet, stylet bend angles, holding the endotracheal tube on the top or in the middle were demonstrated

Table 1 Participant characteristics

Variable	Mean		Standard deviation
Age (years)	38.56	±	5.19
Duration of Practice in the emergency department (years)	12.09	±	5.38
Total	32		
Attending physician	26		
Resident	2		
Nurse practitioner	4		
Height (cm)	169.69	±	6.47
Men:women	27:5		

of banana shape stylets with 28 cm and 26 cm longitudinal distance, holding middle of banana shape stylets with 28 cm and 26 cm longitudinal distance, holding top of straight-to-cuff with 35 degrees and 50 degrees bend angles, holding top of straight-to-cuff with 35 degrees and 50 degrees bend angles were 33.63 ± 33.87 s, 31.91 ± 31.82 s, 30.10 ± 18.73 s, 31.06 ± 24.59 s, 34.81 ± 27.70 s, 28.03 ± 16.36 s, 34.10 ± 32.12 s, 27.53 ± 16.31 s, 23.75 ± 14.24 s, 20.72 ± 6.90 s, respectively; the success rate were 90.63, 93.75, 96.88, 93.75, 93.75, 96.88, 93.75, 96.88, 100, 100%, respectively; the VAS scores were 4.24 ± 2.11 cm, 4.34 ± 2.33 cm, 4.62 ± 1.94 cm, 4.48 ± 2.12 cm, 4.67 ± 2.30 cm, 4.36 ± 2.32 cm, 4.29 ± 4.48 cm, 3.90 ± 2.12 cm, 4.15 ± 2.22 cm, 3.97 ± 2.13 cm, respectively (Table 2).

A Kaplan-Meier plot (Fig. 3) illustrates a significantly shorter time to successful intubation with the two subgroups that performed lifting of the epiglottis with stylets (23.75 ± 14.24 s and 20.72 ± 6.90 s among bend angles of 35° and 50°, respectively) and 100% success rate of intubation. In the Cox regression analysis, only the lifting of the epiglottis was significant ($p < 0.0001$, Table 3).

Based on the results from logistic and linear regression models, VAS was strongly related to intubation time. For each 1 cm increase in the VAS, the odds ratio of success was increased by 0.55, and the intubation time increased by 3.77 s. (Tables 2 and 3, respectively).

Discussion

Levitan et al. found that for bend angles beyond 35°, straight-to-cuff ET can jeopardize the success rate of tracheal intubation and increase the difficulty of passing the ET [4]. However, among difficult airway, such as C-L III, larger angulations might confer some advantage. In our study, the straight-to-cuff and bend angles at 50° exhibited a trend of shorter intubation times and better success rates compared to bend angles at 35°, despite the method of holding the ET parts (97.92% versus 95.83%, 25.43 ± 14.17 versus 30.89 ± 26.05 s, $p = 0.0859$, 95% CI 0.97–1.61, respectively). Participants also felt that intubation was easier if a larger angulation was used (4.08 ± 2.18 versus 4.37 ± 2.20 cm). On the contrary, banana-shaped ET with larger angulations (longitudinal distance of 26 versus 28 cm) did not show any difference in the success rate, intubation time, or VAS score (equally 93.75%, 31.48 ± 28.21 versus 31.86 ± 27.21 s, 4.41 ± 2.21 versus 4.43 ± 2.02 cm, respectively). The banana shape might cross the visual axis twice if the tube axis is parallel to the visual axis. Thus, this method is believed to be unfavorable for intubation. Our results, however, showed no difference between the straight-to-cuff and banana-shaped tubes despite the effect of the bend angles and holding parts of the tube on success rate, intubation time, and subjective difficulty (96.88% versus 93.75%, 28.16 ± 21.10 versus 31.67 ± 27.60 s, 4.22 ± 2.19 versus 4.42 ± 2.11 cm, respectively).

Table 2 Ten different subgroup settings and the results of the duration of intubation, success rate, and visual analogue difficulty scoring

	Manipulation Holding part of tube	Shape	Longitudinal distance (cm) Bend angles (°)	Duration of intubation			Success rate (%)	Visual analogue scale score (cm)
				Mean ± Standard deviation (seconds)	HR	95% CI		
1	Top	Banana	28 cm	33.63 ± 33.87	1.00	1.00	90.63%	4.24 ± 2.11
2	Top	Banana	26 cm	31.91 ± 31.82	1.05	0.60–1.83	93.75%	4.34 ± 2.33
3	Middle	Banana	28 cm	30.10 ± 18.73	1.01	0.63–1.62	96.88%	4.62 ± 1.94
4	Middle	Banana	26 cm	31.06 ± 24.59	1.04	0.68–1.59	93.75%	4.48 ± 2.12
5	Top	Straight-to-cuff	35°	34.81 ± 27.70	0.87	0.55–1.37	93.75%	4.67 ± 2.30
6	Top	Straight-to-cuff	50°	28.03 ± 16.36	1.11	0.68–1.82	96.88%	4.36 ± 2.32
7	Middle	Straight-to-cuff	35°	34.10 ± 32.12	1.00	0.65–1.53	93.75%	4.29 ± 4.48
8	Middle	Straight-to-cuff	50°	27.53 ± 16.31	1.15	0.74–1.78	96.88%	3.90 ± 2.12
9	Lifting of epiglottis	Straight-to-cuff	35°	23.75 ± 14.24	1.54	1.01–2.34	100%	4.15 ± 2.22
10	Lifting of epiglottis	Straight-to-cuff	50°	20.72 ± 6.90	1.85	1.23–2.78	100%	3.97 ± 2.13

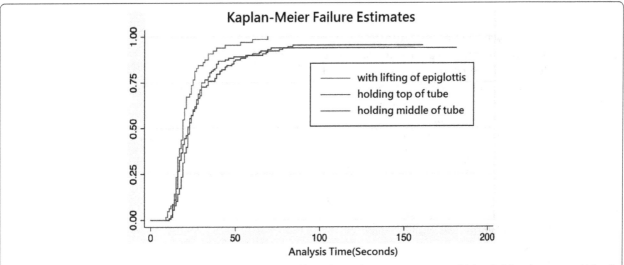

Fig. 3 Kaplan–Meier failure estimate for different intubation postures: lifting the epiglottis was more successful than holding the top or middle of the endotracheal tube ($p < 0.001$)

By holding the top of the ET and flexing the elbow to the chest when the cuff passes the incisors, a larger torque is generated, which might be useful in managing a difficult airway. Compared to holding the middle part of the endotracheal tube, the tilting angle of the ET tip is larger during intubation when holding the top and starting up by the elbow instead of the wrist. However, no significant difference was found between holding the top or holding the middle of the ET on intubation success rates or VAS scores in spite of different bend angles and shapes (32.09 ± 28.04 versus 27.88 ± 20.66 s; 93.75% versus 96.88%; 4.40 ± 2.25 versus 4.23 ± 2.10 cm, respectively). The participants in our study were all inexperienced in holding the ET on the top before our study. Such a condition may lead to a higher failure rate. However, our study showed no evidence that the holding position improved the outcome of the management of the difficult airway.

When only the epiglottis is visible under laryngoscopy (C-L grade III), the ET passing between the vocal cord and trachea cannot be visualized directly and therefore, is considered a blind intubation. The success rate in the first attempt of intubations in C-L grade III was only 44.7% under direct laryngoscopy in one report in an ED setting [5]. When an intubation attempt fails, the practitioner usually will reposition the patient and focus on the left hand go deeper toward the vallecula or lift harder to obtain a better glottic view. However, we often neglect our right hand, which is directly lifting the epiglottis with stylets. This type of manoeuvre can improve the glottic view and allow the practitioner to focus only on the left hand. Nestling the tip of the endotracheal tube under the epiglottis and moving it along the anterior larynx leads to the tracheal inlet. Ueda et al. reported a case wherein lifting of the epiglottis with stylets helped improve the glottic view [3]. In our study, the success rate of intubation with stylet-assisted epiglottis lifting was 100% in contrast to without lifting (94.53%). Lifting of the epiglottis also decreased the mean duration of intubation more than without lifting (22.23 ± 11.20 versus 31.39 ± 25.86 s, respectively). In the survival analysis, lifting of the epiglottis was a strong factor in improving intubation (Fig. 3, $p < 0.0001$). Additionally, lifting the epiglottis with stylets was not considered to be more difficult compared to not lifting the epiglottis (4.06 ± 2.16 cm versus 4.36 ± 2.16 cm, $p = 0.137$, 95% CI -0.80-0.11). Lifting of the epiglottis can accelerate intubation and improve the success rate in difficult intubations without increasing the level of difficulty.

Among the different conditions associated with C-L grade III in our study, holding the top of the endotracheal tube with a straight-to-cuff tube and a bend angle of 35° was considered to be the most difficult intubation performed, followed by holding the middle of the tube with the smaller curvature of the banana-shape (longitudinal distance = 28 cm). In contrast, holding the middle of the ET with the straight-to-cuff tube and a bend angle of 50° was the easiest. The VAS score was directly related to intubation time (odds ratio = 0.55), such that the higher the VAS scores, the longer the intubation duration will be.

Table 3 Analysis of the results of covariates

Variable	HR	95% CI	p-Value
Shapes of stylet (banana vs. straight-to-cuff)	0.99	0.82–1.20	0.950
Lifting of epiglottis	1.68	1.34–2.11	< 0.001
Holding level of tube (middle vs. top)	1.04	0.86–1.26	0.675
Duration of service	1.00	0.96–1.04	0.945
Height of the participant	1.09	0.97–1.05	0.631

Limitations

First, this was a mannequin study. During the intubations, the participants were asked to avoid better glottic visualisation and continue intubating on a simulated C-L defined difficult airway. Such conditions are likely to not occur in the clinical setting. However, we recorded the entire intubation process on video clips and reviewed them with respect to the precise time intervals and C-L grades just before intubation. We found that the participants tended to lift the epiglottis unintentionally, particularly when they repeatedly failed to pass the ET. However, in simulating the clinical setting, prohibiting contact with the epiglottis would not be natural. Although the study was designed to investigate C-L grade III where only the epiglottis was visible, some of the glottic views, as reviewed by the video clips, were grade IIb (3.13%), in which the lower part of the vocal cord might be seen. The inexperience of the participants in 'holding the top' of the ET technique might have reduced the significance of the result in this group. Moreover, the study results were based on direct laryngoscopy on mannequin, further study need to be investigated for the video laryngoscopy and safety on real patients. Finally, this was a convenience sample and may be vulnerable to selection bias. But this study focused on experienced intubation performers that managing difficult airway in their daily practice and the technique of epiglottis lifting still significantly accelerated the intubation process despite their insufficient practice of this new technique.

Conclusions

When tested on a manikin, lifting the epiglottis with stylets as an adjunctive technique can facilitate and improve the success rate of intubation in difficult airway, such as C-L III, under direct laryngoscopy without increasing the difficulty of the intubation. Our study suggests that based on proper laryngoscope management, using the tip of the stylet-equipped ET to lift the epiglottis and following the anterior part of larynx can significantly facilitate tracheal intubation where only the epiglottis is seen.

Abbreviations
C-L: Cormack-Lehane; ED: emergency department; ET: endotracheal; HRs: hazard ratios; VAS: visual analogue scale

Acknowledgements
None

Authors' contributions
TYH and YHY carried out the conceptualization of the investigation. TYH and LWL, YHY, and TFY participated in the design of the study. TYH, LWL, and CHL conceived of the study and participated in its design and coordination. TYH, TFY performed the drift writing. TYH and YCS participated in statistical analysis. TFY carried out the overall supervision. All authors read and approved the final manuscript.

Author details
[1]Department of Biological Science and Technology, College of Biological science and Technology, National Chiao Tung University, NO.75 Po-Ai Street, Hsinchu 30068, Taiwan. [2]Department of Emergency Medicine, Zhong-Xing branch, Taipei City Hospital, Taipei, Taiwan. [3]CrazyatLAB (Critical Airway Training Laboratory), Taipei, Taiwan. [4]Department of Emergency, Shin Kong Wu Ho-Su Memorial Hospital, Taipei, Taiwan. [5]School of Medicine, Fu Jen Catholic University, New Taipei City, Taiwan. [6]School of Medicine, Tzu Chi University, Hualien, Taiwan. [7]Department of Emergency, Dalin Tzu Chi Hospital, Buddhist Tzu Chi Medical Foundation, Chiayi, Taiwan. [8]Graduate Institute of Medical Informatics and Cardiology, Taipei Medical University, Taipei, Taiwan.

References
1. Cormack RS, Lehane J. Difficult tracheal intubation in obstetrics. Anaesthesia. 1984;39:1105–11.
2. Yentis SM, Lee DJ. Evaluation of an improved scoring system for the grading of direct laryngoscopy. Anaesthesia. 1998;53:1041–4.
3. Ueda W, Arai YP. The use of a stylet to aid the lifting of the epiglottis with a video laryngoscope. Anesth Pain Med 2016;6:e38507. eCollection 2016 Aug.
4. Levitan RM, Pisaturo JT, Kinkle WC, Butler K, Everett WW. Stylet bend angles and tracheal tube passage using a straight-to-cuff shape. Acad Emerg Med. 2006;13:1255–8 Epub 2006 Nov 1.
5. Jonathan D. Casey, Matthew W. Semler, David R. Janz, Derek W. Russell, Aaron Joffee, Todd W. Rice Cormack-Lehane grade of view and successful first-pass intubation with vide.

Permissions

All chapters in this book were first published by BioMed Central; hereby published with permission under the Creative Commons Attribution License or equivalent. Every chapter published in this book has been scrutinized by our experts. Their significance has been extensively debated. The topics covered herein carry significant findings which will fuel the growth of the discipline. They may even be implemented as practical applications or may be referred to as a beginning point for another development.

The contributors of this book come from diverse backgrounds, making this book a truly international effort. This book will bring forth new frontiers with its revolutionizing research information and detailed analysis of the nascent developments around the world.

We would like to thank all the contributing authors for lending their expertise to make the book truly unique. They have played a crucial role in the development of this book. Without their invaluable contributions this book wouldn't have been possible. They have made vital efforts to compile up to date information on the varied aspects of this subject to make this book a valuable addition to the collection of many professionals and students.

This book was conceptualized with the vision of imparting up-to-date information and advanced data in this field. To ensure the same, a matchless editorial board was set up. Every individual on the board went through rigorous rounds of assessment to prove their worth. After which they invested a large part of their time researching and compiling the most relevant data for our readers.

The editorial board has been involved in producing this book since its inception. They have spent rigorous hours researching and exploring the diverse topics which have resulted in the successful publishing of this book. They have passed on their knowledge of decades through this book. To expedite this challenging task, the publisher supported the team at every step. A small team of assistant editors was also appointed to further simplify the editing procedure and attain best results for the readers.

Apart from the editorial board, the designing team has also invested a significant amount of their time in understanding the subject and creating the most relevant covers. They scrutinized every image to scout for the most suitable representation of the subject and create an appropriate cover for the book.

The publishing team has been an ardent support to the editorial, designing and production team. Their endless efforts to recruit the best for this project, has resulted in the accomplishment of this book. They are a veteran in the field of academics and their pool of knowledge is as vast as their experience in printing. Their expertise and guidance has proved useful at every step. Their uncompromising quality standards have made this book an exceptional effort. Their encouragement from time to time has been an inspiration for everyone.

The publisher and the editorial board hope that this book will prove to be a valuable piece of knowledge for researchers, students, practitioners and scholars across the globe.

List of Contributors

Axel Schmutz, Thomas Loeffler and Ulrich Goebel
Department of Anesthesiology and Critical Care, Faculty of Medicine, Medical Center - University of Freiburg, University of Freiburg, Hugstetter Strasse 55, 79106 Freiburg im Breisgau, Germany

Arthur Schmidt
Department of Medicine II, Faculty of Medicine, Medical Center - University of Freiburg University of Freiburg, Hugstetter Strasse 55, Freiburg im Breisgau 79106, Germany

Yen-Chu Lin and Yung-Tai Chung
Department of Anesthesiology, Chang Gung Memorial Hospital, No.5, Fuxing St., Guishan Dist., Taoyuan City 333, Taiwan

An-Hsun Cho
Department of Anesthesiology, Chang Gung Memorial Hospital, No.5, Fuxing St., Guishan Dist., Taoyuan City 333, Taiwan
College of Medicine, Chang Gung University, Taoyuan City, Taiwan

Jr-Rung Lin
Department of Anesthesiology, Chang Gung Memorial Hospital, No.5, Fuxing St., Guishan Dist., Taoyuan City 333, Taiwan
Clinical Informatics and Medical Statistics Research Center, Chang Gung University, Taoyuan City, Taiwan
Graduate Institute of Clinical Medical Sciences (Joint Appointment), Chang Gung University, Taoyuan City, Taiwan
College of Medicine, Chang Gung University, Taoyuan City, Taiwan

Yuji Kamimura, Toshiyuki Nakanishi, Eisuke Kako and Kazuya Sobue
Department of Anesthesiology and Intensive Care Medicine, Nagoya City University Graduate School of Medical Sciences, 1 Kawasumi, Mizuho-cho, Mizuho-ku, Nagoya 467-8601, Japan

Aiji Boku Sato
Department of Anesthesiology, Aichi Gakuin University School of Dentistry, 2-11 Suemori-dori, Chikusa-ku, Nagoya 464-8651, Japan

Satoshi Osaga
Clinical Research Management Center, Nagoya City University Hospital, 1 Kawasumi, Mizuho-cho, Mizuho-ku, Nagoya 467-8601, Japan

Yanli Liu
Science and technology department, China Pharmaceutical University, Nanjing, People's Republic of China

Jiashuo Wang
Research Center of Biostatistics and Computational Pharmacy, China Pharmaceutical University, Nanjing, People's Republic of China

Shan Zhong
Department of Anesthesiology, Children's Hospital of Nanjing Medical University, No. 72, Guangzhou Road, Gulou District, Nanjing 210008, People's Republic of China

Go Wun Kim, Jong Yeop Kim, Eun Jeong Park and Sung Yong Park
Department of Anaesthesiology and Pain Medicine, Ajou University School of Medicine, 164, World Cup-ro, Yeongtong-gu, Suwon 16499, Republic of Korea

Soo Jin Kim and Yeo Rae Moon
Office of Biostatistics, Ajou University School of Medicine, Suwon, Republic of Korea

Zhe Mao and Yingqiu Cui
Guangzhou Women and Children's Medical Center, No 9, Jinsui Road, Guangzhou 510623, Guangdong, China

Na Zhang
Guangzhou Women and Children's Medical Center, No 9, Jinsui Road, Guangzhou 510623, Guangdong, China
Department of Anesthesiology, Qilu Hospital of Shandong University (Qingdao), No.758 Hefei Road, Qingdao, People's Republic of China

Bingchuan Liu, Fang Zhou, Hongquan Ji and Yun Tian
Department of Orthopaedics, Peking University Third Hospital, Beijing, China
Beijing Key Laboratory of Spinal Disease Research, Beijing, China

Yanan Song, Kaixi Liu and Yong Zheng Han
Department of Anesthesiology, Peking University Third Hospital, 49 North Garden Rd, Haidian District, Beijing 100191, China

Chunji Han, Ying Guo, Li Sun, Gang Chen, Weidong Mi and Changsheng Zhang
Anesthesia and Operation Center, The First Medical Center of Chinese PLA General Hospital, 28th Fuxing Rd., Haidian District, Beijing 100853, P. R. China

Peng Li
Department of Anesthesia, The Sixth Medical Center of Chinese PLA General Hospital, Beijing, China

Zhenggang Guo
Department of Anesthesiology, Peking University Shougang Hospital, Beijing 100144, China

Xiaojue Qiu
Department of Gastroenterology, The First Medical Center of Chinese PLA General Hospital, Beijing, China

Lorenzo Berra
Department of Anesthesia, Critical Care and Pain Medicine, Massachusetts General Hospital, Boston, MA, USA

Min Suk Chae, Jong-Woan Kim, Hyun Sik Chung, Chul Soo Park, Jong Ho Choi and Sang Hyun Hong
Department of Anesthesiology and Pain medicine, Seoul St. Mary's Hospital, College of Medicine, The Catholic University of Korea, 222, Banpo-daero, Seocho-gu, Seoul 06591, Republic of Korea

Joon-Yong Jung
Department of Radiology, Seoul St. Mary's Hospital, College of Medicine, The Catholic University of Korea, Seoul, Republic of Korea

Ho Joong Choi
Department of Surgery, Seoul St. Mary's Hospital, College of Medicine, The Catholic University of Korea, Seoul, Republic of Korea

Bacha Aberra, Girmay Teklay and Hagos Tasew
Aksum University, Aksum City, Tigray, Ethiopia

Adugna Aregawi
Addis Ababa University, Addis Ababa, Ethiopia

Ping Yi, Zhoujing Yang, Li Cao, Xiaobing Hu and Huahua Gu
Department of Anesthesiology, Huashan Hospital, Fudan University, No.12 Wulumuqi Zhong Road, Shanghai 200040, China

Qiong Li
Department of Anesthesiology, Shanghai Jiahui International Hospital, Shanghai 200000, China

Siyi Yan and Huan Zhang
Department of Anesthesiology, Beijing Tsinghua Chang gung Hospital, No.168, Li Tang Road, Chang Ping District, Beijing, China

Shigekazu Sugino, Daisuke Konno and Masanori Yamauchi
Department of Anesthesiology and Perioperative Medicine, Tohoku University School of Medicine, 2-1, Seiryo-machi, Aoba-ku, Sendai, Miyagi 980-8575, Japan

Norifumi Kuratani
Department of Anesthesia, Saitama Children's Medical Center, 1-2, Shin-toshin, Chuo-ku, Saitama City, Saitama 330-8777, Japan

Hiroshi Sumida
Department of Anesthesiology and Perioperative Medicine, Tohoku University School of Medicine, 2-1, Seiryo-machi, Aoba-ku, Sendai, Miyagi 980-8575, Japan
Department of Anesthesia, Katta General Hospital, 36 Shimoharaoki, Kuramoto, Fukuoka, Shiroishi, Miyagi 989-0231, Japan

Jun-ichi Hasegawa
Department of Anesthesia, Katta General Hospital, 36 Shimoharaoki, Kuramoto, Fukuoka, Shiroishi, Miyagi 989-0231, Japan

Ming Jian Lim
Department of Women's Anesthesia, KK Women's and Children's Hospital, 100 Bukit Timah Road, Singapore 229899, Singapore

Hon Sen Tan, Chin Wen Tan and Ban Leong Sng
Department of Women's Anesthesia, KK Women's and Children's Hospital, 100 Bukit Timah Road, Singapore 229899, Singapore
Duke-NUS Medical School, 8 College Road, Singapore 169857, Singapore

Shi Yang Li and Wei Yu Yao
Department of Anesthesiology and Perioperative Medicine, Quanzhou Macare Women's Hospital, Quanzhou, Fujian Province, China

Yong Jing Yuan
Department of Anesthesiology, Qinghai University Affiliated Hospital, Xining, Qinghai Province, China

Rehena Sultana
Centre for Quantitative Medicine, Duke-NUS Medical School, 8 College Road, Singapore 169857, Singapore

Ulku Ozgul, Feray Akgul Erdil, Mehmet Ali Erdogan, Zekine Begec, Aytac Yucel and Mahmut Durmus
School of Medicine, Department of Anesthesiology and Reanimation, Inonu University, Malatya, Turkey

Cemil Colak
School of Medicine, Department of Biostatistics, and Medical Informatics, Inonu University, Malatya, Turkey

Jun Cao, Xiaoyun Gao, Xiaoli Zhang, Jing Li and Junfeng Zhang
Department of Anesthesiology, Shanghai Jiao Tong University Affiliated Sixth People's Hospital, No. 600, Yishan Rd., Shanghai, China

Ping Huang, Renlong Zhou, Zhixing Lu, Yannan Hang, Shanjuan Wang and Zhenling Huang
Department of Anesthesiology, Renji Hospital, School of Medicine, Shanghai Jiaotong University, Shanghai 200001, China

Wenxi Tang, Penghui Wei, Haipeng Zhou, Jinfeng Zhou, Qiang Zheng and Jianjun Li
Department of Anesthesiology, Qilu Hospital of Shandong University (Qingdao), No.758 Hefei Road, Qingdao, People's Republic of China

Jiapeng Huang
Department of Anesthesia, Jewish Hospital and Department of Anesthesiology & Perioperative Medicine, University of Louisville, Louisville, KY, USA

Zhigang Wang
Department of Neurosurgery, Qilu Hospital of Shandong University (Qingdao), Qingdao, People's Republic of China

Zhuo Liu, Qianqian Jia and Xiaochun Yang
Department of Anesthesiology, The First Hospital of Qinhuangdao, N.O. 258, Wenhua Road, Qinhuangdao, Hebei, China

Michael W. van Emden and Jeroen J. G. Geurts
Department of Anatomy and Neurosciences, Amsterdam UMC, Vrije Universiteit, 1007 MB, De Boelelaan 1117, 1081, HV, Amsterdam, The Netherlands

Patrick Schober and Lothar A. Schwarte
Department of Anaesthesiology, Amsterdam UMC, Vrije Universiteit, De Boelelaan 1117, 1081, HV, Amsterdam, The Netherlands

Kyle M. Behrens
Chicago Medical School, Rosalind Franklin University of Medicine and Science, 3333 Green Bay Road, North Chicago, IL 60064, USA

Richard E. Galgon
Department of Anesthesiology, University of Wisconsin School of Medicine and Public Health, 600 Highland Ave., B6/319, Madison, WI 53792, USA

Xiaohua Wang, Ke Huang, Fei Lan, Dongxu Yao, Yanhong Li, Jixiu Xue and Tianlong Wang
Department of Anesthesiology, Xuanwu Hospital, Capital Medical University, Beijing 100053, China
Institute of Geriatrics, Beijing 100053, China
National Clinical Research Center for Geriatric Disorders, Beijing 100053, China

Hao Yan
Department of Urinary surgery, Xuanwu Hospital, Capital Medical University, Beijing 100053, China

Haozhen Zhu, Jinxing Liu, Lulu Suo, Chi Zhou, Yu Sun and Hong Jiang
Department of Anesthesiology, Shanghai Ninth People's Hospital Affiliated to Shanghai Jiao Tong University School of Medicine, 639 Zhizaoju Road, Shanghai 200011, China

Gang Zheng
Department of Anesthesiology and Perioperative Medicine, The University of Texas MD Anderson Cancer Center, 1515 Holcombe Boulevard, Faculty Center – Unit 409, Houston, TX 77030, USA

Lei Feng
Department of Biostatistics, The University of Texas MD Anderson Cancer Center, FCT4.5047, T. Boone Pickens Academic Tower, 1400 Pressler St, Houston, TX 77030-4008, USA

Carol M. Lewis
Department of Head and Neck Surgery, The University of Texas MD Anderson Cancer Center, Unit 1445, T. Boone Pickens Academic Tower, 1515 Holcombe Blvd, Houston, TX 77030-4009, USA

R. Schiewe, M. Stoeck and B. Bein
Department of Anaesthesiology and Intensive Care Medicine, Asklepios Hospital St. Georg, Lohmuehlenstr. 5, D-20099 Hamburg, Germany

M. Gruenewald and J. Hoecker
Department of Anaesthesiology and Intensive Care Medicine, University Hospital Schleswig-Holstein, Campus Kiel, Schwanenweg 21, D-24105 Kiel, Germany

Yun Jeong Chae, Bokyeong Jun and In Kyong Yi
Department of Anaesthesiology and Pain Medicine, Ajou University School of Medicine, 164, World cup-ro, Yeongtong-gu, Suwon 16499, South Korea

Heirim Lee
Office of Biostatics, Ajou Research Institute for Innovative Medicine, Ajou University Medical Center, 164, World cup-ro, Yeongtong-gu, Suwon 16499, South Korea

Ippei Jimbo, Kohji Uzawa, Joho Tokumine, Shingo Mitsuda, Kunitaro Watanabe and Tomoko Yorozu
Department of Anesthesiology , Kyorin University, School of Medicine 6-20-2 Shinkawa, Mitaka City, Tokyo 181-0004, Japan

Yang Gu, Ruowang Duan, Xin Lv and Jiong Song
The Department of Anesthesiology, Tongji University Affiliated Shanghai Pulmonary Hospital, 507 Zhengmin Rd, Shanghai, China

Hyerim Kim, Jung-Man Lee, Jee-Eun Chang and Dongwook Won
Department of Anesthesiology and Pain Medicine, Seoul Metropolitan Government Seoul National University Boramae Medical Center, 20 Boramae-ro 5-gil, Dongjak-gu, Seoul 07061, Republic of Korea

Jiwon Lee
Department of Anesthesiology and Pain Medicine, Keimyung University Dongsan Medical Center, Keimyung University School of Medicine, 1095 Dalgubeol-daero, Dalseo-gu, Daegu 42601, Republic of Korea

Jin-Young Hwang and Seong-Won Min
Department of Anesthesiology and Pain Medicine, Seoul Metropolitan Government Seoul National University Boramae Medical Center, 20 Boramae-ro 5-gil, Dongjak-gu, Seoul 07061, Republic of Korea
Department of Anesthesiology and Pain Medicine, Seoul National University College of Medicine, 101 Daehak-ro, Jongno-gu, Seoul 03080, Republic of Korea

Hyun-Joung No
Department of Anesthesiology and Pain Medicine, Anesthesia and Pain Research Institute, Yonsei University College of Medicine, 50-1 Yonsei-ro, Seodaemun-gu, Seoul 03722, Republic of Korea

Hyung Sang Row
Department of Anesthesiology and Pain Medicine, Seoul National University Hospital, 101 Daehak-ro, Jongno-gu, Seoul 03080, Republic of Korea

Cristina Monteserín-Matesanz and Tatiana González
Anaesthesia department, Hospital General Universitario Gregorio Marañón, C/ Doctor Esquerdo, N° 46, 28007 Madrid, Spain

María José Anadón-Baselga
Department of Legal Medicine, Psychiatry and Pathology Universidad Complutense, Madrid, Spain

Matilde Zaballos
Anaesthesia department, Hospital General Universitario Gregorio Marañón, C/ Doctor Esquerdo, N° 46, 28007 Madrid, Spain
Department of Legal Medicine, Psychiatry and Pathology Universidad Complutense, Madrid, Spain

Tzu-Yao Hung
Department of Biological Science and Technology, College of Biological science and Technology, National Chiao Tung University, NO.75 Po-Ai Street, Hsinchu 30068, Taiwan
Department of Emergency Medicine, Zhong-Xing branch, Taipei City Hospital, Taipei, Taiwan
CrazyatLAB (Critical Airway Training Laboratory), Taipei, Taiwan

Li-Wei Lin
CrazyatLAB (Critical Airway Training Laboratory), Taipei, Taiwan
Department of Emergency, Shin Kong Wu Ho-Su Memorial Hospital, Taipei, Taiwan
School of Medicine, Fu Jen Catholic University, New Taipei City, Taiwan

Yu-Hang Yeh and Chieh-Hung Lin
Department of Emergency Medicine, Zhong-Xing branch, Taipei City Hospital, Taipei, Taiwan

Yung-Cheng Su
School of Medicine, Tzu Chi University, Hualien, Taiwan
Department of Emergency, Dalin Tzu Chi Hospital, Buddhist Tzu Chi Medical Foundation, Chiayi, Taiwan

Ten-Fang Yang
Department of Biological Science and Technology, College of Biological science and Technology, National Chiao Tung University, NO.75 Po-Ai Street, Hsinchu 30068, Taiwan
Graduate Institute of Medical Informatics and Cardiology, Taipei Medical University, Taipei, Taiwan

Index